Yatdjuligin

Aboriginal and Torres Strait Islander Nursing and Midwifery Care

Third Edition

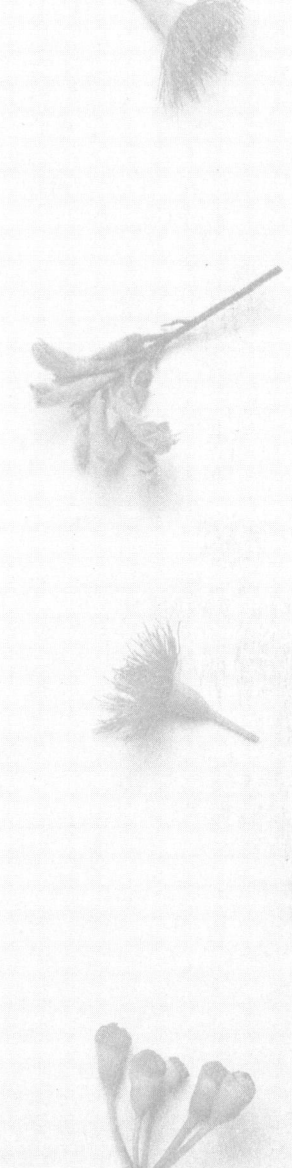

Yatdjuligin: Aboriginal and Torres Strait Islander Nursing and Midwifery Care introduces students to the fundamentals of healthcare of Indigenous Australians, encompassing the perspectives of both the client and the health practitioner. Written for all nurses and midwives, this book addresses the relationship between Aboriginal and Torres Strait Islander cultures, mainstream health services and Aboriginal Community Controlled Health Organisations. It introduces readers to historical and contemporary approaches to practice and research in a variety of healthcare contexts.

This edition has been fully updated to reflect current research and documentation, with an emphasis on cultural safety and culturally safe practice underpinning each chapter. Three new chapters cover social and emotional wellbeing in mainstream mental health services, quantitative research and Torres Strait Islander health and wellbeing. Chapter content is complemented by case study scenarios, reflection questions and authors' reflections on their own professional experiences. These features illustrate historical and contemporary challenges, encourage students to reflect on their own attitudes, values and beliefs and provide strategies to deliver quality, person-centred healthcare.

With contributions from leading Aboriginal and Torres Strait Islander academics, researchers and practising nurses and midwives, this essential resource will equip all students with the knowledge and tools to prepare them for practice with clients and colleagues across a range of health services and settings.

Odette Best is Professor in the School of Nursing and Midwifery at the University of Southern Queensland. She is the School's Associate Head: Indigenous Research and Community Engagement.

Bronwyn Fredericks is Professor and Pro-Vice-Chancellor (Indigenous Engagement) at the University of Queensland.

Cambridge University Press acknowledges the Australian Aboriginal and Torres Strait Islander peoples of this nation. We acknowledge the traditional custodians of the lands on which our company is located and where we conduct our business. We pay our respects to ancestors and Elders, past and present. Cambridge University Press is committed to honouring Australian Aboriginal and Torres Strait Islander peoples' unique cultural and spiritual relationships to the land, waters and seas and their rich contribution to society.

Yatdjuligin

Aboriginal and Torres Strait Islander Nursing and Midwifery Care

Third Edition

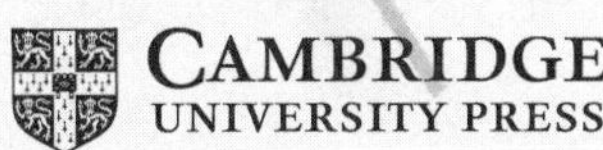

CAMBRIDGE UNIVERSITY PRESS

Edited by Odette Best & Bronwyn Fredericks

CAMBRIDGE
UNIVERSITY PRESS

University Printing House, Cambridge CB2 8BS, United Kingdom

One Liberty Plaza, 20th Floor, New York, NY 10006, USA

477 Williamstown Road, Port Melbourne, VIC 3207, Australia

314–321, 3rd Floor, Plot 3, Splendor Forum, Jasola District Centre, New Delhi – 110025, India

79 Anson Road, #06–04/06, Singapore 079906

Cambridge University Press is part of the University of Cambridge.

It furthers the University's mission by disseminating knowledge in the pursuit of education, learning and research at the highest international levels of excellence.

www.cambridge.org
Information on this title: www.cambridge.org/9781108794695

First published 2014

Second edition 2018

Third edition 2021

Cover designed by Leigh Ashforth, watershed art + design
Typeset by Integra Software Services Pvt. Ltd
Printed in Malaysia by Vivar Printing, May 2021

A catalogue record for this publication is available from the British Library

A catalogue record for this book is available from the National Library of Australia

ISBN 978-1-108-79469-5 Paperback

Additional resources for this publication at
https://www.cambridge.org/highereducation/isbn/9781108794695/resources

Please be aware that this publication may contain several variations of Aboriginal and Torres Strait Islander terms and spellings; no disrespect is intended. Please note that the terms 'Indigenous Australians', 'Aboriginal and Torres Strait Islander peoples' and 'First Nations peoples' may be used interchangeably in this publication.

Foreword

The World Health Organization designated 2020 as the International Year of the Nurse and Midwife in recognition of the many roles nurses and midwives fill and the outstanding contribution they make to global healthcare. This international celebration was the perfect backdrop to meet the request for a third edition of this highly regarded textbook, *Yatdjuligin: Aboriginal and Torres Strait Islander Nursing and Midwifery Care.*

For this new edition, the editors, Professor Odette Best and Professor Bronwyn Fredericks, as well as other leading Aboriginal and Torres Strait Islander contributors, responded to feedback and developments in healthcare. The response necessitated a chapter on social and emotional wellbeing within mainstream health organisations and another about quantitative research methods to complement the qualitative research methods chapter and enhance research led by Indigenous nurses. The updates did not stop there, with the inclusion of a chapter specifically about Torres Strait Islander health written by Torres Strait Islander nurses.

This new edition is timely. The release of the Australian Nursing and Midwifery Council's Registered Nurse Accreditation Standards 2019 and the Midwife Accreditation Standards and Essential Evidence 2020 has mandated once again that nursing and midwifery programs include Aboriginal and Torres Strait Islander peoples' history, culture and health as a discrete subject, and that content relevant to health outcomes of Aboriginal and Torres Strait Islander peoples is to be embedded throughout the programs. The Standards also require the inclusion of cultural safety, which *Yatdjuligin* now has proudly done for all three of its editions. As an accompaniment to the Nursing and Midwifery Aboriginal and Torres Strait Islander Health Curriculum Framework, *Yatdjuligin* provides the knowledge and understanding required by current and future nurses and midwives. The comprehensive nature of *Yatdjuligin* extends beyond a discrete subject and will influence many other subjects in nursing and midwifery programs. Additionally, it follows the National Aboriginal and Torres Strait Islander Health Plan 2013–2023, which places great emphasis on building pathways into the health professions for Aboriginal and Torres Strait Islander people. One definite pathway is access to this esteemed textbook, which speaks directly to and about Indigenous Australians.

As this edition goes to print, the world is experiencing a pandemic. Anxiety levels are high – but no higher than in and for Indigenous communities. The *Closing the Gap Report 2020* identified the health disparities between Indigenous and non-Indigenous populations and the limited progress made to address that gap. Not only are there poor maternal health outcomes for Indigenous mothers and children, but high prevalence rates of chronic circulatory, endocrine, mental and cancer diseases remain in the broader Indigenous population. A rampant coronavirus outbreak would have devastating effects across Indigenous communities across Australia. The need for well-prepared nurses and midwives to manage coronavirus and other public health emergencies has never been greater, and this textbook is an invaluable resource.

Yatdjuligin is seminal literature – the Uluru Statement from the Heart permeates every page. That this is the third edition of *Yatdjuligin* speaks to its relevance: it encapsulates Indigenous and Torres Strait Islander knowledges and practice as it relates, applies and drives nursing and midwifery care for, with and by Indigenous people.

Christine Neville PhD RN
Professor of Nursing
Head of School
School of Nursing and Midwifery
University of Southern Queensland
January 2021

Contents

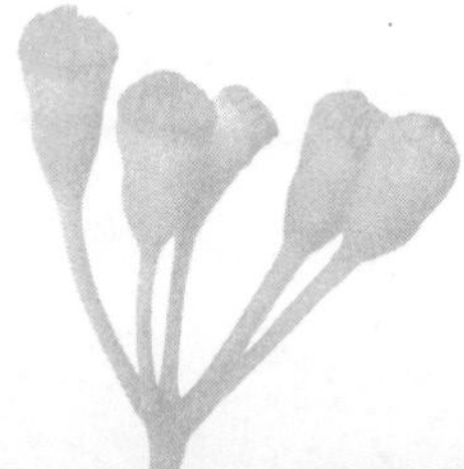

Contributors

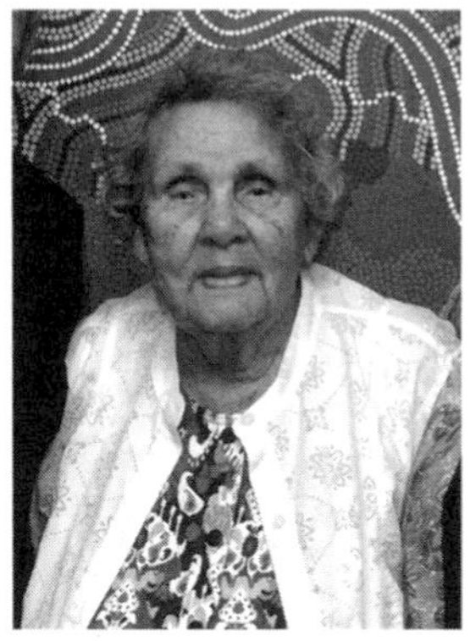

Ivy Molly Booth (nee Darby) (gifter of language) is the Elder of the Wakgun people of the Gurreng Gurreng Nation. She was born at Camboon Station and removed to Taroom Aboriginal Settlement in the early 1920s, before again being removed to Woorabinda Mission on its inception in 1927. Well over 100 years of age, she is the only surviving original dormitory girl of Woorabinda. At Woorabinda, Ivy Booth met and married her husband, Clancy Booth, a Boonthamurra man. Ivy Booth is great-great-grandmother to a large and extended family across Woorabinda and Rockhampton in Queensland and further afield in New South Wales, Canberra and Victoria. Ivy Molly Booth gifted the editors of this text the name *Yatdjuligin*.

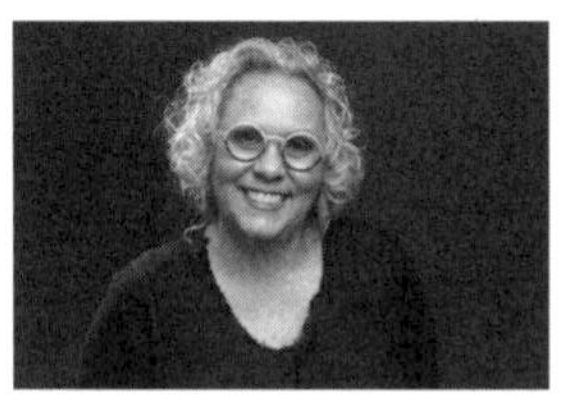

Odette Best is a Wakgun clan member of the Gurreng Gurreng Nation and holds a Boonthamurra bloodline with adoption ties to the Koomumberri, Yugambeh people. Odette is Professor and Associate Head: Indigenous Research and Community Engagement, School of Nursing and Midwifery at the University of Southern Queensland (Ipswich Campus). She commenced her training at the Princess Alexandra Hospital in the late 1980s, and holds a Bachelor of Health Sciences (double major in Aboriginal Health and Community Development), a Master of Philosophy and a PhD. Odette has worked for 30 years in Indigenous health. Clinically, she worked for a decade as sexual health coordinator at the Brisbane Aboriginal and Islander Community Health Service and within the women's and youth prison systems across Brisbane. In 2000, she moved into discipline teaching within nursing in the tertiary sector. Odette's leadership in Indigenous health and Indigenous nursing research is acknowledged globally, and she is a Fellow of the American Academy of Nursing (the only Aboriginal Australian nurse), a Churchill Fellow (the first Aboriginal Australian nurse) and a Fellow of the Congress of Aboriginal and Torres Strait Islander Nurses and Midwives. As an historian of Aboriginal nurses and midwives, Odette is passionate about uncovering and documenting the experiences of Aboriginal nurses and midwives and saving them from historical oblivion. Odette is Ivy Molly Booth's granddaughter.

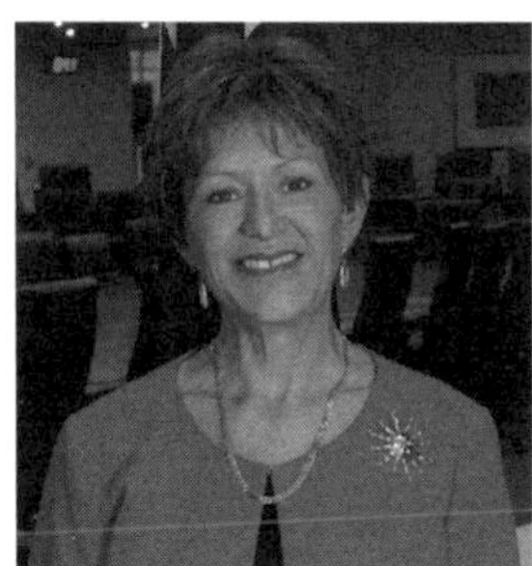

Bronwyn Fredericks an Indigenous woman from South-East Queensland with over 30 years' experience working in and with the tertiary sector, state and federal governments, and Aboriginal and Torres Strait Islander community-based organisations. She is a Professor and the Pro-Vice-Chancellor (Indigenous Engagement) at the University of Queensland, and still maintains an active research program. Bronwyn is a member of the Australian Institute of Aboriginal and Torres Strait Islander Studies

(AIATSIS) Research Advisory Committee (RAC), the Beyond Blue National Research Advisory Committee and the Australian Research Council (ARC) College of Experts. In 2016, Bronwyn was appointed as a Commissioner with the Queensland Productivity Commission (QPC) (one of only two appointments) to lead the Inquiry into Service Delivery in Queensland's Remote and Discrete Indigenous Communities. In 2018, she was again appointed to work on Queensland's Inquiry into Imprisonment and Recidivism, which was completed in 2019.

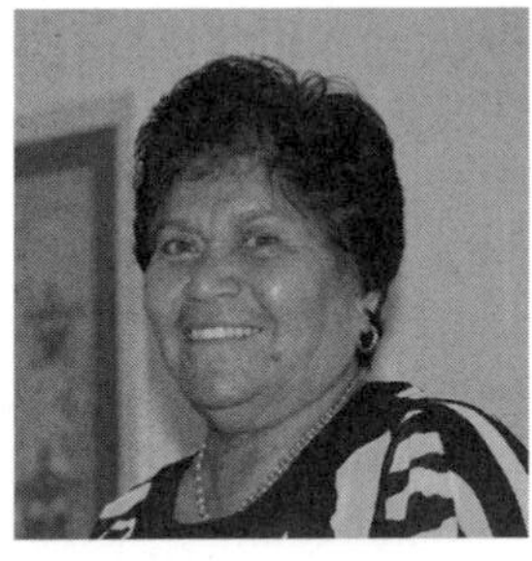

Gracelyn Smallwood is a Birrigubba, Kalkadoon and South Sea Islander woman originating from Townsville. She is Professor of Nursing and Midwifery/Community Engagement at Central Queensland University in Townsville. She is a Registered Nurse and a Registered Midwife. In 1986, Gracelyn was awarded Queensland Aboriginal of the Year and in 1992 she was awarded an Order of Australia for services to public health, particularly HIV-AIDS education. In 1993, she became the first Indigenous Australian to receive a Master of Science in Public Health from James Cook University. Gracelyn is a member of numerous healthcare boards and councils around the world. In 2007, she was awarded the Deadly Award for Outstanding Lifetime Achievement in Indigenous Health. In 2013, she was awarded the United Nations Association of Australia Queensland Community Award – Individual. In 2014, she received the NAIDOC Person of the Year award. She was awarded the Lifetime Achievement Award by the Congress of Aboriginal and Torres Strait Islander Nurses and Midwives (CATSINaM).

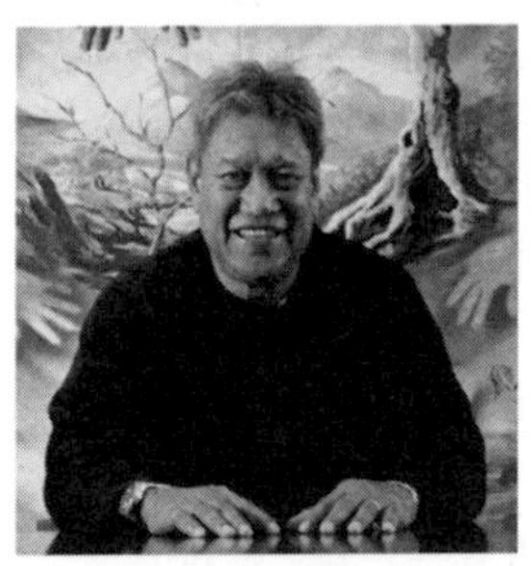

Mick Adams is a descendent of the Yadhiagana/Wuthathi peoples of Cape York Peninsula in Queensland (on his father's side), and has traditional family ties with the Gurindji people of Central Western Northern Territory (on his mother's side) and extended family relationship with the people of the Torres Strait, Warlpiri (Yuendumu) and East Arnhem Land (Gurrumaru) communities. He is a Senior Research Fellow with the Australian Indigenous HealthInfoNet at Edith Cowan University in Perth, Adjunct Professor in the School of Public Health, Queensland University of Technology and a member of the National Indigenous Research and Knowledges Network (NIRAKN). Mick holds a Master of Arts (Indigenous Research and Development), Bachelor of Social Work and Bachelor of Applied Science (Aboriginal Community Management and Development). His PhD is to date the only research study conducted with Aboriginal and Torres Strait Islander males on sexual and reproductive health. Mick is recognised as a respected Elder within Aboriginal and Torres Strait Islander communities. He has been involved in advocating to improve the status of the health and wellbeing of Aboriginal and Torres Strait Islander people for over 30 years, having served in various national organisations and on a number of committees. He was awarded the Queensland University of Technology 2010 Chancellor's Outstanding Alumnus Award and the Queensland University of Technology 2010 Faculty of Health Outstanding Alumnus Award, and recently received an Elders award from the Aboriginal and Torres Strait Islander Higher Education Advisory Council.

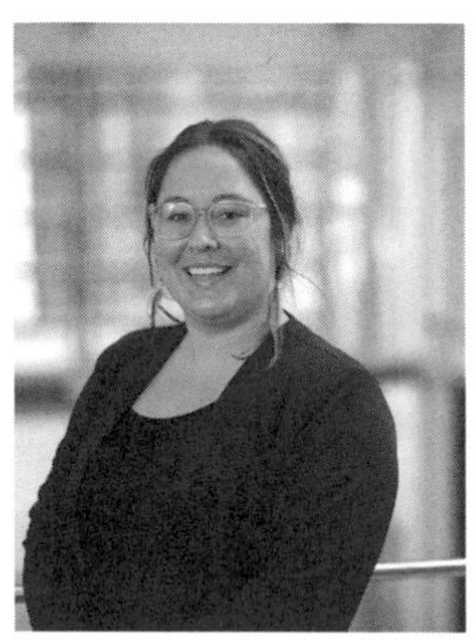

Jessica Bennett (nee Taggart) (RN, M Clinical Nursing (NICU), PhD candidate) is a proud Gamilaroi Yinarr from Tamworth. Jessica is a Registered Nurse who has specialised in the world of neonatal intensive care in a metropolitan children's hospital in New South Wales. She is a young academic at the University of Newcastle, lecturing on Aboriginal health and cultural capability to undergraduate health professionals as part of the Thurru-Indigenous Health Unit team. Jessica has recently become a PhD candidate, and is driven to explore and empower Indigenous families in the neonatal setting and support their social and emotional wellbeing from Indigenous cultural ways of doing, being and knowing.

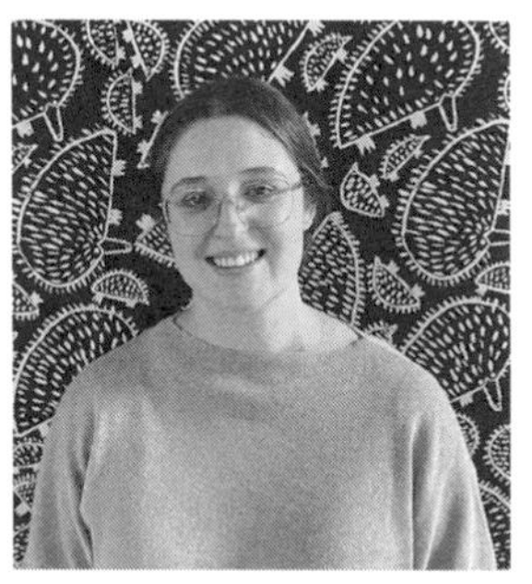

Makayla-May Brinckley is a Wiradjuri woman. She is a 2018 Bachelor of Science (Psychology)/Bachelor of Arts, and 2019 Psychology Honours graduate from the Australian National University (ANU). She is currently working as a research assistant across various projects in the Aboriginal and Torres Strait Islander Health Program at the National Centre for Epidemiology and Population Health (NCEPH), ANU. She is passionate about Aboriginal and Torres Strait Islander mental health and wellbeing.

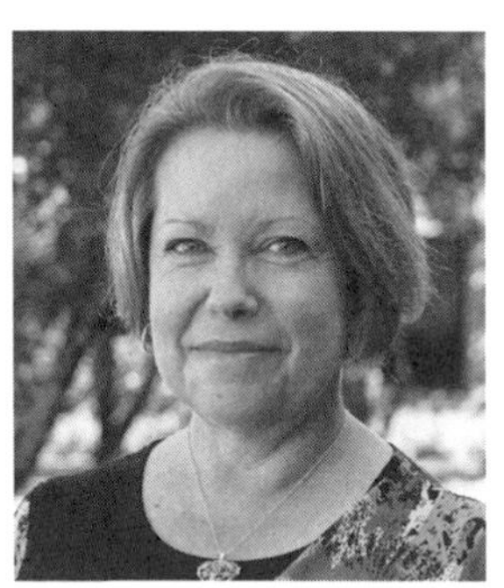

Linda Deravin (RN, PhD, MHM, Grad Cert in L&T in Higher Ed, Grad Cert Anaes & Rec Room Nurs, Grad Dip Gerontology, Grad Cert E Health, BN, FCHSM) identifies as a Wiradjuri woman and is the course director for the School of Nursing, Midwifery and Indigenous Health at Charles Sturt University. Throughout her nursing career, she has worked as a clinician, educator, senior nurse and health manager in a variety of settings. She has a research interest in Indigenous health, chronic care and nursing workforce issues.

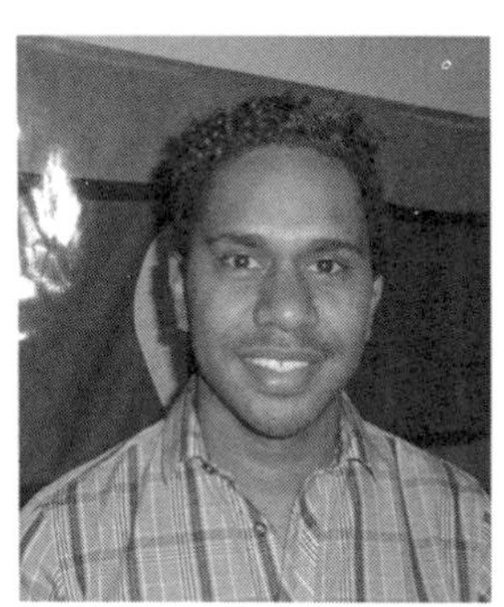

Ali Drummond grew up on Thursday Island. His people are the Meriam le of the Murray Islands and the Wuthathi people of northern Queensland. He is a senior lecturer in QUT's School of Nursing and the Research and Education Manager at the Southern Queensland Centre of Excellence in Aboriginal and Torres Strait Islander Primary Health Care in Inala. Ali is a registered nurse, whose fifteen years of experience span clinical nursing (primary health care and orthopaedics), Aboriginal and Torres Strait Islander health and nursing policy, education and research. He completed his Bachelor of Nursing at James Cook University as one of the three inaugural graduates of the Thursday Island campus. Ali also holds a Graduate Certificate in Academic Practice, a Masters of International Public Health, and is a Fellow of Advanced Higher Education. Ali is currently a PhD candidate investigating the experiences of Indigenous and non-Indigenous nurse academics tasked with developing, delivering and evaluating Aboriginal and Torres Strait Islander health curricula in partnership with Aboriginal and Torres Strait Islander peoples.

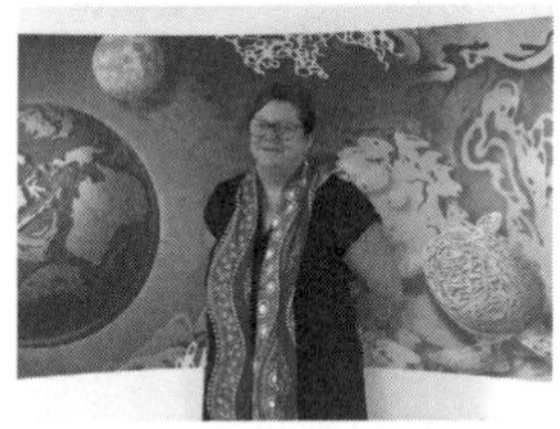

Donna Hartz (RN, RM, M Mid, PhD, Fellow ACM) identifies as a descendant of her grandmother's people, Kamilaroi (Gomeroi). Donna is a midwife and nurse with 39 years' experience as a clinician, educator, lecturer, manager, consultant and researcher. Currently, she is an Adjunct Associate Professor at the Molly Wardaguga Research Centre at Charles Darwin University (CDU) and the School of Nursing and Midwifery, Western Sydney University. She also holds an associate position with Burbangana Group, a wholly Aboriginal owned consultancy company supporting the wellbeing of Aboriginal communities. Most recently, she was the Associate Professor on Midwifery and Associate Dean Indigenous Leadership in the College of Nursing and Midwifery at CDU. Prior to this, she was the Acting Director and Academic Lead in the University of Sydney's National Centre of Cultural Competence (NCCC). She has held senior midwifery consultant roles in northern Sydney and south-western Sydney, focusing on clinical governance, midwifery practice development, clinical redesign and translation of evidence into policy and practice. She has been a lecturer, tutor or examiner in substantive and honorary positions in midwifery, nursing or medicine at six Australian universities, including the University of Newcastle, University of Sydney, University of Technology Sydney (UTS), University of New South Wales (UNSW), Western Sydney University and CDU. Her main research focus has been in the clinical redesign and evaluation of maternity and midwifery models of care. Her current foci are on birth on Country models of care for Aboriginal and Torres Strait Islander women and babies (she is currently a chief investigator on a two NHMRC grants); Aboriginal Child Protection; community-derived programs underpinned by Aboriginal cultural healing models; and midwifery and nursing education pathways and support for Aboriginal and Torres Strait Islander people.

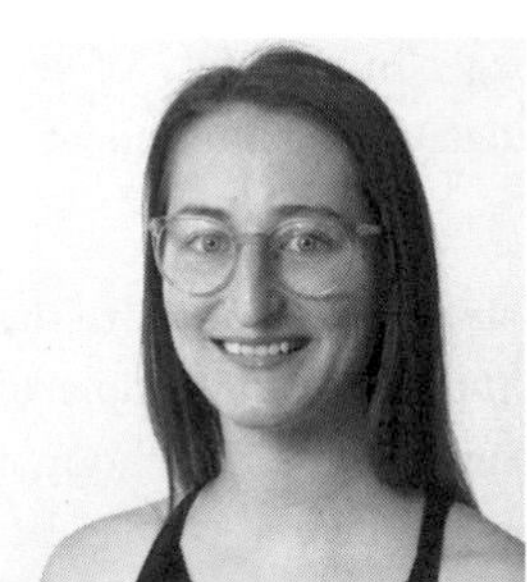

Roxanne Jones is a Palawa woman, PhD candidate and research associate at the Australian National University (ANU), and holds an NHMRC postgraduate scholarship. Roxy is an epidemiologist and Registered Nurse with a passion for Aboriginal and Torres Strait Islander child and infant health. Roxy has postgraduate qualifications in epidemiology and Indigenous research, as well as undergraduate qualifications in nursing and health sciences (paramedics).

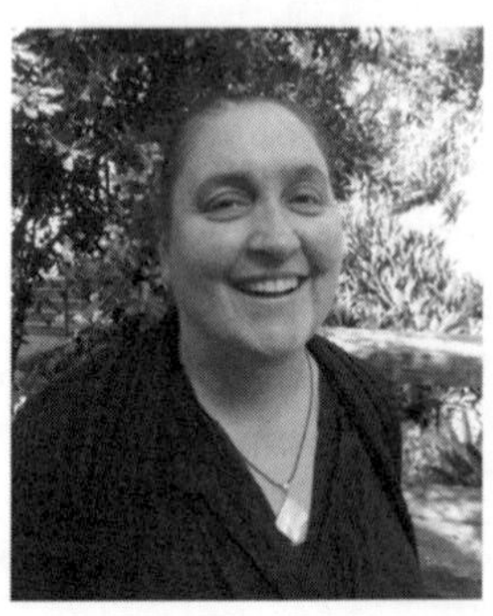

Machellee Kosiak is a Wiradjuri woman whose family ties are in country New South Wales. Machellee is a Registered Nurse and practising Endorsed Registered Midwife, and has worked in a variety of maternity settings over 25 years. She is a midwifery academic and course adviser for the Away from Base Bachelor of Midwifery program at the Australian Catholic University in Brisbane. She holds a Bachelor of Nursing and is undertaking a Masters of Midwifery (Research), with a research program entitled 'Facilitators and Challenges Faced by Indigenous Bachelor of

Midwifery Students'. Machellee's postgraduate rotations were in intensive care, emergency, surgical and oncology wards, where she observed how Indigenous women and women from other cultures were treated. She helped establish the Murri Clinic at the Mater Mothers Public Hospital in Brisbane (the first midwifery-led, all-risk antenatal clinic for Aboriginal and Torres Strait Islander women) and the Indigenous birthing service at Caboolture, named by the Aunties as *Ngarrama*. Machellee is an inaugural board member of the Rhodanthe Lipsett Indigenous midwifery trust. She has been involved with the working party for Birthing on Country in our Community, and has published research articles on this topic.

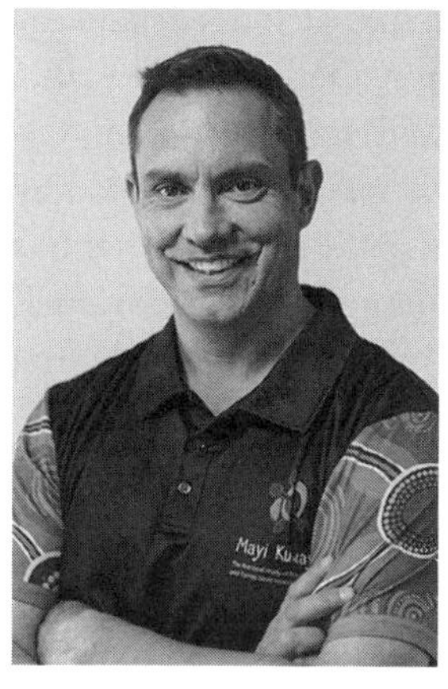

Ray Lovett is of the Ngiyampaa/Wongaibon people. He is a research fellow at the National Centre for Epidemiology and Population Health at the Australian National University, where he continues to work on large-scale cohort studies with the aim of improving care delivery in Aboriginal and Torres Strait Islander health. Ray also supports and supervises other Aboriginal and Torres Strait Islander scholars at the Australian National University (ANU). Ray holds a Bachelor of Nursing, Bachelor of Health Science (Public Health), a Master of Applied Epidemiology and a PhD in epidemiology. He has practised across the spectrum of the health system, including in the emergency department, and in neurosurgery and coronary care. He has also worked in rural hospitals and as an Aboriginal health worker in community health and in aged care. Ray has moved into primary healthcare, and specifically into Aboriginal community controlled health, where he has worked as a Registered Nurse and administrator.

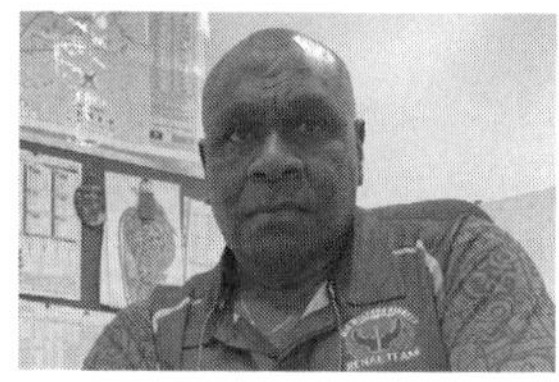

Sam Mills is a Nagilgal from Naghir Island of the Kulkalgal nation – he is intrinsically linked through his mother to Mer and the Dauareb tribe of Zenath Kes (Torres Strait). Sam's vision is to develop Torres Strait Islanders as world citizens who are able to govern and navigate their own affairs. Sam's experiences of working both in the hospital ward and chronic disease care in the community setting over the last 21 years, since graduating with a Bachelor of Nursing Studies from the University of New England, have fostered a passion for innovative primary healthcare models that embrace corporate responsibility as a solid foundation for improving the social status, and thus meaningful improvements in the health status, of Torres Strait Islander and Aboriginal people.

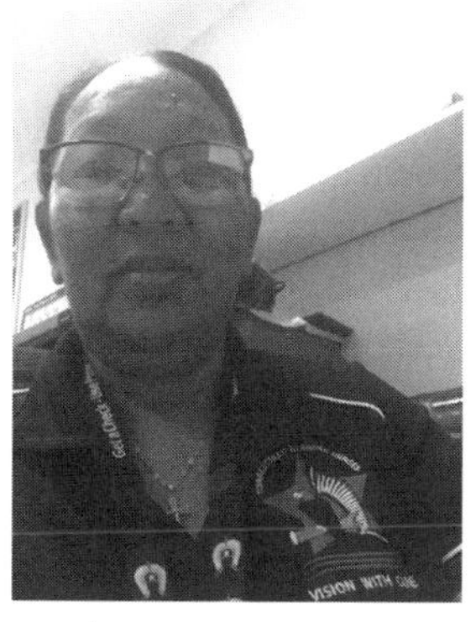

Yoko Mills was born and grew up on Thursday Island. Her father is Japanese and her mother's family connections are from the bottom Western and Eastern Islands of the Torres Strait. Yoko is a Clinical Nurse Consultant in Sexual & Reproductive Health on Thursday Island. Her nursing career takes her back to 1977, working as an assistant in nursing. She was one of the first graduates from a small cohort of students to complete the Enrolled Nurse training at the School of Nursing, Thursday Island Hospital, which commenced in 1981. In 1985 she worked as a sole practitioner for three years in the clinic previously called Special

Services, which was focused predominantly on sexual and women's health. Prior to commencing her degree in nursing, she completed a Diploma in Sexual Health Counselling through the Australasian College of Venereologist. In 2004 she completed her Bachelor of Nursing Studies at the University of New England in Armidale and returned to work in sexual health in 2005 at the Primary Health Care Centre on Thursday Island. Being passionate about sexual and reproductive health, in 2012 Yoko graduated with a Masters of Nurse Practitioner Studies – Young People's Health.

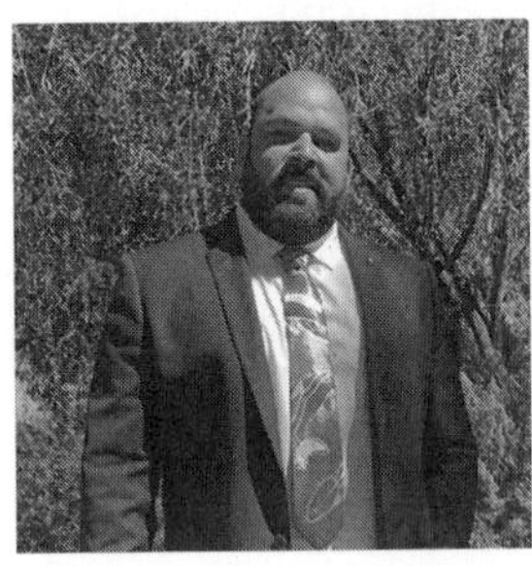

Francis Nona is a Torres Strait Islander employed in the School of Public Health at the University of Queensland, as a lecturer and researcher. He grew up in Brisbane and Saibai in the Torres Strait and is an initiated Badulaig man. His work is informed by his strong cultural training, balanced by his role as a Registered Nurse. As a Registered Nurse, he has undertaken previous roles as clinic manager for an Aboriginal community controlled health service, working in residential aged care, rural hospital and a youth detention centre. The research grant projects to which he is currently contributing include strategies to embed Aboriginal and Torres Strait Islander ways of knowing into public health teaching curricula, food sustainability for people in the Torres Strait, the health impacts of climate change on people in the Torres Strait, community understanding of impacts of COVID-19 on Aboriginal and Torres Strait Islander people and an evaluation of an Aboriginal and Torres Strait Islander healthy lifestyle program. Francis is very passionate about culturally appropriate healthcare for Aboriginal and Torres Strait Islander people. He was first inspired to become a Registered Nurse by observing the compassionate care his mother received in palliative care.

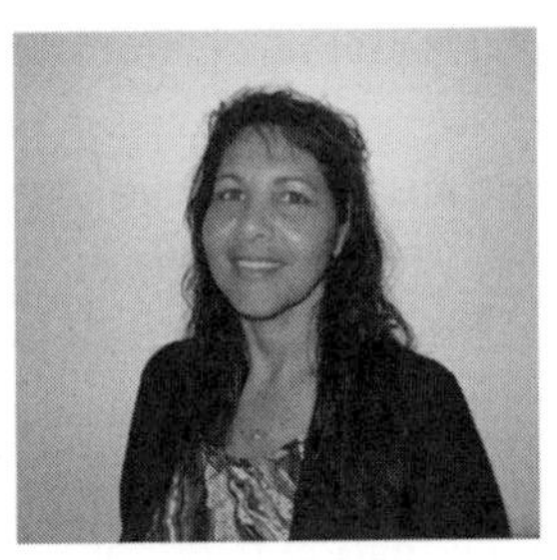

Nicole Ramsamy is an Aboriginal and Torres Strait Islander woman raised in Cairns. Her maternal side is the Kuku Yalanji from Bloomfield, Far North Queensland and her paternal family is from Boigu Island in the Torres Strait. Nicole is the Nurse Practitioner at the Weipa Integrated Health Service in a remote mining town and remote Aboriginal community. She is a Registered Nurse, Endorsed Registered Midwife and Nurse Practitioner, endorsed in rural and remote nursing. For most of her nursing career, she has lived in remote communities, and has worked for Queensland Health as a clinical nurse and clinical nurse-consultant; she has also relieved in the Director of Nursing and Midwifery role.

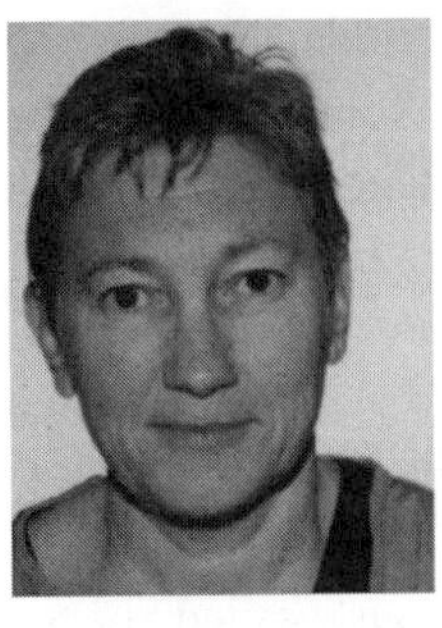

Juanita Sherwood is a proud Wiradjuri woman. She is Pro-Vice-Chancellor of Indigenous Engagement at Charles Sturt University. She is a Registered Nurse, teacher, lecturer, researcher and manager with a depth of working experiences of some 30 years in Aboriginal and Torres Strait Islander health and education. She has a PhD from the University of New South Wales, and has previously worked in lecturing, research, management and consultative roles in health, education and Indigenous studies.

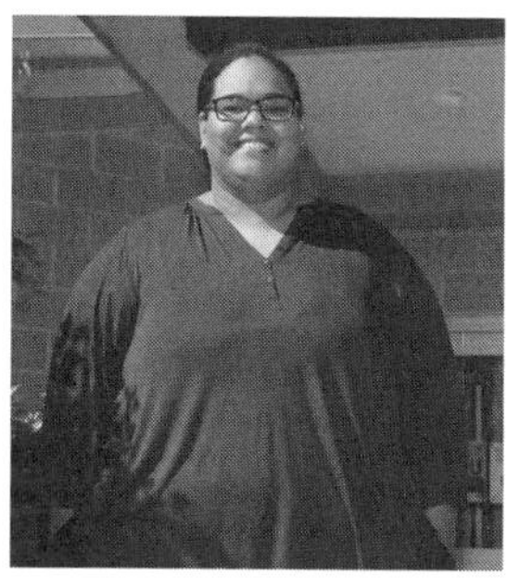

Kristin Waqanaviti is a clinical psychiatric nurse of mixed heritage from Far North Queensland. On her maternal great grandmother's side, she is connected to the Waanyi people and her maternal grandparents are of Torres Strait Islander descent. Kristin's father is an Indigenous Fijian, an iTaukei of the Naocodogo people and Kauna Clan of Rewa and Suva region. Kristin was raised in Cairns, Townsville and Brisbane, and spent time in rural Fiji and Alice Springs. Kristin is an Authorised Mental Health Practitioner currently working for Queensland Health and attained her undergraduate degree in Registered Nursing through Deakin University's Institute of Koorie Education. She has worked in aged care and acute settings before discovering her niche in a Medium Secure Psychiatric Unit in the Townsville Hospital. Kristin completed her Masters of Mental Health Nursing at the University of Newcastle and is currently working towards her next postgraduate qualification with the aim of effecting change for Aboriginal and Torres Strait Islander people experiencing mainstream service delivery in Queensland.

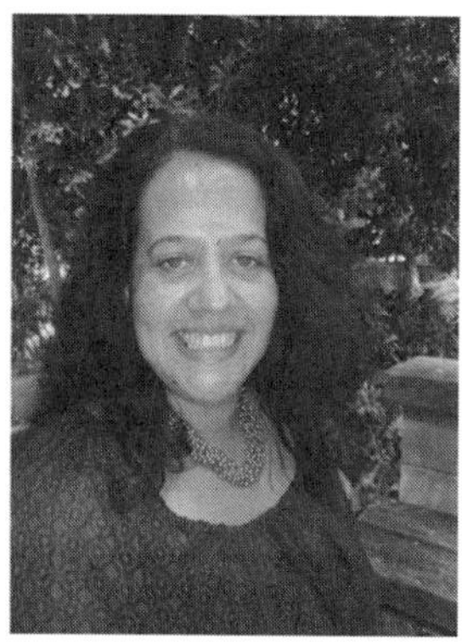

Raelene Ward (nee McKellar, Monaghan) is an Aboriginal woman of the Kunja traditional owner group of Cunnamulla and surrounding areas on her grandfather's side, and on her grandmother's side is a descendant of the Kooma people. both originating from south-west Queensland. Raelene received her PhD in 2019. She has been a practising nurse for just over 30 years, focusing on clinical work, lecturing and research on suicide, suicide prevention, Aboriginal health, social and emotional wellbeing and mental health, determinants of Aboriginal health, and broader areas of social justice. Her research efforts and impact in the Indigenous health space is evident in her career trajectory over the last 20+ years. Her research practice is Aboriginal nurse-led, and informed by community through effective and culturally appropriate consultation and engagement principles. It is recognised both nationally and internationally – particularly in the context of suicide prevention, Indigenous health and social and emotional wellbeing. Prior to that, she worked extensively in a variety of positions across a number of sectors: universities; rural, remote and regional communities; government organisations and the Aboriginal community controlled health sector (at state level and nationally). For the last 13 years, in the university context, Raelene has progressed through positions as project coordinator, research fellow, senior lecturer and associate professor with key leadership roles in the College for Indigenous Studies, Education and Research. Raelene is an academic in the University of Southern Queensland Nursing program, involved in leading curriculum reform in the context of Indigenous health, teaching at undergraduate and postgraduate levels, developing courses and course materials, engaging with Indigenous communities in the context of teaching and research initiatives, and supporting students.

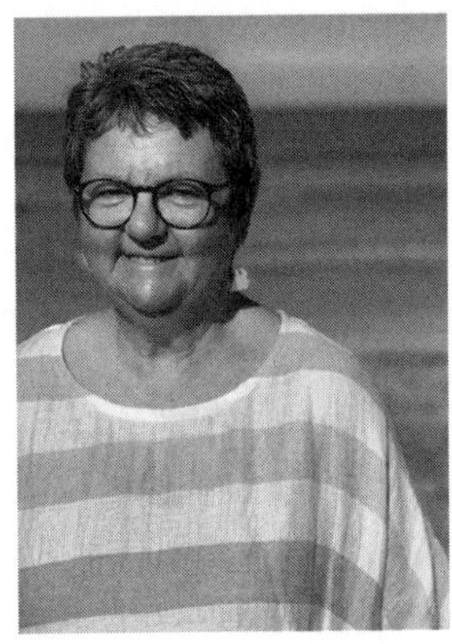

Rhonda L. Wilson PhD is a descendent of the Wiradjuri people on her grandmother's side. She was born and raised on Aniawan Land, a place and people for which she has a deep and enduring respect. Having lived in many places, with many cultures, she now lives respectfully on Darkinjung Country. Rhonda is an internationally recognised mental health nursing scientist with a research focus on digital health interventions. She has published widely in journals and books, and delivered conference presentations throughout the world. She is Professor of Nursing, and Deputy Head of School (Central Coast Campus), and Head of Indigenous in the School of Nursing and Midwifery at the University of Newcastle. Concurrently, she holds an external fractional appointment as a Professor of Nursing at Massey University, New Zealand. She is a Registered Nurse and a Credentialled Mental Health Nurse in Australia. She has worked across a variety of roles as a clinical nurse, researcher and academic in Australia, Denmark and New Zealand over the past 34 years. In addition, she is an experienced scientific assessor for the National Health and Medical Research Council (NHMRC) and the European Research Council. Most of her career has been in rural and regional locations across eastern Australia. Rhonda returned to Australia in 2019 after living and working in Denmark (University of Southern Denmark – SDU) where she was employed as Associate Professor of E Mental Health and Director of a Telepsychiatric Research Centre in the (health) Region of Southern Denmark (RSD), and affiliated with the Center for Psychiatric Nursing Research Denmark.

Acknowledgements

As is custom, we begin by acknowledging the Indigenous custodians across this nation, now known as Australia. We honour our collective Elders, past and present and emerging. We hope that they find this work honourable and join with us in seeing this as a contribution to the continuity of Indigenous knowledges and peoples.

We offer our deepest respect and appreciation to Wakgun Elder Ivy Molly Booth as the gifter of language for this textbook. Her gift enabled all of us to maintain a focus on the goal and the process of learning and talking in a good way.

A special thank you to the Cambridge University Press team for believing that this textbook was needed and for commitment to working with us in a way that did not diminish the voices of Aboriginal and Torres Strait Islander nurses, midwives and health specialists. The team enabled and supported our collective voices to bring this text to fruition, to fill the identified gap within the nursing and midwifery curriculum.

Odette and Bronwyn wish to thank all of the authors for their dedicated time and commitment to not only creating the first text of its kind in Australia, but also for realising the effect this textbook will have on the gap in life differentials that remain between Indigenous and non-Indigenous Australians. A special mention to their families and communities for supporting them and for allowing them the space to produce this work and to be part of this book.

We thank each other for sharing the dream, the belief that we could do it, the laughs, tears, the joy in seeing it realised. *Yatdjuligin* fills a gap and we understand its capacity to make a difference, both now and into the future.

We are grateful to the following individuals and organisations for permission to use their material in *Yatdjuligin*.

Figure 2.1: based on data © Commonwealth of Australia 2020. Licensed under Attribution 4.0 International (CC BY 4.0), https://creativecommons.org/licenses/by/4.0; **2.2:** based on data © Commonwealth of Australia 2019 and 2020. Licenced under Creative Commons Attribution 4.0 International licence (CC BY 4.0): https://creativecommons.org/licenses/by/4.0; **2.3**: based on data © Commonwealth of Australia 2016, 2017, 2019, 2020 and © Australian Institute of Health and Welfare. Licenced under Creative Commons Attribution 3.0 Australia licence: https://creativecommons.org/licenses/by/3.0/au/deed.en and Creative Commons Attribution 4.0 International licence: https://creativecommons.org/licenses/by/4.0; **2.4** based on data © Commonwealth of Australia 2016, 2017, 2019 and 2020. Licenced under Creative Commons Attribution 3.0 Australia licence: https://creativecommons.org/licenses/by/3.0/au/deed.en and Creative Commons Attribution 4.0 International licence: https://creativecommons.org/licenses/by/4.0; **3.1**: Reproduced with permission; **4.1**: Reproduced from image © Torres Strait Regional Authority; **4.2**: based on data from ABS (2017). © Commonwealth of Australia. Licensed under Attribution 4.0 International (CC BY 4.0), https://creativecommons.org/licenses/by/4.0; **6.1**: © Australian

Institute of Health and Welfare 2015. Licenced under Creative Commons Attribution 3.0 Australia (CC BY 3.0) licence: https://creativecommons.org/licenses/by/3.0/au; **7.1**, **7.2**, **14.2**: © Commonwealth of Australia. Licenced under Attribution 4.0 International (CC BY 4.0): https://creativecommons.org/licenses/by/4.0; **7.3**, **7.4**: © Australian Institute of Health and Welfare 2020. Licensed under Attribution 3.0 Australia (CC BY 3.0 AU), https://creativecommons.org/licenses/by/3.0/au; **7.5**, **7.6**, **16.1**: © Australian Institute of Health and Welfare. Licenced under Attribution 3.0 Australia (CC BY 3.0): https://creativecommons.org/licenses/by/3.0/au; **10.2**, **10.3**: © NATSIHWA. Reproduced with permission; **10.4**, **10.5**: © 2020 AHPRA. Reproduced with permission; **11.1**: © 2013 National Collaborating Centre for Aboriginal Health. Reproduced with permission; **11.2**: © Commonwealth of Australia 2018. Licenced under Creative Commons CC BY 4.0 licence: https://creativecommons.org/licenses/by/4.0; **12.2**: adapted from material © Curtin University of Technology 2015. Reproduced with permission: https://bcec.edu.au/assets/bcec-community-wellbeing-from-the-ground-up-a-yawuru-example.pdf; **14.1**: © CBPATSISP. Reproduced with permission; **14.4**: based on data © Commonwealth of Australia. Adapted under Creative Commons Attribution 4.0 International Licence: https://creativecommons.org/licenses/by/4.0.

Table 12.2: adapted from material © Curtin University of Technology 2015. Reproduced with permission: https://bcec.edu.au/assets/bcec-community-wellbeing-from-the-ground-up-a-yawuru-example.pdf; **12.3**: reproduced from material © 2018 by the authors. Licensee MDPI, Basel, Switzerland. This article is an open access article distributed under the terms and conditions of the Creative Commons Attribution (CC BY) license (http://creativecommons.org/licenses/by/4.0/); **Box 16.3**: © The State of Queensland (Children's Health Queensland) 2020, Queensland Government. Licenced under Creative Commons Attribution 4.0 International licence (CC BY 4.0): https://creativecommons.org/licenses/by/4.0/deed.en.

Extract from Face the Facts: © Australian Human Rights Commission 2012.

Extract from Uluru Statement of the Heart © Commonwealth of Australia 2017. Licenced under Creative Commons Attribution 4.0 International licence: https://creativecommons.org/licenses/by/4.0/legalcode.

Extracts from Jones et al (2018), Associations between Participation in a Ranger Program and Health and Wellbeing Outcomes among Aboriginal and Torres Strait Islander People in Central Australia: A Proof of Concept Study, *International Journal of Environmental Research and Public Health*: Copyright © 2018 by the authors. Licensee MDPI, Basel, Switzerland. This article is an open access article distributed under the terms and conditions of the Creative Commons Attribution (CC BY) license (http://creativecommons.org/licenses/by/4.0).

Extracts from *National Strategic Framework for Aboriginal and Torres Strait Islander Peoples' Mental Health and Social and Emotional Wellbeing*: © Commonwealth of Australia 2017. Licenced under Creative Commons Attribution 4.0 International licence (CC BY 4.0): https://creativecommons.org/licenses/by/4.0/deed.en.

Every effort has been made to trace and acknowledge copyright. The publisher apologises for any accidental infringement and welcomes information that would rectify the situation.

Acronyms and abbreviations

AAQA	Australian Aged Care Quality Agency
ABS	Australian Bureau of Statistics
ACCHO	Aboriginal Community Controlled Health Organisation
ACCHS	Aboriginal Community Controlled Health Service
ACHT-CACHS	Aboriginal Child Health Team – Child and Adolescent Community Health Service
ACM	Australian College of Midwives
ACSCDS	Aged Care Sector Committee Diversity Sub-group
ACSQHC	Australian Commission on Safety and Quality in Health Care
AECG	Aboriginal Education Consultative Group
AH & MRCNSW	Aboriginal Health and Medical Research Council of New South Wales
AHCSA	Aboriginal Health Council of South Australia
AHMAC	Australian Health Ministers Advisory Council
AHPRA	Australian Health Practitioner Regulations Agency
AHRC	Australian Human Rights Commission
AHWLO	Aboriginal Health Worker and Liaison Officer
AIATSIS	Australian Institute of Aboriginal and Torres Strait Islander Studies
AICCHS	Aboriginal and Islander community controlled health services
AIFS	Australian Institute of Family Studies
AIHW	Australian Institute of Health and Welfare
AIPA	Australian Indigenous Psychologists Association
ALRC	Australian Law Reform Commission
ALS	advanced life support
AMCHS	Aboriginal Maternal and Child Health Services
AMS	Aboriginal Medical Service
AMSANT	Aboriginal Medical Services Alliance Northern Territory
ANAO	Australian National Audit Office
ANFPP	Australian Nurse Family Partnership Program
ANMAC	Australian Nursing and Midwifery Accreditation Council
APA	American Psychiatric Association
ARHD	acute rheumatic heart disease
ATSICHS	Aboriginal and Torres Strait Islander Community Health Service
ATSIHP	Aboriginal and Torres Strait Islander health practitioner
ATSIHPBA	Aboriginal and Torres Strait Islander Health Practice Board of Australia

ATSISPEP	Aboriginal and Torres Strait Islander Suicide Prevention Evaluation Project
AWHN	Australian Women's Health Network
AWHN-TC	Australian Women's Health Network Talking Circle
BATSIHS	Brisbane Aboriginal and Torres Strait Islander Health Service
BMA	Body Mass Index
CAAC	Central Australian Aboriginal Congress
CARPA	Central Australian Rural Practitioner Association
CATSINaM	Congress of Aboriginal and Torres Strait Islander Nurses and Midwives
CBPATSISP	Centre of Best Practice in Aboriginal and Torres Strait Islander Suicide Prevention
CCHS	community controlled health service
CDEP	Community Development Employment Project
CEE	Centre for Epidemiology and Evidence
CEO	chief executive officer
CHQHHS	Children's Health Queensland Hospital and Health Service
CLC	Central Land Council
COAG	Council of Australian Governments
CRANA	Council of Remote Area Nurses of Australia
CRCAH	Cooperative Research Centre for Aboriginal Health
CSDH	Commission on Social Determinants of Health
CVD	cardiovascular disease
CWA	Country Women's Association
DAA	Department of Aboriginal Affairs
DATSIPD	Department of Aboriginal and Torres Strait Islander Policy and Development
DFAT	Department of Foreign Affairs and Trade
DHA	Department of Health and Ageing
DHAC	Department of Health and Aged Care
DHWA	Department of Health Western Australia
DIISRTE	Department of Industry, Innovation, Science Research and Tertiary Education
DMF	Decision-making Framework for Nursing and Midwifery
DOGIT	Deed of Grant in Trust
DPMC	Department of the Prime Minister and Cabinet
EDIS	Emergency Department Information System
ENT	Ear Nose and Throat
ERP	Estimated Resident Population
FASD	Foetal Alcohol Spectrum Disorder
FCAATSI	Federal Council for the Advancement of Aborigines and Torres Strait Islanders
GDM	gestational diabetes mellitus (GDM)
GP	general practitioner
HACC	Home and Community Care
HPF	Health Performance Framework

HREC	Human Research Ethics Committee
HREOC	Human Rights and Equal Opportunity Commission
HRSCAA	House of Representatives Standing Committee on Aboriginal Affairs
HWA	Health Workforce Australia
IAHA	Indigenous Allied Health Australia
ICN	International Council of Nurses
ICU	intensive care unit
IHP	Indigenous health practitioner
IHW	Indigenous health worker
ILO	Indigenous Liaison Officer
IMHW	Indigenous Mental Health Worker
IPCC	Intergovernmental Panel on Climate Change
IT	information technology
IUIH	Institute for Urban Indigenous Health
IV	intravenous
K5	five-item Kessler Psychological Distress Scale
KHRCDU	Koori Health Research and Community Development Unit
LBW	low birthweight
LGBTIQ	lesbian, gay, bisexual, transgender, intersex and queer
LMS	London Missionary Society
MHCNSW	Mental Health Commission of New South Wales
MPS	Multi-Purpose Service
MSM	men who have sex with men
NACCHO	National Aboriginal Community Controlled Health Organisation
NAHSWP	National Aboriginal Health Strategy Working Party
NATSIFACP	National Aboriginal and Torres Strait Islander Flexible Aged Care Program
NATSIHC	National Aboriginal and Torres Strait Islander Health Council
NATSIHMS	National Aboriginal and Torres Strait Islander Health Measures Survey
NATSIHP	National Aboriginal and Torres Strait Islander Health Plan 2013–2023
NATSIHWA	National Aboriginal and Torres Strait Islander Health Worker Association
NCCAH	National Collaborating Centre for Aboriginal Health
NCD	neurocognitive disorder
NCHWS	National Child Health and Wellbeing Subcommittee
NCNZ	Nursing Council of New Zealand
NGO	non-government organisation
NHMRC	National Health and Medical Research Council
NIRAKN	National Indigenous Researchers and Knowledge Network
NMBA	Nursing and Midwifery Board of Australia
NMHC	National Mental Health Commission
NMHWG	National Mental Health Working Group
NRAS	National Registration and Accreditation Scheme

NSLHD	Northern Sydney Local Health District
OM	otitis media
PALS	paediatric life support
PAR	participatory action research
PCCM	Primary Clinical Care Manual
PHCC	Primary Health Care Centre
PHTLS	pre-hospital trauma life support
PNG	Papua New Guinea
PTSS	Patient Travel Subsidy Scheme
QAIHC	Queensland Aboriginal and Islander Health Council
QAIHF	Queensland Aboriginal and Islander Health Forum
QPC	Queensland Productivity Commission
RAICCHO	Regional Aboriginal and Islander Community Controlled Health Organisation
RAN	remote-area nurse
RFDS	Royal Flying Doctor Service
RHSQ	Royal Historical Society of Queensland
RIPERN	Remote Isolated Practice Endorsed Registered Nurse
RN	Registered Nurse
SAAHP	South Australian Aboriginal Health Partnership
SAHMRI	South Australian Health & Medical Research Institute
SCRGSP	Steering Committee for the Review of Government Service Provision
SEWB	social and emotional wellbeing
SHRG	Social Health Reference Group
SIDS	Sudden Infant Death Syndrome
SLQ	State Library of Queensland
SNAICC	Secretariat of National Aboriginal and Islander Child Care
SPA	Suicide Prevention Australia
STI	sexually transmitted infection
TCHHS	Torres and Cape Hospital and Health Services
TNCC	trauma nursing core course
TSIMA	Torres Strait Islander Media Association
TSMPHC	Torres Strait Model for Primary Health Care
TSRA	Torres Strait Regional Authority
UHCW	unregulated healthcare worker
VACCHO	Victorian Aboriginal Community Controlled Health Organisation
VAHS	Victorian Aboriginal Health Services
WHO	World Health Organization

Introduction

Gracelyn Smallwood

This edition of *Yatdjuligin* was written in 2020, the Year of the Nurse and Midwife. It was also written during the first global pandemic for more than 100 years – COVID-19. In this year, while the professions of nursing and midwifery were celebrated, the reality was that nurses and midwives were working in unprecedented times on the front line across the globe.

COVID-19 impacted many of the authors of this textbook. Some of them continued to work on the front line in remote Indigenous communities as they were placed under Biosecurity Acts; other authors had family members who became ill with COVID-19; while yet others navigated the new online realm of nursing and midwifery education. The single goal, however, was to remain focused on producing this textbook to guide the teaching and learning of all student nurses and midwives.

It has been a year of reflection for many. I have been a practising nurse and midwife and retired after 50 years in September 2020. I am a Birrigubba, Kalkadoon and Australian South Sea Islander woman. I grew up in Townsville in a tin shack with hessian bag curtains and a dirt floor with no electricity. I had eighteen siblings. I finished Year 10 and decided to go nursing because nursing was one of the things that was available to Aboriginal people. I completed my four years of general nursing in 1972, then a one-year midwifery course at the Townsville Base Hospital.

My mother and father were both activists. To be an activist is to invite suspicion from white Australia. I have been engaged in a lifelong struggle for my people, the First Peoples of Australia. This book, *Yatdjuligin*, doesn't take the easy path, and reading it isn't always comfortable. It embodies what *Yatdjuligin* means, challenging stereotypes and historically ingrained and accepted ways of working with and caring for Aboriginal and Torres Strait Islander people within health environments. *Yatdjuligin* breaks new ground, and is part of a new activism – one that engages Indigenous nursing and health scholars in shaping what is known about us through the academy.

I encourage you as a student to read the words and savour the knowledge shared through *Yatdjuligin*, then to use it to challenge yourself and others to do your best in your work with Aboriginal and Torres Strait Islander people. Remember that activism does invite suspicion, but know that it is better to challenge and work for change than to see the continued discrimination and injustices faced by my people. I thank you in anticipation.

Nursing Aboriginal and Torres Strait Islander peoples: Why do we need this text?

Within the curriculum for students of nursing and midwifery, learning about the specific health needs of Australia's Aboriginal and Torres Strait Islander peoples is still in its infancy. However, the need for improved approaches to addressing the health needs of Indigenous Australians is not new. Practising Aboriginal and Torres Strait Islander nurses and people who work in the Aboriginal and Torres Strait Islander health sector have long recognised the critical need for improved health outcomes for Indigenous Australians. As far back as the 1940s, Aboriginal midwife Sister Muriel Stanley articulated the need for non-Indigenous nurses and midwives to learn about the health crisis facing Indigenous peoples.

As you will read below, the Australian Nursing and Midwifery Accreditation Council has made strong statements about the nursing and midwifery curriculum and content relevant to the health issues of Aboriginal and Torres Strait Islander people. *Yatdjuligin* is now in its third edition and is the only text for nursing and midwifery students entirely authored by Indigenous Registered Nurses and Midwives and Indigenous health authors focusing on the health needs of Indigenous people. Collectively, the authors have more than 200 years of clinical practice experience.

I have waited a long time for a text like this, which provides practical information for student nurses and midwives about working with Aboriginal and Torres Strait Islander clients. I am excited about this text and respectful of the many Aboriginal and Torres Strait Islander nurses and midwives who have come before me. I honour their commitment to the education of nursing and midwifery students.

Gifting of the book's title: *Yatdjuligin*

The name *Yatdjuligin* was gifted to the authors to use as the title of this textbook by Aboriginal Elder Ivy Molly Booth, who is the grandmother of Odette Best.

Yatdjuligin is from the dialect of the Wakgun Clan group of the Gureng Gureng Nation. These clan lands are in the south-western part of the Gureng Gureng Nation in Queensland, and extend north of the Burnett River, west as far as Mundubbera, north to Eidsvold along the Dawes Range to Cania Gorge, then east to Miriamvale and Baffle Creek and south to Mt Perry and the Burnett River. These boundaries are in the stories and songlines of the Gureng Gureng Nation.

Yatdjuligin translates to 'talking in a good way'. For Wakgun people, the process of *Yatdjuligin* is deeply embedded in learning. It belongs to a two-part process in the traditional passing on of knowledge about Country, its resources and their uses. Wakgun people's knowledge of traditional medicines (pharmacopoeia) is well established and continues to be widely practised.

This passing on of knowledge includes you, as student nurses, in your journey to become Registered Nurses and/or Midwives. As students, you will undergo instruction in a range of skills vital to your work as Registered Nurses and/or Midwives. You will be shown these skills, with explanations of why and how to use them. You will participate in laboratory sessions, where you will mimic what you have learnt. The process of your learning links the theory you are taught to your practice.

Importantly, *Yatdjuligin* can be confronting. Passing on knowledge can sometimes be difficult, for many reasons – the knowledge itself may be difficult to understand, people may not want to know it, or they may not be ready to learn it. Learning can cause discomfort. And discomfort should be expected within this textbook. The health of Aboriginal and Torres Strait Islander people historically has been excluded from the nursing curriculum (and education more broadly), and you may find that learning about the health of Indigenous Australians is confronting and perplexing. This experience of discomfort is essential within *Yatdjuligin* and should not be shunned. While learning the knowledge may cause discomfort, there is safety in the process within which it occurs. I hope that you are able to embrace the new knowledge contained in this text and incorporate it into your practice.

Chapter 1: Historical and current perspectives on the health of Aboriginal and Torres Strait Islander peoples provides the historical context of the life-expectancy gap between Indigenous and non-Indigenous Australians and the health differential crisis that continues today. It emphasises the need for nurses to critically appraise the role of the nurse and midwife as change agents in the field of Indigenous health.

Chapter 2: A history of health services for Aboriginal and Torres Strait Islander people discusses what is known about the pre-invasion health system and the health status of Indigenous Australians. It considers health service provision during the contact period and health status during the separation and protection periods. It also highlights the outcomes for Indigenous health. The chapter discusses the rise of the Aboriginal community controlled health services system. Importantly, each section of this chapter is, where possible, framed within the prism of nursing: it examines the role of nurses historically in the health system and in healthcare delivery.

Chapter 3: The cultural safety journey: An Aboriginal Australian nursing and midwifery context explores the concept of cultural safety as it applies to the Australian nursing and midwifery setting. This chapter discusses ways to understand cultures, with a particular emphasis on encouraging nursing and midwifery students to examine their own beliefs, attitudes and views. The chapter highlights the multiplicity of each individual's cultures and encourages students to consider the potential effects of their cultures while they are caring for Indigenous Australians.

Chapter 4: Torres Strait Islander health and wellbeing critically explores the health and wellbeing needs of Torres Strait Islanders. Aligned with the principles of cultural safety, this chapter uncovers the historical, social and political determinants of health for Torres Strait Islanders, including the ongoing impacts of colonisation and racism. Contemporary health and wellbeing issues for the Torres Strait region are also explored, including climate change and its impact on the social determinants of health, and its role in increasing the risk of some communicable diseases.

Chapter 5: Indigenous gendered health perspectives explores the unique perspectives of what Aboriginal and Torres Strait Islander communities across Australia commonly call 'women's business' and 'men's business'. It breaks down the nuances between men's and women's health, and offers an insight into appropriate nursing and midwifery care. It also explores 'sister girls' within the context of the health needs of Aboriginal and Torres Strait Islander people, and the need for the delivery of healthcare to be underpinned by cultural safety.

Chapter 6: Community controlled health services: What they are and how they work explores the important role of Aboriginal Medical Services in improving health outcomes for Aboriginal and Torres Strait Islander people. The chapter explains the complex development of the sector, explores how the services were conceived and established, and discusses the political reality faced by Aboriginal and Torres Strait Islander people at that time.

Chapter 7: Midwifery practices and Aboriginal and Torres Strait Islander women: Urban and regional perspectives outlines the experiences and needs of urban Indigenous women during pregnancy and birthing. It challenges conventional views about urban Indigenous families and highlights the many issues relevant to understanding the needs of urban Aboriginal and Torres Strait Islander families during pregnancy, birth and early parenting.

Chapter 8: Indigenous birthing in remote locations: Grandmothers' Law and government medicine encourages students to consider the complex issues relevant to midwifery practice in remote areas, both past and present. It questions how current hospital birthing services affect the wellbeing of Aboriginal and Torres Strait Islander women from remote areas who leave their communities to give birth away from Country. This chapter contextualises the effects of the clash between Grandmothers' Law and government medicine on women from remote communities.

Chapter 9: Remote-area nursing practice provides a positive perspective of remote lifestyles and the healthcare needs of Aboriginal and Torres Strait Islander people who live in remote communities. The chapter helps students to evaluate the scope of practice and educational needs required to work as a remote-area nurse. It also describes some of the dynamics in remote communities that influence the ways in which healthcare services are organised and delivered by remote-area nurses.

Chapter 10: Working with Aboriginal and Torres Strait Islander health workers and health practitioners outlines the integral role of Aboriginal and Torres Strait Islander health workers in Indigenous healthcare across the country. Aboriginal and Torres Strait Islander health workers seek to meet the primary healthcare needs of Indigenous Australians. This chapter describes the historical development of the health worker role and helps nursing and midwifery students to understand how to work and collaborate with and delegate to Aboriginal and Torres Strait Islander health workers.

Chapter 11: Indigenous-led qualitative research explores Aboriginal and Torres Strait Islander approaches to research. Research has the potential to support improvements in Aboriginal health by informing and changing both policy and practice. Historically, most research was conducted on, not with, Aboriginal communities. Too often, research was not respectful, did not address Aboriginal priorities and was of no benefit to participating communities. This chapter describes current approaches to Aboriginal and Torres Strait Islander health research and explains the ethical principles that underpin it. It discusses ways in which researchers can develop shared values and priorities, and bring direct health benefits to both Aboriginal and Torres Strait Islander people and to the wider Australian population.

Chapter 12: Aboriginal and Torres Strait Islander quantitative research examines quantitative research methodologies in the Aboriginal and Torres Strait Islander context. It examines the methodological approaches that underpin Indigenous research, with a particular emphasis on quantitative research. The chapter outlines key terms and definitions associated with research and the key differentiations between research methodology and methods. The authors outline what Indigenous methodologies are and how these can be incorporated into research. The theories presented in this chapter are supported by case examples of appropriate quantitative research being undertaken with Aboriginal and Torres Strait Islander people.

Chapter 13: Navigating First Nations social and emotional wellbeing in mainstream mental health services presents an introduction intended to help students understand the main principles related this complex topic area. It explores the harmful effects of exposure to racism, trauma and inequality, and discusses how these can erode the integrity of positive individual, intergenerational and community social and emotional wellbeing, resulting in a deterioration of mental health, and leading to mental illness for some First Nations people. It also presents some practical guidance related to providing culturally appropriate person-centred and trauma-informed mental healthcare to First Nations people.

Chapter 14: Cultural understandings of Aboriginal suicide from a social and emotional wellbeing perspective discusses the differences between mental health and social and emotional wellbeing. It does this through exploring the historical and contemporary perspectives of social and emotional wellbeing. It offers alarming statistics about suicide in Indigenous communities across Australia and offers some understanding of the contributing factors. Further, it discusses the needs for culturally safe service provision for Indigenous people's social and emotional wellbeing.

Chapter 15: Indigenous child health helps to provide an understanding of cultural and social considerations in assessing and caring for Aboriginal and Torres Strait Islander children. It explores the issues and impacts of birth registrations and Aboriginal and Torres Strait Islander identification. It further provides the current and historical health status of Aboriginal and Torres Strait Islander children. Importantly, it also engages the student in understanding culturally safe health screening and initiatives aimed at promoting Aboriginal and Torres Strait Islander children's health.

Chapter 16: Caring for our Elders begins by exploring the situations that face Aboriginal and Torres Strait Islander people as they age, including the early onset of chronic disease, a shorter lifespan and the increasing need for aged care packages. The chapter discusses the need for culturally safe aged care. It discusses options for palliative care and explains the cultural reasons why Aboriginal and Torres Strait Islander people may choose to disengage from treatment and return to their home communities.

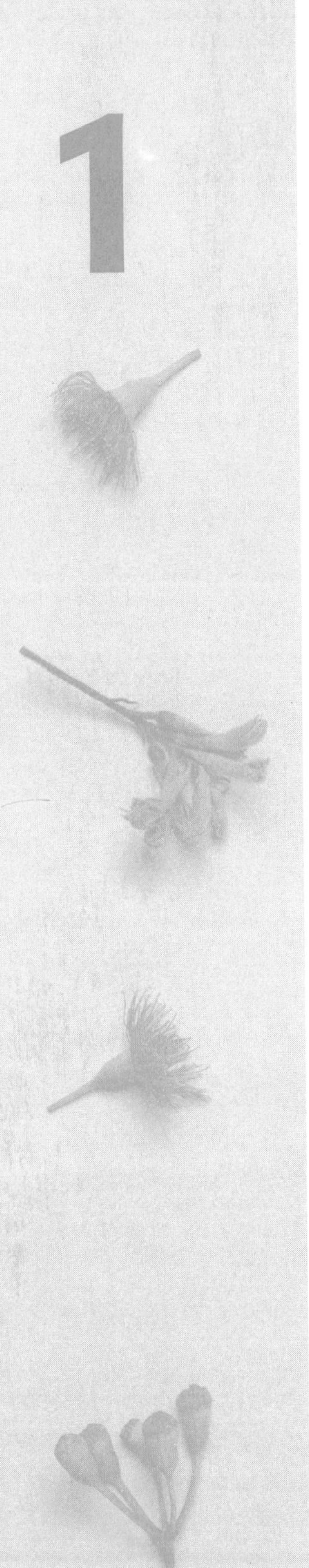

1 Historical and current perspectives on the health of Aboriginal and Torres Strait Islander peoples

Juanita Sherwood

With acknowledgement to Lynore K. Geia

LEARNING OBJECTIVES

This chapter will help you to understand:

- How Aboriginal and Torres Strait Islander health is portrayed
- The key events in Australian history that have influenced the health of Aboriginal and Torres Strait Islander peoples, Australia's First Nations peoples
- The health gap that exists between Aboriginal and Torres Strait Islander peoples and non-Indigenous Australians
- The current health of Aboriginal and Torres Strait Islander peoples, as well as the policies, and environmental and historical factors, that affect Indigenous health outcomes today
- The role of nurses and midwives as change agents in the field of Australia's First Nations peoples' health

KEY WORDS

Australian Charter of Healthcare Rights
Closing the Gap
colonisation
health gap
racism
social determinants of health
social justice
Stolen Generations
worldview

Introduction

The health of Australia's First Nations peoples – Aboriginal and Torres Strait Islander peoples – is critically poor and requires urgent and informed attention at both state and national levels. The early days of contact between colonial forces and First Nations peoples saw the onset of the health catastrophe that continues to engulf Australia's Aboriginal and Torres Strait Islander peoples today. This is a catastrophe of death, disease and entrenched social disadvantage. This crisis is real, and it is complicated by our history and the many factors that shape Australia today.

Prior to 1788, there were at least 500 language groups living as autonomous nations across the land that we now call Australia. Australia is now recognised to be the home of the oldest living and surviving cultural groups in the world. They traded with each other and maintained social and educational systems. Archaeological evidence confirms at least 120,000 years of permanent residence in Australia (Broome, 2002). Prior to **colonisation**, each nation lived separately, each with its own language and cultural traditions. But with invasion and subsequent colonisation, the origins of the First Nations peoples and their names for themselves were dismissed as irrelevant (Smith, 1999). Culturally specific, self-assigned names were replaced with the global terms 'Aboriginal' or 'Indigenous', which were from the Western tradition. Colonising forces named the country and named the people who lived there (Smith, 1999).

colonisation In Australia, a political, economic and social system of British imperialism to seize and establish control over land by force. Colonisation is a continuous and ongoing process and impacts every Australian's life through the production of dominant knowledge systems based on a Western worldview and informed by Western interests. (Sherwood, 2010, p. 140)

This chapter provides a perspective on the current health issues facing First Nations peoples in Australia, placed within their historical context. It explores some of the historical factors that underpin the gap between the health of Indigenous and non-Indigenous Australians. It describes the policy environment that established the **Closing the Gap** campaign, and challenges nurses and midwives to consider their personal responsibility for closing the health gap.

The authors of this chapter are Aboriginal women who have worked or are working as nurses and midwives. We specialise in Aboriginal and Torres Strait Islander health and have been privileged to gain and develop our knowledge and expertise in various sectors of Aboriginal and Torres Strait Islander health. We have used our nursing skills and cultural knowledge to advocate for better and more appropriate health services for Australia's First Nations peoples. We are interested in a range of healthcare environments, from community health clinics to hospitals.

We argue that Aboriginal and Torres Strait Islander health is the business of *every* health professional in Australia. We believe that health professionals need to be familiar with the history of Australia's Aboriginal and Torres Strait Islander peoples. Understanding of the historical context helps to put current healthcare needs into perspective. Understanding something about the Country on which you are working and the custodians who care for it is a critical step in working with Aboriginal and Torres Strait Islander peoples towards building a healthier Australia.

The narrative of Aboriginal and Torres Strait Islander health

racism Expressing overt and covert prejudice, discrimination and/or hostility towards people based on the belief that their race, including their cultural worldview and knowledge systems, is inferior to the race, cultural worldview and/or knowledge systems of the person and/or system with the discriminatory gaze.

social determinants of health Defined by the World Health Organization (WHO) as 'the conditions in which people are born, grow, live, work and age. These circumstances are shaped by the distribution of money, power and resources at global, national and local levels.' (WHO, 2020)

Deficit discourse is the construction of a narrative that portrays Indigenous peoples in a negative way. In Indigenous health, many health providers treat Australia's First Nations peoples with discrimination and **racism**, believing that their poor health status is a result of their lack or failure to maintain wellbeing. This is not the case. **Social determinants of health** within the context of ongoing colonisation are key players in health and are often excluded from the discourse because it is always easier to blame the victim.

The dominant public story of Aboriginal and Torres Strait Islander health status is a 'bad news story', or 'a problem to be solved' (Saggers & Gray, 1991). Media stories portray examples of appalling health, social breakdown, housing crises and wasted money. The dominant story is based on its Western truth, so governments continue to make the same decisions in developing policy, programs and services for Australia's First Nations peoples and their communities, and health improvements often do not occur.

The dominant Western perspective has resulted from a lack of balance in presenting the experiences of Australia's First Nations peoples since invasion. Many health professionals have had little opportunity to gain access to this knowledge because, until very recently, it has not been taught in schools or universities. They also have little opportunity to learn and understand the different worldviews and cultures of Aboriginal and Torres Strait Islander peoples. Further, they often don't have an understanding of their own worldviews, unconscious bias and cultures as non-Indigenous Australians, which is crucial for being culturally safe practitioners.

Policy decisions about Aboriginal and Torres Strait Islander peoples' health continue to be made without community partnership. Geia (2012, p. 20) argues that her community commonly sees governments undergoing a repeated process of policy and program development, but presenting it as though it were new:

> New ways of government 'doing consultation' with Aboriginal communities still appear as interventions for purely political ends that are at most culturally inappropriate and inaccessible for Aboriginal families and bearing little sense of ownership by the Aboriginal people because their participation in policy development is at best given lip service. Again it is policy done to Aboriginal people and not genuine partnerships with Aboriginal people.

Government policy-makers and many health professionals fail to appreciate that by continuing the same old policy practices and program development, little will be gained. It is time that health professionals listened to their clients informing them about their health needs and responded appropriately. The prospect of progress and being effective in improving the lives of the people in communities remains, at best, a pipe dream (Geia, 2012, p. 20). The same outcomes continue to be seen, and the burden of ill-health experienced by Aboriginal and Torres Strait Islander peoples continues to grow.

The stories that health practitioners learn about Aboriginal and Torres Strait Islander people's health – whether through the media or through school, families or connection to communities – influence the ways in which they work with Aboriginal and Torres Strait Islander clients. At the level of patient care, the ways in which nurses and midwives think about, talk about and deliver care to Aboriginal and Torres Strait Islander people will depend on the narrative being played in their heads. Is that story positive or negative? Is it one of hope or hopelessness?

On the whole, these health stories are explored through the narrative of a deficit discourse:

> 'Deficit discourse' is a mode of thinking that frames and represents Aboriginal and Torres Strait Islander people in a narrative of negativity, deficiency and failure (Fforde et al., 2013). It particularly occurs when discussions about disadvantage become so mired in reductionist narratives of failure that Aboriginal and Torres Strait Islander peoples themselves are seen as the problem.
>
> These discussions thus become a continuation of the pejorative and patronising race-based discourses that have long been used to represent Aboriginal and Torres Strait Islander people. Deficit discourse is both a product of, and reinforces, the marginalisation of Aboriginal and Torres Strait Islander people's voices, perspectives and world-views.
>
> It appears likely that deficit discourse impacts on the health and wellbeing of Aboriginal and Torres Strait Islander people in multiple ways. It contributes to forms of external and internalised racism, and shades out solutions that recognise strengths, capabilities and rights.
>
> (Fogarty et al., 2018, p. xi)

We know that nurses and midwives do make value judgements about their clients – whether they intend to or not – and these judgements have invariably been informed through a 'deficit discourse', which will influence the ways in which they deliver patient care (Jongen et al., 2018). It is vital that we all become aware of and reflect upon what messaging we are working from. Is it well informed through an evidence-based First Nations health collaboration or is it furthering discriminatory agendas fuelled by institutional and personal racism?

Knowing the ancient story

Australia's First Nations peoples believe they did not travel to this continent, but originated from their distinct Country. Archaeological evidence suggests that Aboriginal peoples have lived on and cared for the Australian continent for between 60,000 and 120,000 years – a land tenure that outdates that of any other civilisation in the world (Sherwood, 2013). Bruce Pascoe (2014) has researched and delivered an extremely informative text that further substantiates the extensive economies and sophisticated technologies used for the continent's First Nations peoples well before – sometimes many thousands of years before – other civilisations across the world had drawn their first breaths.

Prior to the British invasion, occupation and settlement of Australia in 1788, Aboriginal Australians lived a lifestyle that enhanced their physical, mental, emotional and spiritual wellbeing (Gammage, 2012). First Nations peoples were self-determined, with each nation group in control of their lives and sovereignty of their Country. They were economically independent and practised a lifestyle focused upon sustainability and balance. Lore and Law were and are intrinsically connected to Country and recognised the value of all living and non-living beings and matter. The laws facilitated reciprocal, sharing relationships.

Food was hunted and gathered, with some farming (Gammage, 2012). The nutritional content of food was rich. Varied food sources, seasonal farming practices and trade enabled a wide-ranging diet (Reid & Lupton, 1991). Early writings of people on the First Fleet to Australia reported that the First Nations peoples appeared to be very healthy and strong looking (Saggers & Gray, 1991). This was a reference to the First Nations peoples of the Eora, Tharawal and Darug Nations, who were and continue to be the traditional custodians and owners of what is now known as Sydney.

The history that most Australians have not been told

In 1770, Lieutenant James Cook claimed the eastern side of Australia as a British possession. In 1788, British settlers and convicts arrived on the First Fleet under the command of Captain Arthur Phillip. 'Invasion' and 'settlement' are the terms that best describe what occurred once Phillip and the British Army arrived (Connor, 2003, p. xi):

> 26th January 1788 the colony of New South Wales was established and thereafter other parts of Australia were declared colonies, eventually six in all. Aboriginal societies and their territories were overrun by settlers, and in many parts of the continent and its islands, if they survived at all, they did so in much-reduced and horrible circumstances.
>
> (Langton, 2010, p. xvi)

The British claimed Australia under *terra nullius* (land belonging to no one) (Behrendt, 2012) and immediately commenced their dispossession of the First Nations peoples from their land. British colonial policy handed land that had been Country to countless generations of Aboriginal peoples over to settlers and pardoned convicts. In many circumstances, these were violent colonial acts, undertaken without the consent of Aboriginal Australians. To this day, Aboriginal peoples continue to state that sovereignty of Aboriginal land was never ceded to the British forces. Invasion was followed by frontier warfare over land, which erupted between the British settlers and the Aboriginal peoples. This lasted until 1838, although massacres of large groups of Aboriginal people persisted until the 1930s (Connor, 2003).

Dispossession and ongoing warfare took its toll on the population of Aboriginal peoples. They were also hit hard by diseases that had previously been unknown to them. Since they had had no exposure to these diseases prior to invasion, their immune systems were highly susceptible; infections and disease resulted in the deaths of many. At the same time, the significant disruption in access to traditional foods, Country and traditional practices (such as their ability to undertake vital societal, legal and religious obligations) played heavily upon the First Nations peoples' health and wellbeing (Dudgeon et al., 2014).

As a direct result of the stress of invasion, many Aboriginal peoples died – due to diseases, starvation, poisoning, torture or warfare (Franklin & White, 1991; Reynolds, 1987; Saggers & Gray, 1991). Behrendt (2012, p. 117) notes that historians 'have estimated that in Queensland alone the Aboriginal population was reduced from 120,000 to 20,000, with accusations that the expansion of the pastoral industry in the state accounted for at least 10,000 direct killings':

> It may be stated broadly that the advance of settlement has, upon the frontier at least, been marked by a line of blood. The actual conflict of the two races has varied in intensity and in duration, as the various native tribes have themselves in mental and physical character ... But the tide of settlement has advanced along an ever widening line, breaking the tribes with its first waves and overwhelming their wreck with its flood.
>
> (Fison & Howitt, 1880, cited in Reynolds, 1987, p. 4)

Colonial policy and practice continued to influence the health and wellbeing of Aboriginal and Torres Strait Islander peoples. Since 1788, Aboriginal and Torres Strait Islander peoples have been described as a 'problem' requiring a Western solution (Geia, 2012; Geia, Hayes & Usher, 2011; Sherwood, 2010). Colonisation is universally recognised as a critical determinant of the health and wellbeing of Indigenous peoples (Durie, 2003).

Acknowledging colonisation as a determinant of health requires an appreciation that it is not a 'finished project' (Czyzewski, 2011, p. 10). Data describing the health of Australia's First Nations peoples demonstrate that there has been and continues to be inequity in healthcare (Holland, 2016). Colonisation has left an unrelenting legacy upon Aboriginal and Torres Strait Islander peoples through their continuing economic, social, political and educational marginalisation and its profound effect on their health and wellbeing, and that of their communities (Zubrick et al., 2010).

Protectionism and the 'doomed race'

Implementation of colonial policies that targeted Aboriginal and Torres Strait Islander peoples resulted in significant physical, emotional and spiritual ill-health and the death of many. On hearing of the maltreatment of Aboriginal peoples in the early years of Australian settlement, in 1838 the British Parliament passed a Bill to protect the Aboriginal peoples who were being slaughtered by settlers. Aboriginal Protection Boards were created to oversee the treatment of Aboriginal peoples under the Aboriginal Protection Policy. However, the Bill and its policy failed to be implemented in the manner intended by the British government. Instead, the policy became a notorious outcome of colonialism, which 'mandated total control over Aboriginal peoples' (Sherwood, 2010, p. 45). The policy controlled where Aboriginal peoples could live and enforced restrictions on mobility, employment, marriage, education and nutrition (Sherwood, 2010).

Reserves and missions established under the Aboriginal Protection Policy became the enforced new homes of First Nations Australians. They were placed in overcrowded, poor housing, and diseases flourished. Food rations were provided to some people, generally consisting of flour, sugar and tea. This was a very different from Indigenous people's traditional diet of 'bush food' (Sherwood, 2010).

Health research from this era promoted a 'doomed race theory'. In 1928, tropical health specialist Dr Bruce Cleland claimed that all full-blood Aboriginal peoples would become extinct (Mitchell, 2007). Government underfunding of missions and reserves ensured malnutrition and high rates of infant mortality. Individuals who were observed to be suffering from smallpox, leprosy or syphilis were regarded as threatening the health of non-Indigenous Australians. They were chained by their necks and limbs, then forced to walk great distances to lock hospitals, where they were left to die (Grant & Wronski, 2008, pp. 1–28). (Lock hospitals are discussed in Chapter 2.)

A hint of a turn in the road

In 1938, Aboriginal activists William Ferguson and John Patten paved the way for a pivotal change in the way First Nations Australians engaged with the wider Australian population. Ferguson and Patten gave voice to the silent cries of Aboriginal and Torres Strait Islander peoples by challenging the notion that Australia Day should be celebrated. They declared that First Nations Australians would not rejoice on 26 January 1938; rather, they announced it as a Day of Mourning:

> These are hard words, but we ask you to face the truth of our accusation. If you openly admit that the purpose of your Aborigines legislation has been, and now is, to exterminate the Aborigines completely so that not a trace of them or their descendants remains, we could describe you as brutal, but honest. But you dare not admit openly that your hope and wish is for our death! You hypocritically claim that you are trying to 'protect' us; but your modern policy of 'protection' (so-called) is killing us off just as surely as the pioneer policy of giving us poisoned damper and shooting us like dingoes ... The arbitrary treatment which we receive from the Aborigines Protection Board reduces our standards of living below life-preservation point, which suggests that the intention is to exterminate us. In such circumstances, it is impossible to maintain normal health. So the members of our community grow weak and apathetic, lose desire for education, become ill and die while still young.
>
> (Ferguson & Patten, 1938, pp. 54–6)

The concerns raised by Ferguson and Patten went unheard by both federal and state governments. In 2017, many years later, a coming together of our peoples in Uluru resulted in the development of *Makarrata* as a statement of for action. It is known as 'The Uluru Statement from the Heart', and it reads:

> We, gathered at the 2017 National Constitutional Convention, coming from all points of the southern sky, make this statement from the heart:
>
> Our Aboriginal and Torres Strait Islander tribes were the first sovereign Nations of the Australian continent and its adjacent islands, and possessed it under our own laws and customs. This our ancestors did, according to the reckoning of our culture, from the Creation, according to the common law from 'time immemorial', and according to science more than 60,000 years ago.
>
> This sovereignty is a spiritual notion: the ancestral tie between the land, or 'mother nature', and the Aboriginal and Torres Strait Islander peoples who were born therefrom, remain attached thereto, and must one day return hither to be united with our ancestors. This link is the basis of the ownership of the soil, or better, of sovereignty. It has never been ceded or extinguished, and co-exists with the sovereignty of the Crown.
>
> How could it be otherwise? That peoples possessed a land for sixty millennia and this sacred link disappears from world history in merely the last two hundred years?

With substantive constitutional change and structural reform, we believe this ancient sovereignty can shine through as a fuller expression of Australia's nationhood.

Proportionally, we are the most incarcerated people on the planet. We are not innately criminal people. Our children are alienated from their families at unprecedented rates. This cannot be because we have no love for them. And our youth languish in detention in obscene numbers. They should be our hope for the future.

These dimensions of our crisis tell plainly the structural nature of our problem. This is the torment of our powerlessness.

We seek constitutional reforms to empower our people and take a rightful place in our own country. When we have power over our destiny our children will flourish. They will walk in two worlds and their culture will be a gift to their country.

We call for the establishment of a First Nations Voice enshrined in the Constitution.

Makarrata is the culmination of our agenda: *the coming together after a struggle.* It captures our aspirations for a fair and truthful relationship with the people of Australia and a better future for our children based on justice and self -determination.

We seek a Makarrata Commission to supervise a process of agreement-making between governments and First Nations and truth-telling about our history.

In 1967 we were counted, in 2017 we seek to be heard. We leave base camp and start our trek across this vast country. We invite you to walk with us in a movement of the Australian people for a better future.

https://ulurustatement.org/the-statement

Forced removal: The Stolen Generations

The workings of colonisation and the implementation of the Aboriginal Protection Policy produced overwhelming trauma in Aboriginal and Torres Strait Islander families and their communities. It was a devastating betrayal of Aboriginal protection. The forced removal of children is perhaps the most critical betrayal of all.

Records from New South Wales show that from the very first weeks of colonial invasion in January 1788, Aboriginal children were taken from their families under the guise of being 'civilised'. Children were kidnapped and 'exploited as slaves and guides' for settlers (Ella et al., 1998, p. 29). In 1890, the NSW Aboriginal Protection Board authorised the removal of children so they could be apprenticed and trained in state-run institutions. The *Aborigines Protection Act 1909* (NSW) enabled the Aboriginal Protection Board to remove any Aboriginal child from their family and place the child in an institution. In 1937, the Aboriginal Protectors from Western Australia, South Australia and the Northern Territory decided that it was their duty to remove Aboriginal children from their families if they believed the children were the offspring of Aboriginal and non-Aboriginal parents. They justified these removals on the basis of neglect. Recent estimates suggest that between 20,000 and 25,000 children were removed from their families under this policy (AHRC, 2012).

Removed children were often placed in state-run homes. Historian and scholar Dr Rosalind Kidd (2000) describes these homes as generally uncaring institutions where many hundreds of children died due to physical abuse, starvation and psychological neglect. The *Bringing Them Home* report (HREOC, 1997) provides detailed narratives of people's experiences of removal and life after their removal. Some of these stories describe the children's treatment at the hands of the Aboriginal

Stolen Generations Aboriginal and Torres Strait Islander children who were targeted by government agencies and forcibly removed en masse from their families to provide a basic workforce to the settler population, under the guise that governments were caring for these children by removing them from their families.

Protector. Many of the survivors of the **Stolen Generations** reported to the Inquiry that they had been forbidden to speak their own language, were told that their parents did not want them, experienced neglect and abuse (physical, emotional and sexual), received little or no education and were refused contact with their families (HREOC, 1997):

> Separating Aboriginal and Torres Strait Islander children from their parents and communities has been demonstrated to have serious long-term impacts on their safety, well-being, mental health, cultural identity and development. In many cases, the forced removal of members of the 'Stolen Generations' from their families and communities has prevented them from acquiring language, culture and the ability to carry out traditional responsibilities. It has also made it difficult for these individuals to establish their genealogical links. Most forcibly removed children were denied the experience of being parented or at least cared for by a person to whom they were attached; for many, this was the most significant of all the major consequences of the removal policies. Forcible removal also had long term impacts on the physical and mental health of people removed, and long term problems with substance abuse and imprisonment. In 2008, of those who had experienced removal from their natural family, 35% assessed their health as fair or poor and 39% experienced high or very high levels of psychological distress, compared with 21% and 30% of those not removed. The *Bringing Them Home* report details the intergenerational consequences and effects of removal. Many members of the 'Stolen Generations' still have not been reunited with their families. The legacy of forcible removal remains in the lives of Aboriginal and Torres Strait Islander individuals and communities today and contributes to their continued disadvantage. The *Bringing Them Home* report recommended that reparations be made in response to the gross violations of human rights that occurred as a result of the forcible removals. In addition to acknowledgement and an Apology, the Report recommended that reparations should include guarantees against repetition, restitution, rehabilitation and monetary compensation.
>
> (AHRC, 2012, 1.13)

In 1938, the Western Australian Aboriginal Protector, A.O. Neville, asked his Aboriginal Protector colleagues:

> Are we going to have a population of 1000,000 blacks in the Commonwealth, or are we going to merge them into our white community and eventually forget that there ever were any Aborigines in Australia?
>
> (cited in Bennett, 2013, p. 12)

The Northern Territory Aboriginal Protector, Dr Cecil Cook, responded: 'Every endeavour is being made to breed out the colour' (cited in Bennett, 2013, p. 12).

The Stolen Generations policies were overt attempts at state-sanctioned genocide that occurred within living memory. The impact of these genocidal acts have injured children and their families, and have caused a sustained intergenerational trauma. First Nations people's attempts to deal with this ongoing legacy of trauma are often observed as a deficit discourse. Families are blamed for their own distress and are further harmed by acts of ongoing forced removal.

The Stolen Generations continue

Many Australians are surprised to hear or read that the Stolen Generations is a story that continues in Australia today. The Apology made in the Commonwealth Parliament in 2008 by the then Prime Minister Kevin Rudd was greatly appreciated but did not stop the high numbers of First Nations children being removed from their families. Twelve years later, in February 2020, the Secretariat of National Aboriginal and Islander Child Care (SNAICC) reported:

> There are 17,979 Aboriginal and Torres Strait Islander children living in out-of-home care [Australia-wide] (an increase of 39% from last year's Review on Government Services report). This number does not include large numbers of children on permanent care orders or who have been adopted so the actual number of Aboriginal and Torres Strait Islander children who have been removed from their families is far higher. Our children are now 10.6 times more likely to be removed from their families than non-Indigenous children. If urgent action is not taken, that rate is projected to double in the next 10 years.
>
> (SNAICC, 2020)

This evidence backs up the concerns of many Aboriginal and Torres Strait Islander families, who claim that there are more children being removed today than in the past. The Stolen Generations continue.

In 2017, the *Family Matters Report* (SNAICC, 2017) alerted government bodies that there was an over-representation of Australia's First Nations children in out-of-home-care – meaning not living with biological and extended family. The report showed that in 2015–16, Australia's First Nations children were 5.1 times more likely to be reported to child protection services than other children, 6.3 times more likely to be investigated by child protection and 9.8 times more likely to be living in out-of-home-care than non-Indigenous children – rates have been increasing progressively over the last ten years (SNAICC, 2017, p. 28).

Key issues that impact the over-notification are connected to ongoing socioeconomic marginalisation, hyper-surveillance of First Nations families by colonial agencies such as the police and the discriminatory characterisation of Aboriginal communities as 'problem groups' – another deficit discourse (Libesman, 2014, p. 174).

Cunneen and Libesman (2002) undertook a review of the NSW government agency with the responsibility for child removals. Their findings showed that, 'While the Department had a commitment to appropriate service provision to Indigenous families, it failed to translate this policy into practice' (Libesman, 2014, p. 64). Some of the reasons for this lack of a culturally safe approach were the result of a lack of funding of this service as well as the failure of case workers to respect cultural differences:

> Limited departmental resources and the individual case method resulted in a crisis style response to particular incidents with a failure to meet the family's circumstances holistically, in a community or historical context, or to deal with underlying issues.
>
> (Libesman, 2014, p. 64)

In many files assessed by this research, 'there seemed to be an abandonment of any real commitment to assisting the child or family' (Libesman, 2014, p. 64).

QUESTION FOR REFLECTION

How do contemporary child removal practices and the current out-of-home-care system resemble the Stolen Generations policies of the past?

CASE STUDY

Collective parenting

Aunty Gladys is a grandmother of six beautiful grandchildren. (Note that it is a sign of cultural respect to refer to Elders as Uncle or Aunty.) Sometimes her grandchildren will come and live with her, as collective parenting is a strong part of Aboriginal culture and it is important for grandchildren to learn from their Elders. Keeping family together is very important to Aunty Gladys because her mother was a survivor of the genocidal policies of the Stolen Generations.

Growing up, Aunty Gladys heard many stories about her mother's suffering, the racism she endured, how First Nations peoples were not even considered human before the 1967 referendum. Aunty Gladys knows many people in her family and community who were stolen and forced to live and work in institutions or with white people who would exploit, neglect and abuse them.

Aunty Gladys has inherited the sadness, pain and anger of her mother's and her people's experience of colonisation as well as an inherent distrust of colonial systems such as the police, welfare and public health. She has spent her whole life dealing with racism and trying to heal herself and her family from the crimes of past governments and colonial systems.

One day, her grandson is playing in a tree and falls to the ground, injuring his arm. Aunty Gladys takes him to the hospital. A white nurse takes them into triage. When Aunty Gladys explains the situation, the nurse treats them with suspicion and begins to ask about whether there is any domestic violence at home. Despite Aunty Gladys giving clear information about the circumstances in which the injury occurred, the nurse assumes the worst and says she will need to involve welfare. Aunty Gladys expresses anger at the nurse's overt racism and becomes deeply afraid that her grandson will be removed as she has heard many stories of Aboriginal children being taken during visits to hospital. She leaves the hospital with her grandson in a state of extreme distress.

QUESTIONS FOR REFLECTION

- Why is it important that nurses and midwives are aware of the ongoing impacts of colonial policies and systems on Australia's First Nations peoples?
- Intergenerational trauma is fundamentally a health issue. What are the factors at play in this situation that are contributing to Aunty Gladys's distress?
- How would a deficit lens interpret this situation? How would a culturally safe lens interpret this situation?

Creating the health gap

The stories described in this chapter provide a very brief overview of the government policies and practices that have influenced the health of First Nation Australians. From the time of colonisation, First Nation peoples have not enjoyed the health and social equity that many non-Indigenous Australians have had. This situation continues today. Government policies and practices over the past 200 years, including specific polices targeting Aboriginal and Torres Strait Islander peoples, have contributed greatly to what is now known as the **health gap**.

health gap the disparity in health outcomes experienced by different groups in society. In Australia, there are significant health and life-expectancy gaps between Aboriginal and Torres Strait Islander peoples and other Australians.

In correspondence to the Secretary General of the United Nations as far back as 1970, The Aborigines Advancement League wrote:

> This is an urgent plea of several hundred thousand so-called 'Aborigines' of Australia that the United Nations uses its legal and moral powers for the vindication of our rights to the lands which we have traditionally occupied. We make this plea under the Item 55 of the General Assembly, which deals with the elimination of all racial discrimination for its only racial discrimination which can explain the refusal of the Government to grant us, and us alone, our rights …
>
> We must emphasise: FROM THE TIME OF THE FIRST SETTLELMENT IN 1788 TO DATE THE CROWN HAS NEVER USED EVEN ITS CLAIMED POWER TO TAKE OUR LAND, EITHER BY TREATY OR BY PURCHASE. THE CROWN HAS BLATANTLY TAKEN OUR LAND WITHOUT TREATY, WITHOUT PURCHASE, AND WITHOUT COMPENSATION OF ANY KIND.
>
> We, the Aborigines of Australia whom the invaders have not yet succeeded in wiping off the face of the earth, are the owners of the land of Australia in equity, in the eye of any system of civilised law and in justice and yet we have no share in the great mineral, agricultural and pastoral wealth of our country.
>
> (cited in Reynolds, 1989, p. 87)

Aboriginal historian and Distinguished Professor Marcia Langton offered a personal perspective of Australian history that has significantly impacted the creation of a health gap:

> History was for me a terrible burden because it was in this class that I learnt that people like me were hated, and that the only stories told about us provided a steady stock of evidence about our supposedly shockingly violent tendencies, savagery and, most importantly, our innate tendency to steal and pilfer.
>
> (Langton, 2010, pp. ix–x)

The current health story

First Nations health today is a story informed by history, policies, warfare, Western medicine and press bias. It is important to recognise that the poor health status experienced by Australia's First Nations peoples did not simply just occur; it is the result of past events. We believe it is vital that all health professionals gain a deep appreciation of the current health status of Aboriginal and Torres Strait Islander peoples. Health professionals need to recognise that the appalling health outcomes experienced by First Nations peoples are the direct result of colonisation (not only in Australia, but also experienced by Indigenous peoples worldwide) (CSDH, 2007; Czyzewski, 2011; Giroux & Giroux, 2008).

At the end of June 2016, the Australian population of Aboriginal and Torres Strait Islander peoples was recorded to be 798,400 (ABS, 2018). New South Wales has the largest population, with about 33 per cent of the national Aboriginal and Torres Strait Islander population living in the state. The Northern Territory has the highest percentage of First Nations peoples, with 30 per cent of the population being Aboriginal or Torres Strait Islander (ABS, 2018).

Recent health data indicate that there is a significant difference in morbidity and mortality between First Nations Australians and the general population (AIHW, 2015). Australia is considered a developed nation, so Indigenous health must be seen as a social justice issue (CSDH, 2008). As Adelson (2005) notes, disparities in health are markers of a disproportionate suffering of disease within a population. Figures from the Australian Institute of Health and Welfare (AIHW) and the Australian Health Ministers' Advisory Council (AHMAC, 2017) indicate that:

- In 2011, First Nations Australians experienced a burden of disease that was 2.3 times the rate of non-Indigenous Australians (AIHW, 2016).
- In the period 2011–15, the leading cause of death for First Nations Australians (24 per cent of deaths) was circulatory disease.
- Cancer death rates for First Nations communities increased by 21 per cent between 1998 and 2015, while rates for non-Indigenous Australians declined in the same period (by 13 per cent).
- There was no improvement in mortality rates for diabetes or injury between 1998 and 2015, and there was a significant increase in the Indigenous suicide rate (32 per cent). In 2012–13, 11 per cent of Indigenous adults had diabetes (three times the non-Indigenous rate) and the incidence rate of end-stage kidney disease for Indigenous Australians was seven times the rate for non-Indigenous Australians in 2012–14.
- On a more positive note, there was a significant decline in the mortality rate for Indigenous Australians (15 per cent) between 1998 and 2015. Major contributors to this decline included circulatory diseases (43 per cent decline), respiratory disease (24 per cent decline) and kidney disease (47 per cent decline between 2006 and 2015).

There is some evidence that the overall story about the health of Aboriginal and Torres Strait Islander peoples may not be entirely accurate. Despite improvements in data collection specifically focused upon First Nations peoples across Australia, there continues to be a deficit in the reporting of deaths, cancers and disease (MacRae et al., 2013). It is important that we capture health data effectively, so an accurate story can inform policy for health service providers. This is something that has not been done well in Australia. The Australian Bureau of Statistics and the AIHW often warn health planners that the data they report are not entirely valid due to poor documentation of Indigenous status by health professionals across the nation.

CASE STUDY

Making assumptions about health

Lorri is a 34-year-old woman with three children. The eldest is twelve, the second is eight and her third is just two years old. Lorri has just started back at university to complete her studies after a break following the birth of her last child. She arrives at accident and emergency at 10 p.m. She presents with a headache and slightly slurred speech, unsteady on her feet. Because her husband was working, Lorri had to wake up her children to bring them with her to the hospital and as a result they are tired and cranky and the baby is crying.

The triage nurse is about to finish her shift and is not happy about this late arrival. The nurse assumes the slurred speech is a result of Lorri being drunk, so does not bother to triage her, leaving her for the next shift to delegate. The nurse details this assumption in her handover to the next triage nurse starting her shift. As a consequence, Lorri has been left in the waiting room for four hours without any observations being taken. The children have settled, sleeping on their mother.

The children are woken when Lorri falls to the floor. The nurse says, 'Typical – she's just come in to sleep this one off'. The children scream with worry as their mother is now unconscious and the eldest demands that their mother be seen by a doctor. Because they are terrified, the children make a lot of noise until this happens.

The doctor and nursing staff bring the mother and children into the A&E triage rooms and commence emergency treatment. The doctor smells her breath and immediately recognises that she is a diabetic and not drunk. Lorri is in fact suffering from a hypoglycaemic event.

Lorri had been suffering from undiagnosed diabetes since her third pregnancy. She was told she was diabetic when she was pregnant and that it would be all okay once she had the baby. However, 18 months after Lorri had her baby, she started to have symptoms such as headaches and tiredness, which she put down to simply being a mum and studying again.

Lorri was seriously injured in her fall, and – worse – could have died as a result of the delay in her treatment. Her case was taken up by a human rights lawyer, and the A&E and the nursing staff were found to be negligent. The hospital had to pay a considerable amount in compensation to Lorri and her traumatised children.

QUESTIONS FOR REFLECTION

- Lorri's situation – a mother with children requiring emergency healthcare – is not uncommon. What should the triage nurse on duty have done?
- It was physically obvious that Lorri was an Aboriginal woman. Why do you think the staff failed to diagnose her diabetic status?
- Why do you think it was assumed that Lorri would be a drinker?
- How differently would you have managed this case?

Indigenous ways of knowing about health

worldview The paradigms that guide and determine how people see the world. Worldviews influence the ways people make sense of their world through their systems of knowledge. They describe what can be known and the systems of knowing that relate people to their environment, cultures and experiences.

Aboriginal and Torres Strait Islander people view health from a **worldview** that is significantly different from the biomedical model. Understanding and appreciating this different way of viewing health and life is fundamental to providing healthcare for Aboriginal and Torres Strait Islander peoples. Worldviews are important because:

> Each culture's worldview is self-contained and adequate in the sense that it provides a coherent view of reality as *perceived and experienced* by the cultural group under consideration … Thus – allowing for the principles of modification in each culture, and varying degrees of openness to change – each culture's worldview is adequate for *that culture* and thus valid *in its own terms.*
>
> (Jenkins, 2006, cited in Ranzijn, McConnochie & Nolan, 2009, p. 17)

The National Aboriginal Health Strategy Working Party (NAHSWP) describes the health worldview of Aboriginal and Torres Strait Islander peoples in this way:

> Health is not just the physical well-being of the individual, but the social, emotional and cultural well-being of the whole community. This is a whole of life view and it also includes the cycle of life–death–life.
>
> (NAHSWP, 1989, p. ix)

The definition provides health professionals with a valuable tool with which to approach Indigenous health. The following definition is also helpful:

> [The] Aboriginal concept of health is holistic, encompassing mental health and physical, cultural and spiritual health. Land is central to wellbeing. This holistic concept does not merely refer to the 'whole body' but in fact is steeped in the harmonised interrelations which constitute cultural wellbeing. These inter-relating factors can be categorised largely as spiritual, environmental, ideological, political, social, economic, mental and physical. Crucially it must be understood that when the harmony of these inter-relations is disrupted, Aboriginal ill-health will persist.
>
> (Swan & Raphael, 1995, p. 13, cited in Taylor & Guerin, 2010, p. 90)

Taylor and Guerin (2010) explore this view as a social health model. Unfortunately, this social approach to health has not influenced how federal and state governments respond to the health of Aboriginal and Torres Strait Islander people. Importantly:

> The widespread failure of governments to engage in socially constructive dialogue concerning the health and welfare of their minority, disadvantaged or marginalised population groups has led to an interest in utilising human rights discourse as a framework for arguing that governments have international obligations to take proactive steps to improve the health and well-being of these groups.
>
> (Gray, 2007, p. 253)

social justice A concept that is about acknowledging inequity and disadvantage and attempting to alleviate it through proactive policies, rights, positive discrimination and appropriate services.

Health as a social justice issue

The health of Aboriginal and Torres Strait Islander people is increasingly being recognised as a **social justice** issue.

Michael Dodson, who was the first Indigenous Social Justice Commissioner for Human Rights and Equal Opportunity, affirmed:

> Social justice is what faces you when you get up in the morning. It is awakening in a house with an adequate water supply, cooking facilities and sanitation. It is the ability to nourish your children and send them to school where their education not only equips them for employment but reinforces their knowledge and appreciation of their cultural inheritance. It is the prospect of genuine employment and good health: a life of choices and opportunity, free from discrimination.
>
> (HREOC, 1993, p. 4)

In 2005, the then Social Justice Commissioner, Tom Calma, took a proactive step in setting a challenge to the federal, state and territory governments:

> **The Indigenous Health Challenge**
> I am recommending that the governments of Australia commit to achieving equality of health status and life expectation between Aboriginal and Torres Strait Islander and non-Indigenous people within 25 years.
>
> (Calma, 2005, p. 1)

More than fifteen years have passed since Tom Calma issued this Indigenous health challenge, and the health gap between First Nations Australians and other Australians remains unacceptably wide. Funding cuts to essential Indigenous services have been systematic at all levels of government over the past decade, neglecting the very social determinants of this health gap. First Nations Australians do not have the same access to primary healthcare and health infrastructure as non-Indigenous Australians, including access to safe drinking water and food supplies, healthy housing, effective sewerage systems and rubbish-collection services. Unless these social determinants of health are addressed, programs that target specific diseases and conditions are not likely to bring about any lasting or sustainable change.

Indigenous health needs to be addressed from a holistic perspective, with a strong focus on social justice. Federal, state and territory governments must commit to working together and taking a whole-of-government approach. Most importantly, they need to do this in partnership with Aboriginal and Torres Strait Islander peoples.

A human rights approach to health

The *Social Justice Report* (Calma, 2005) proposes a human rights-based campaign to address the health inequality of Australia's First Nations peoples. Crucially, the report asks governments to commit within a set timeframe to addressing both the health inequality and the inequality of opportunity to be healthy. It also calls on governments to commit increased funding – to levels that match the needs of Aboriginal and Torres Strait Islander communities. The report states that Aboriginal and Torres Strait Islander peoples have a *right* to health.

The approach advocated in the *Social Justice Report* acknowledges that Aboriginal and Torres Strait Islander peoples do not currently have an equal opportunity to be healthy. Addressing the underlying issues that influence health is an essential foundation to the campaign for health equality.

Australian Charter of Healthcare Rights Describes the rights of patients, consumers and other people using the Australian healthcare system.

Launched in 2019, the **Australian Charter of Healthcare Rights** describes the rights of patients, consumers and other people using the Australian healthcare system. These rights relate to the following seven key areas: access, safety, respect, communication, participation, privacy and comment. These rights are considered essential to the provision of high quality and safe healthcare (ACSQHC, 2019).

The Closing the Gap initiative

Closing the Gap A federal government policy that aims to close the gaps that exist between Aboriginal and Torres Strait Islander and other Australians in health, education and employment.

One of Australia's more recent health policies targeting Aboriginal and Torres Strait Islander health is the campaign for Indigenous health equality known as **Closing the Gap**. Since 2006, key Indigenous and non-Indigenous health bodies have worked with government and non-government service providers in a spirit of cooperation to provide health equality and equity services. Their goal is to bring Aboriginal and Torres Strait Islander health and life expectancy to the level enjoyed by non-Indigenous Australians (Holland, 2016). The Closing the Gap campaign was launched by the federal government in 2008:

> The campaign's goal is to close the health and life expectancy gap between Aboriginal and Torres Strait Islander peoples and non-Indigenous Australians within a generation. The campaign is built on evidence that shows that significant improvements in the health status of Aboriginal and Torres Strait Islander peoples can be achieved within short time frames. By joining our efforts we can make sure that by 2030 any Aboriginal or Torres Strait Islander child born in this country has the same opportunity as other Australian children to live a long, healthy and happy life.
>
> (AHRC, 2013)

In 2007, the Council of Australian Governments (COAG) developed measurable targets to track the health and wellbeing of First Nations Australians. They included achieving health equality within a generation and halving the mortality rate gap for children under five years old within a decade. Closing the Gap is not restricted to the health sector: it has a wider agenda of reconciliation between Aboriginal and Torres Strait Islander people and non-Indigenous Australians. Every year, a Closing the Gap report is submitted to parliament to detail the progress on the targets alongside a report by the Close the Gap Steering Committee specifically focused on the two health-related targets as well as recommendations to the government. The message of Closing the Gap has permeated all levels of healthcare. It challenges orthodox health systems to change the way they have always done business and to look for ways of developing services that are culturally accessible to Aboriginal and Torres Strait Islander people.

Despite these efforts, over twelve years later in 2020, there had been no significant improvement on any of the measurable targets. The *Closing the Gap Report 2020* indicates that life expectancy is still significantly lower for First Nations Australians compared with other Australians. In 2015–17, life expectancy at birth was 71.6 years for Indigenous males (8.6 years less than non-Indigenous males) and 75.6 years for Indigenous females (7.8 years less than non-Indigenous females) (DPMC, 2020). In 2018, the Indigenous child mortality rate was 141 per 100,000 – twice the rate for non-Indigenous children (67 per 100,000). Since the 2008 target baseline, the Indigenous child mortality rate has improved slightly; however, the mortality rate for non-Indigenous children has improved at a faster rate, so the gap has actually widened (DPMC, 2020).

Significant work has been done in recent years to hold governments accountable to their commitments in addressing Aboriginal and Torres Strait Islander health inequality through initiatives such as the Primary Health Care Access Program and the National Aboriginal and Torres Strait Islander Health Plan 2013–2023 (Commonwealth of Australia, 2013). The latter was specifically developed in response to the Closing the Gap campaign and recognises the fundamental need for a coordinated effort from all levels of government in partnership with health organisations using 'a long-term, evidence-based policy framework' (Commonwealth of Australia, 2013, p. 4). In order to undertake this process and the actions required, the following strategies were set to:

- continue working across governments and sectors to close the gap in Aboriginal and Torres Strait Islander disadvantage
- invest in making health systems accessible, culturally safe, effective and responsive for all Aboriginal and Torres Strait Islander people, and
- support good health and wellbeing across the life-course, and continue to target risk factors at key life stages (Commonwealth of Australia, 2013, p. 5).

The outcomes of the measurements have indicated that Closing the Gap remains an elusive goal. The lack of adequate funding has ensured that the set targets have not been met. The Aboriginal community controlled health services sector and other health services have argued for greater funding to directly target the discrepancies. In 2018, the chairperson of the National Aboriginal Community Controlled Health Organisation (NACCHO), John Singer, said more needed to be done because, despite ten years of this campaign, 'the gap in life expectancy between Aboriginal and Torres Strait Islander peoples and non-Indigenous Australians is widening, not closing' (NACCHO, 2018).

Closing the Gap can be personal – and we argue that, for nurses and midwives, it should be. Nurses and midwives are in a prime position to use their personal and professional knowledge and skills towards Closing the Gap for Aboriginal and Torres Strait Islander peoples. Hospitals and community health services are major government healthcare systems that constantly engage with Aboriginal and Torres Strait Islander communities. First Nations people walk through the doors of health services and hospitals every day, and many have little experience of hospital stay and care. Closing the Gap begins when a client meets health service staff – for example, in the way nurses and midwives approach their care of an Aboriginal or Torres Strait Islander client from the moment they meet.

QUESTIONS FOR REFLECTION

- How might nurses and midwives take steps to Closing the Gap in their personal and professional lives?
- What does Closing the Gap look like to you?
- How might you, as a nurse or midwife, Close the Gap on your first encounter with an Aboriginal or Torres Strait Islander client?
- What difference can you make to your patient's stay on your ward or in your health service?
- What experience of your nursing or midwifery care would you like an Aboriginal or Torres Strait Islander client to take with them upon discharge from hospital or when leaving your health service?

Our personal stories of how nurses and midwives can make a difference

First Nation nurses and midwives have been making a difference to healthcare, research, treatment, health policy and social justice since the days of the 1967 Referendum and the First Aboriginal Medical Service in Redfern, Sydney. We want to tell our stories here, to reflect on our own nursing and midwifery.

When you read these stories, examine them critically as examples that indicate how to provide best practice in health and nursing care. Ask yourself: Can I as a nurse or midwife make a difference?

Lynore's story

I am a Bwgcolman woman. I was born on Palm Island in Queensland, on what was then known as the Palm Island Aboriginal Reserve (under the policy of the *Aboriginals Protection and Restriction of the Sale of Opium Act 1897*). Palm Island is 65 kilometres north-east of Townsville. The community was established by the Queensland government almost one hundred years ago as a penal reserve for 'problem' Aboriginal people. Six generations of Palm Island (Bwgcolman) families have survived the harrowing history of dispossession and child removal under the complete control of state government policy and practices. Today, Palm Island continues to challenge the prevailing attitudes of both the Australian and Queensland Governments' policies as well as sectors of the wider Australian society.

My decision to enter nursing began during a school career week in the 1970s, when I visited the then Townsville General Hospital. I was fifteen years old and very naïve, and I thought nursing sounded like a good idea. Little did I know where my decision to join the nursing profession would lead me! My nursing journey began in practice in 1975, as an assistant to Registered Nurse Sister Betty Sawyers, who was a child health nurse on Palm Island.

It was in the environment of my own community, learning about nursing and the life of mothers and babies, that my desire to help my own people began to grow. Under the tutelage, mentorship and friendship of Sister Sawyers, I was able to confidently take my initial steps into the unknown world of nursing. I repeated Year 12 mathematics, as I needed to improve my maths knowledge in order to do the calculations required for drug administration.

I entered into nursing training in March 1977, the only Aboriginal nurse in my group. Life as a trainee nurse was enjoyable, particularly my new-found independence, only a few years out from under the *Aboriginal Protection Act*. I threw myself into my theory and practical nursing, making friends and earning my first professional salary (which at that time was under $20,000 in the first year). I was well accepted by my nursing colleagues and patients alike.

I vividly recall two negative experiences in my early years of nursing. The first was when my acceptance into nursing training was cast in doubt by nursing management because of my Aboriginal identity and my origins on Palm Island. The second negative experience took place in a private ward when I was the Registered Nurse in charge on my shift and I accompanied a private consultant on his ward round. The consultant was very reluctant for me to accompany him because he believed I was not a 'real nurse' (he really said this!). I knew at that moment that he was referring to my Aboriginality and my ability to perform my professional duty.

Notwithstanding these two events, my nursing training was an experience of friendship and laughter with my nursing peers. At the ward and patient-care level, I knew that my presence as an Aboriginal nurse created a positive healing environment for the Aboriginal and Torres Strait Islander patients and their families in the wards on which I worked. Nursing was filled with camaraderie, as we banded together to help each other complete our shift tasks – from taking patient observations to tidying and buffing up the bed pans until we could see our reflections in the cold metal (we planned our social life in the pan room!).

When I completed my training in 1980, I left Australia with a nursing friend to travel. After a whirlwind European tour, I settled into nursing in Lewisham Hospital in south-east London. It was in England that my confidence as a black nurse took an exponential rise. I was surrounded by black Registered Nurses and Midwives from across the nations of the world. For once in my life, I felt I was a member of a majority people. It was an empowering experience, both personally and professionally.

I remained in London for just over three years, undertaking midwifery training at Lewisham Hospital. I returned to Australia and to Palm Island at the end of 1983, in response to what I believe was a spiritual call to return home and work with my own people. Nursing on Palm Island was not in a hospital setting. I was employed by the then Palm Island Council to set up the first childcare centre in a Queensland Aboriginal community, where I worked as the director. For me, nursing involved family and child healthcare in a community setting.

During this time on Palm Island, I fell in love with a beautiful non-Aboriginal man whose professional superiors did not take kindly to us 'stepping out together' in the community. Black and white coupling was not well tolerated in those years; consequently, this young man was transferred from the community within a matter of hours. With our relationship torn apart, I embarked on twelve years of nursing and midwifery in Aboriginal health in Central Australia.

Nursing in Central Australia opened my eyes even more to the plight of Aboriginal Australians and the inequity in health that they experience on a daily basis. I became involved in the politics of health at the territory, state and national levels under the leadership and mentorship of many gifted and insightful Aboriginal leaders. These leaders worked in Aboriginal health organisations such as the Nganampa Health Council, Central Australian Aboriginal Congress, Congress Alukura by the Grandmothers' Law, the National Aboriginal Community Controlled Health Organisation (NACCHO) and the Aboriginal Medical Services Alliance Northern Territory (AMSANT). I was privileged to learn from well-known health and community luminaries such as the late Dr Arnold (Puggy) Hunter and Ms Pat Anderson.

During those twelve years, my nursing career was strengthened in community practice and engagement in partnership with Central Australian Aboriginal communities. Politics and health service delivery went hand in glove. Back then, the notion of 'Closing the Gap' in Aboriginal health was an immense political struggle as Aboriginal community controlled health services pushed boundaries to secure a place at the government negotiating tables. Arguments and submissions were placed on the table, vying for health dollars to keep Aboriginal health programs running. Significant inroads were made in addressing the healthcare needs of Aboriginal people; good healthcare access and health equity was something that became tenable.

My role as a nurse and midwife was expanded and enriched. I particularly focused on the idea of holistic healthcare, delivered in the Aboriginal way, under Aboriginal control. My nursing and midwifery experience in Central Australia was formative in establishing and developing my professional reputation as a nurse, midwife, advocate and social justice worker. Nursing became so much more than just the beds in hospital wards.

I returned to Queensland in 1999 as a single mother, to work in my own community of Palm Island. Working for Queensland Health again was difficult after working in Aboriginal community controlled organisations for over a decade. In 2000, I completed the Master of Public Health and Tropical Medicine program at James Cook University in Townsville. Six years later, I embarked on a Doctor of Philosophy program in nursing (completed in December 2012).

Between 1999 and 2012, I was fortunate to advocate for health for Aboriginal communities through work in and with government and non-government organisations at the federal and state government levels. Nursing has provided a way for me to engage at various levels of government and community, and to contribute to discussion about health changes that will affect Aboriginal people and their communities. I have been involved in work that empowers people to take a step forward towards their vision of health equity. This is just a part of the bigger picture in Aboriginal and Torres Strait Islander health in Australia. There is still so much more to be done to close the gap, and nursing provides a professional pathway and ladder to ascend to places where my voice as an Aboriginal nurse can make a difference for Aboriginal health.

Juanita's story

I am a Wiradjuri woman born in Sydney. My family was taken off Country three generations ago.

When I was sixteen years old, I was a patient in a Sydney hospital for ten days. It was several hours' drive from home, and I was admitted over Christmas and the school holidays. I was in hospital for major surgery – a cholecystectomy for the removal of my gall bladder and gallstones. The surgery involved a laparotomy, not a laparoscopy.

I woke up after the surgery, feeling rather groggy and in agony, to the attentions of a nurse whose caring approach cut through my pain, anguish and shame. I thought she was an angel. The nurse assisted me in post-operative care, and was sensitive and thoughtful towards a very scared, lonely and vulnerable teenager. Her attentive and kind manner immediately relaxed me, and I felt safe and secure under her care. It was then that I realised my desire to make others feel that way. I knew what I wanted to be: a nurse.

Over my many days in the hospital, separated from family and friends, I observed closely how the health professionals treated me. There were nurses who were abrupt and impersonal, and made me worry. There were nurses who shared their stories with me and made me laugh. This was who I wanted to be: a nurse who made people feel safe, shared stories and could laugh.

Only a few years later, I got the opportunity to follow my heart and take up nursing. I trained at St Vincent's in Darlinghurst, and successfully graduated as a Registered

Nurse. My training provided me with skills that I have valued ever since, and built my confidence in communicating with people and providing safety and security to my patients/clients.

Some time later, I decided to complete a primary school teaching diploma, which I was able to do full-time for three years while nursing part-time. The two professions opened the door for me to step into child and family health in the community health setting, another aspiration I had held for many years. I loved working in community health. I became a member of an outreach child and family multidisciplinary team and learnt a great deal from the people with whom I worked – both peers and community members.

This working experience was one of the most enriching in my life. Although I remember being told by a psychology lecturer that my professional choices of nursing and teaching would be ineffective, I fortunately had different ideas. I came alive and reawakened in Redfern, where I worked until I gave birth to my son in late 1992. During that time, I became a clinical nurse specialist in Aboriginal health and Nursing Unit Manager for child health in the eastern arm of Central Sydney Health Services.

While working in child health, my nursing and teaching foundations were to prove very important. During my teaching training, we learnt about specific health issues that affect learning, including hearing loss, which was considered to be a significant problem for classroom learning. In my work in child health, I was able to improve students' opportunities to learn in the classroom. I screened children's vision, hearing, speech and anything else that parents specifically wanted me to review.

The screening work uncovered a very high rate of children with hearing loss in many of the schools. My job was to inform parents and refer the children to local doctors for further management. Parents and teachers were often surprised to find out that their child had a significant hearing loss, but then understood some of the common behaviours of not listening, and were keen to have their child reviewed and supported.

The high rates of hearing loss had considerable implications for education in the community and needed to be addressed. A community meeting was held with parents, teachers, community members and the NSW Aboriginal Education Consultative Group (AECG) to explore ways of improving awareness of this health and education issue. The group recommended a research project to examine the incidence of hearing loss. This was 1989, and it was the beginning of my research journey. I was accompanied by another Indigenous nurse, Sister Jennifer Bush, and Doctor Terry Nienhuys from the Menzies Centre for Health Policy. Researchers at the Menzies Centre knew a lot about otitis media (OM) in Aboriginal populations, but were surprised by our findings. Our research showed that 85 per cent of students in the inner city suffered from an educationally significant hearing loss. Prior to this study, it was thought that OM was a health issue that only affected remote communities.

The NSW Education Minister took up the findings of our study and immediately responded with teaching support for students with conductive hearing loss. This was another first, and a result of the research and community advocacy. The minister also funded further research to explore what other states and territories were doing to improve opportunities for Indigenous students with OM. The research went out to tender, and I applied and won the tender and took up the research project. This research journey brought up many important findings and established a national network of health and educational professionals working together.

For that project, I interviewed an audiologist working in Alice Springs in 1991, who was from the United States and had worked in schools with high levels of OM. He had designed a classroom system that amplified the volume of the teacher's voice, so all the students could hear the teacher better. Through the support of the Australian hearing services and Lou, the audiologist, classroom amplification systems were designed and purchased by schools across the state and country. This strategy was successful and quite inexpensive. The completed research recommended and established in New South Wales the first-ever intersectoral government committee to address the implications of OM.

In 1994, a national conference on OM was hosted by the national AECG. I convened the conference, which was held in Alice Springs. It allowed us to share resources and publish strategies for dealing with OM. It also led to a new direction in dealing with OM for governments across the country. The federal government funded Aboriginal medical services across the country to screen children and adults for OM.

In 1994, I started work in the Aboriginal Health Branch at NSW Health, and it was this branch that established the first OM strategy for the state. In 1996, I worked with the NSW Health Department and a team of health professionals to develop and produce the first-ever medical guidelines for the management of OM. This was another very important step in addressing the health and educational implications of OM.

I have been very fortunate to have been involved in the development of many strategies, policies and guidelines that aim to improve the health and education of our peoples.

Conclusion

Nurses and midwives have the potential to be agents of change for future nursing and midwifery practice. However, to be an agent of change one must have knowledge about what needs to change and a desire to put that knowledge into practice. This means that future change in Aboriginal and Torres Strait Islander health requires today's nursing and midwifery students to expand their knowledge of Australia's colonial history and the contemporary issues of colonial legacy that affect Aboriginal and Torres Strait Islander peoples and the way they access healthcare services.

How might you, as a nurse, contribute to Closing the Gap? You can do so by being an agent of change through respectful and genuine partnership with Aboriginal and Torres Strait Islander peoples. You could engage in research that is relevant to improving nursing and midwifery practice. You could practise nursing and/or midwifery with intention when you are caring for First Nation Peoples, and build on the strengths that already exist in individuals and communities. You could critically reflect on theory and how it is relevant to your practice. Above all, you can treat Aboriginal and Torres Strait Islander peoples in the way that you would want to be treated if the roles were reversed. Afford respect and dignity to your clients and you will succeed in being an agent of change as you take steps to Close the Gap in health status faced by Aboriginal and Torres Strait Islander peoples. Nursing and midwifery are important professions, and nurses and midwives do make a difference. Closing the Gap is every nurse and midwife's business.

Learning activities

1. Consider the effect on people of the introduction of new diseases, frontier warfare and being taken away from Country to which they have been connected for millennia. What are the likely effects on the health and wellbeing of communities and families?
2. How has colonisation affected the health of Aboriginal and Torres Strait Islander peoples?
3. How has colonisation continued to affect the health and wellbeing of Indigenous Australians?
4. Consider the life and times of eighteenth-century Australia, compared with that of twenty-first century Australia. What factors have influenced the development of Australia? How do these factors affect Aboriginal and Torres Strait Islander peoples and their health?
5. Explain the importance of finding out about the Country, the history and the peoples where you are working. Why is this relevant to your healthcare provision?
6. What is your personal view of Aboriginal and Torres Strait Islander peoples and health? How will your personal view affect your nursing practice with Aboriginal and Torres Strait Islander clients?
7. How might you personally and professionally contribute to Closing the Gap?

FURTHER READING

Burgess, P.C., Johnston, H.F., Bowman, S.D. & Whitehead, J.P. (2005). Healthy country: Healthy people? *Australian and New Zealand Journal of Public Health*, 29(2), 117–22.

Calma, T. (2008). Achieving Aboriginal and Torres Strait Islander health equality within a generation. *Australian Journal of Human Rights*, 14(1), 21–39.

Cox, L. (2007). Fear, trust and Aborigines: The historical experience of state institutions and current encounters in the health system. *Health and History*, 9(2), 1–13.

Davis, M. (2019). *Family is Culture Review Report 2019: Independent Review of Aboriginal Children and Young People in OOHC*. Canberra: AIFS. Retrieved from www.familyisculture.nsw.gov.au/__data/assets/pdf_file/0011/726329/Family-Is-Culture-Review-Report.pdf

Dean, A. (2018). *The Growing Over-representation of Aboriginal and Torres Strait Islander Children in Care*. Canberra: AIFS. Retrieved from https://aifs.gov.au/cfca/2018/05/07/growing-over-representation-aboriginal-and-torres-strait-islander-children-care

Pascoe, B. (2014). *Dark Emu*. Broome, W.A.: Magabala Books.

Sherwood, J. (2013). Colonisation – It's bad for your health: The context of Aboriginal health. *Contemporary Nurse*, 46(1), 28–40.

SNAIC (2017). *The Family Matters Report 2017: Measuring Trends to Turn the Tide on the Over-representation of Aboriginal and Torres Strait Islander Children in Out-of-home Care in Australia*. Melbourne: SNAICC. Retrieved from www.familymatters.org.au/family-matters-state-2017

Steering Committee for the Review of Government Service Provision (2017). *Report on Government Services 2017*. Canberra: Productivity Commission. Retrieved from www.pc.gov.au/research/ongoing/report-on-government-services/2017

Visit the companion website at www.cambridge.org/highereducation/isbn/9781108794695/resources to see further online resources.

REFERENCES

ABS (2018). *Estimates of Aboriginal and Torres Strait Islander Australians*. Canberra: ABS. Retrieved from www.abs.gov.au/statistics/people/aboriginal-and-torres-strait-islander-peoples/estimates-aboriginal-and-torres-strait-islander-australians/latest-release

ACSQHC (2019). *Australian Charter of Healthcare Rights*. Retrieved from www.safetyandquality.gov.au/consumers/working-your-healthcare-provider/australian-charter-healthcare-rights

Adelson, N. (2005). The embodiment of inequity. *Canadian Journal of Public Health*, 96(2), 45–61.

AHMAC (2017). *Aboriginal and Torres Strait Islander Health Performance Framework – 2017 Report*. Canberra: AHMAC. Retrieved from www.niaa.gov.au/sites/default/files/publications/2017-health-performance-framework-report_1.pdf

AHRC (2012). *Face the Facts*. Retrieved from www.humanrights.gov.au/our-work/race-discrimination/publications/2012-face-facts

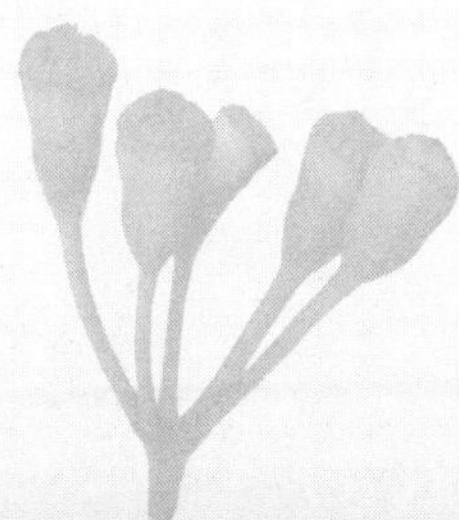

AHRC (2013). *Close the Gap: Campaign for Indigenous Health Equality.* Retrieved from www.humanrights.gov.au/close-gap-indigenous-health-campaign.

AIHW (2015). *The Health and Welfare of Australia's Aboriginal and Torres Strait Islander Peoples: 2015.* Canberra: AIHW. Retrieved from www.aihw.gov.au/publication-detail/?id=60129550168

AIHW (2016). *Australian Burden of Disease Study: Impact and Causes of Illness and Death in Aboriginal and Torres Strait Islander People 2011.* Canberra: AIHW. Retrieved from www.aihw.gov.au/reports/burden-of-disease/illness-death-indigenous-australians/contents/summary

Behrendt, L. (2012). *Indigenous Australia for Dummies.* Brisbane: Wiley.

Bennett, B. (2013). The importance of Aboriginal and Torres Strait Islander history for social work students and graduates. In B., Bennett, S. Green, S. Gilbert & D. Bessarab (eds), *Our Voices: Aboriginal and Torres Strait Islander Social Work.* Melbourne: Palgrave Macmillan.

Broome, R. (2002). *Aboriginal Australians: Black responses to white dominance 1788–2001* (3rd edn). Sydney: Allen & Unwin.

Calma, T. (2005). *Social Justice Report 2005: The Indigenous Health Challenge.* Retrieved from www.humanrights.gov.au/publications/social-justice-report-2005-indigenous-health-challenge

Commonwealth of Australia (2013). *National Aboriginal and Torres Strait Islander Health Plan 2013–2023.* Canberra: Commonwealth of Australia. Retrieved from www1.health.gov.au/internet/main/publishing.nsf/content/B92E980680486C3BCA257BF0001BAF01/$File/health-plan.pdf

Connor, J. (2003). *The Australian Frontier Wars 1788–1838.* Sydney: UNSW Press.

CSDH (2007). *Social Determinants and Indigenous Health: The International Experience and its Policy Implications.* Adelaide: CSDH.

CSDH (2008). *Closing the Gap in a Generation: Health Equity Through Action on the Social Determinants of Health. Final Report of the Commission on Social Determinants of Health.* Geneva: WHO.

Cunneen, C. and Libesman, T. (2002). Removed and discarded: The contemporary legacy of the Stolen Generations. *Australian Indigenous Law Reporter* 7(4), 1–26.

Czyzewski, K. (2011). Colonialism as a broader social determinant of health. *The International Indigenous Policy Journal*, 2(1/5), 1–14.

DPMC (2020). *Closing the Gap Report.* Canberra: DPMC. Retrieved from https://ctgreport.niaa.gov.au/sites/default/files/pdf/closing-the-gap-report-2020.pdf

Dudgeon, P., Wright, M., Paradies, Y., Garvey, D. & Walker, I. (2014). Aboriginal social, cultural and historical contexts. In P. Dudgeon, H. Milroy & R. Walker (eds), *Working Together: Aboriginal and Torres Strait Islander Mental Health and Wellbeing Principles and Practice*, Canberra: DPMC, pp. 3–24.

Durie, M. (2003). The health of indigenous peoples [editorial]. *British Medical Journal.* 326, 510–11.

Ella, R., Smith, P., Kellaher, M., Bord, S. & Hill, T. (1998). *Securing the Truth: NSW Government Submission to the Human Rights and Equal Opportunity Commission Inquiry into the Separation of Aboriginal and Torres Strait Islander Children from their Families.* Sydney: Department of Aboriginal Affairs.

Ferguson, W. & Patten, J. (1938). Cries from the heart: Aborigines claim citizens' rights! In I. Moores (ed.), *Voices of Aboriginal Australia Past Present Future.* Springwood, NSW: Butterfly Books, pp. 54–61.

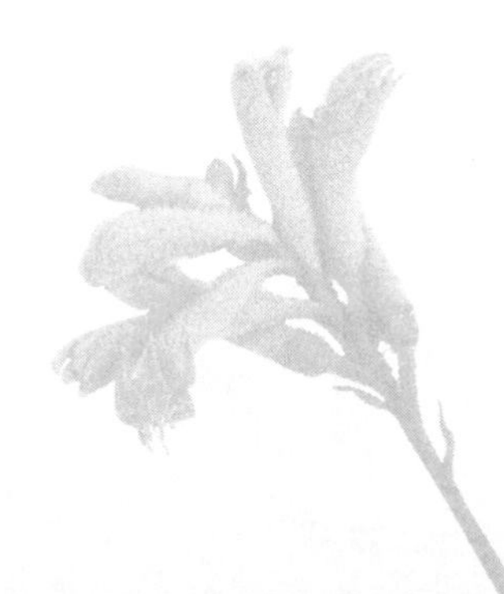

Fforde, C., Bamblett, L., Lovett, R., Gorringe, S. & Fogarty, B. (2013). Discourse, deficit and identity: Aboriginality, the race paradigm, and the language of representation in contemporary Australia, *Media International Australia*, 149, 162–73.

Fogarty, W., Bulloch, H., McDonnell, S. & Davis, M. (2018). *Deficit Discourse and Indigenous Health: How Narrative Framings of Aboriginal and Torres Strait Islander People are Reproduced in Policy*. Melbourne: Lowitja Institute. Retrieved from www.lowitja.org.au/page/services/resources/Cultural-and-social-determinants/racism/Deficit-Discourse-and-Indigenous-Health

Franklin, M.-A. & White, I. (1991). The history and politics of Aboriginal health. In J. Reid & P. Trompf (eds), *The Health of Aboriginal Australia*. Sydney: Harcourt Brace Jovanovich.

Gammage, B. (2012). *The Biggest Estate on Earth: How Aborigines Made Australia*. Sydney: Allen & Unwin.

Geia, L.K. (2012). First steps, making footprints: Intergenerational Palm Island families' Indigenous stories (narratives) of childrearing practice strengths. Unpublished PhD thesis, James Cook University.

Geia, L.K., Hayes, B. & Usher, K. (2011). A strengths based approach to Australian Aboriginal childrearing practices is the answer to better outcomes in Aboriginal family and child health. *Collegian*, 18(3), 99–100.

Giroux, H. & Giroux, S. (2008). Challenging neoliberalism's New World Order: The promise of critical pedagogy. In N. Denzin, Y. Lincoln & L. Smith (eds), *Handbook of Critical and Indigenous Methodologies*. Thousand Oaks, CA: Sage, pp. 181–90.

Grant, M. & Wronski, I. (2008). Aboriginal health and history. In S. Couzos & R. Murray (eds), *Aboriginal Primary Health Care: An Evidenced-based Approach*. Melbourne: Oxford University Press, pp. 1–28.

Gray, N. (2007). Human rights. In B. Carson, T. Dunbar, R.D. Chenall & R. Bailie (eds), *Social Determinants of Indigenous Health*. Sydney: Allen & Unwin, pp. 253–70

Holland, C. (2016). *Close the Gap: Progress and Priorities Report 2016*. Canberra: Close the Gap Campaign Steering Committee for Indigenous Health Equality.

HREOC (1993). *Social Justice Report*. Sydney: Commonwealth of Australia.

HREOC (1997). *Bringing Them Home: Report of the National Inquiry into the Separation of Aboriginal and Torres Strait Islander Children from Their Families*. Sydney: HREOC.

Jongen, C., McCalman, J., Bainbridge, R. & Clifford, A. (2018). *Cultural Competence in Health: A Review of the Evidence*. Singapore: Springer.

Kidd, R. (2000). *Black Lives, Government Lies*. Sydney: UNSW Press.

Langton, M. (2010). Prologue. In R. Perkins & M. Langton (eds), *First Australians* (2nd edn). Melbourne: Miegunyah Press, pp. ix–xxvi.

Libesman, T. (2014). *Decolonising Indigenous Child Welfare: Comparative Perspectives*. London: Routledge.

MacRae, A., Thomson, N., Burns, A.J. ... Urquhart, B. (2013). *Overview of Australian Indigenous Health Status 2012*. Perth: Australian Indigenous HealthInfoNet, Edith Cowan University.

Mitchell, J. (2007). History. In B. Carson, T. Dunbar, R.D. Chenall & R. Bailie (eds), *Social Determinants of Indigenous Health*. Sydney: Allen & Unwin, pp. 41–62.

NACCHO (2018). Increased support to Aboriginal community controlled health organisations needed to Close the Gap in life expectancy gap. Media release.

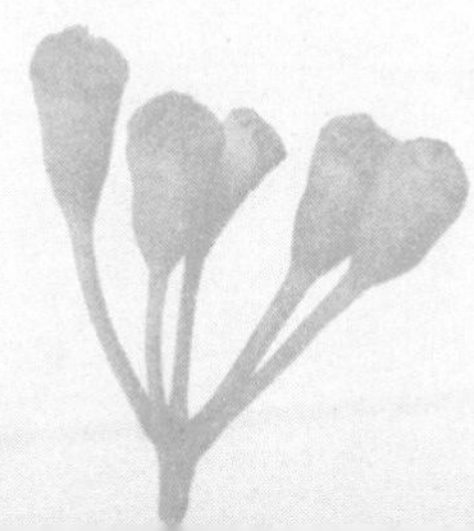

Retrieved from www.naccho.org.au/increased-support-to-aboriginal-community-controlled-health-organisations-needed/#:~:text=%E2%80%9CBut%20ten%20years%20on%20the,Australians%20is%20widening%2C%20not%20closing.

NAHSWP (1989). *National Aboriginal Health Strategy*. Canberra: Commonwealth of Australia.

Pascoe, B. (2014). *Dark Emu*. Broome: Magabala Books.

Ranzijn, R., McConnochie, K. & Nolan, W. (2009). *Psychology and Indigenous Australians: Foundations of Cultural Competence*. Melbourne: Palgrave Macmillan.

Reid, J. & Lupton, D. (1991). Introduction to the health of Aboriginal Australia. In J. Reid & P. Trompf (eds), *The Health of Aboriginal Australia*. Sydney: Harcourt Brace Jovanovich, pp. xi–xxi.

Reynolds, H. (1987). *Frontier: Aborigines, Settlers and Land*. Sydney: Allen & Unwin.

Reynolds, H. (1989). *Dispossession: Black Australians and White Invaders*. Sydney: Allen & Unwin.

Saggers, S. & Gray, D. (1991). *Aboriginal Health & Society: The Traditional and Contemporary Aboriginal Struggle for Better Health*. Sydney: Allen & Unwin.

Sherwood, J. (2010). Do no harm: Decolonising Aboriginal health research. Unpublished PhD thesis, University of New South Wales.

Sherwood, J. (2013). Colonisation – It's bad for your health: The context of Aboriginal health. *Contemporary Nurse* 46(1), 28–40.

Smith, L.T. (1999). *Decolonizing Methodologies*. Dunedin: University of Otago Press.

SNAICC (2017). *The Family Matters Report 2017: Measuring Trends to Turn the Tide on the Over-representation of Aboriginal and Torres Strait Islander Children in Out-of-home Care in Australia*. Melbourne: SNAICC. Retrieved from www.familymatters.org.au/family-matters-state-2017

SNAICC (2020). Removal of Aboriginal and Torres Strait Islander children continues 12 years after the Apology. Media release, 13 February. Retrieved from www.snaicc.org.au/media-release-removal-of-aboriginal-and-torres-strait-islander-continues-12-years-after-the-apology

Taylor, K. & Guerin, P. (2010). *Health Care and Indigenous Australians: Cultural Safety in Practice*. Melbourne: Palgrave Macmillan.

Uluru Statement (2017). *The Uluru Statement from the Heart*. Retrieved from https://ulurustatement.org/the-statement

WHO (2020). *Social Determinants of Health*. Geneva: WHO. Retrieved from www.who.int/gender-equity-rights/understanding/sdh-definition/en/#:~:text=Social%20determinants%20of%20health%E2%80%93The,global%2C%20national%20and%20local%20levels

Zubrick, R.S., Dudgeon, P., Gee, G., … Walker R. (2010). Social determinants of Aboriginal and Torres Strait Islander social and emotional wellbeing. In N. Purdie, P. Dudgeon and R. Walker (eds), *Working Together: Aboriginal and Torres Strait Islander Mental Health and Wellbeing Principles and Practice*. Canberra: DPMC, pp. 98–112.

LEGISLATION CITED

Aboriginals Protection and Restriction of the Sale of Opium Act 1897 (Qld)

Aborigines Protection Act 1909 (NSW)

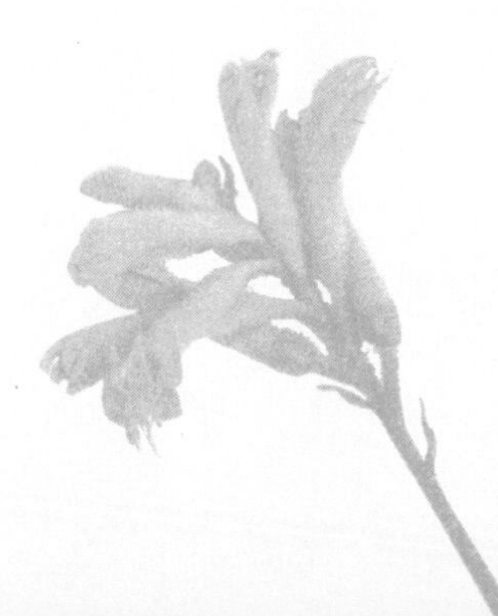

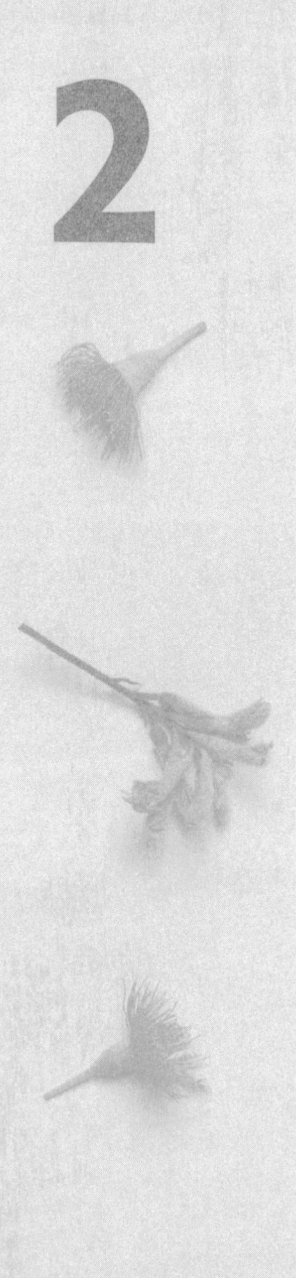

2 A history of health services for Aboriginal and Torres Strait Islander people

Ray Lovett and Makayla-May Brinckley

LEARNING OBJECTIVES

This chapter will help you to understand:

- The defining Indigenous health periods and systems
- The varied history of health service provision to Aboriginal and Torres Strait Islander peoples
- The history of Aboriginal and Torres Strait Islander peoples' health in Australia
- The link between self-determination, community control and improved health outcomes
- How the history of health service provision to Aboriginal and Torres Strait Islander peoples relates to contemporary health outcomes

KEY WORDS

Aboriginal community controlled health services (ACCHSs)
cultural determinants of health
lock hospitals
self-determination

Introduction

Contemporary understandings of Aboriginal and Torres Strait Islander health are framed largely by an understanding of the social determinants of health: the economic, social, political and environmental conditions that influence an individual's health status. These social determinants are the conditions in which people are born, grow, live, work and age. They are shaped by the distribution of money, power and resources at the global, national and local levels (WHO, 2020).

Social determinants are the primary cause of health inequities, which are demonstrated through the unfair and avoidable differences in health status within and between countries (Solar & Irwin, 2010). The social determinants of health also influence the health outcomes of different groups within a country, as demonstrated by the disparate health outcomes evident across Australia. An historical perspective of the social determinants of health reveals the thinking and actions that influenced Aboriginal and Torres Strait Islander health policies and practices that have contributed to devastating inequities in health and social outcomes for Indigenous Australians.

This chapter offers an historical examination of Aboriginal and Torres Strait Islander healthcare from a nursing viewpoint. It considers how the current shape of Aboriginal and Torres Strait Islander health has been formed by actions taken since European colonisation. It discusses the status of Aboriginal and Torres Strait Islander health during different historical periods, including what is known about the pre-invasion health system and health service provision during the periods of initial contact, separation and protection. Finally, the chapter discusses the rise of the Aboriginal and Torres Strait Islander community-controlled health system and contemporary choices for Aboriginal and Torres Strait Islander people in the delivery of healthcare and health outcomes. Each section of this chapter is, where possible, framed within the prism of nursing, exploring the role of nursing in health systems and the delivery of healthcare.

Pre-contact health status and the health system

There are limited recordings of the health status, health practices and care of Aboriginal and Torres Strait Islander people prior to invasion. This section relies on the early accounts of observers and archaeological evidence from bones and tools (Smith, 2011). This evidence offers a glimpse into the health conditions of Indigenous Australians prior to colonisation.

Health status pre-invasion

Accounts of the health status of Aboriginal and Torres Strait Islander people prior to invasion vary greatly. An early explorer of the Australian continent, William Dampier, who landed on the west coast of Australia in 1688, is said to have described Aboriginal people as the 'most miserable people in the world' due to great plagues of flies prevalent for about three-quarters of the year (Bates, 1985). It is likely that the flies, wind, dust and sand caused 'sandy-blight', a condition that results in weeping eyes and trachoma (Bates, 1985).

In contrast, many other early accounts (including pictorial evidence) described how healthy, lean and fit Aboriginal and Torres Strait Islander people were. For example, one account stated that 'they were of a middle stature straight bodied and slender-limb'd the colour of wood soot or of dark chocolate ... their features are far from disagreeable' (Clark, 1966, p. 51). Other accounts, such as those of Cleland (1928), Hamilton (1981) and Stone (1974) drew similar conclusions.

While it appears likely that Aboriginal and Torres Strait Islander people were healthy before invasion, some common diseases and conditions were known, including yaws and trachoma (Smith, 2011). Yaws is an infectious disease characterised by skin lesions and is highly transmissible through personal contact. Trachoma is a disease that affects the mucous membrane of the eye and cornea. The symptoms cause pain and weeping from the eye and light sensitivity. It is spread predominantly by flies and is likely to be what Dampier described in 1688 on Australia's west coast.

In addition to documented observation, bone and fossil records have been used to examine health status. Evidence from skeletal remains uncovered in various parts of Australia indicates that congenital abnormalities were present, such as premature fusion of bones in the skull, arms and legs (Smith, 2011). Neural tube defects were also present.

One study of the skeletal remains of over 1000 Aboriginal people from between the lower Murray and the south-east coastal regions found that the right tibial bone showed prevalence of *Harris lines* in between 8 and 33 per cent of people (the study assumed that all the people had died before the 1788 invasion). Harris lines, or growth arrest lines, are lines of increased bone density that show the position of the growth plate at the time growth stopped. They are only visible by radiograph or in cross-section. The lines are thought to be caused by periods of acute malnutrition in children under the age of five years, with the lines present for the remainder of the person's life. The rate of these lines is indicative of malnutrition occurring among people who have survived periods of food insecurity. It is likely that, due to extreme seasonal variations, many of the young population would have perished during periods of famine (Smith, 2011).

Another major source of morbidity and mortality from this period would have been trauma – either inflicted or accidental. Studies of bones from various regions of Australia show a relatively high incidence of fractures. Among one group in Central Australia, a high rate of fracture of the long bones of the leg suggests that accidents often occurred during travel or hunting excursions (Smith, 2011). Among another group from the Murray River region north of Adelaide, fracture of the left ulna was observed as a common feature, perhaps indicating the blocking or parrying of blows sustained during conflict. A study by D.G. Knuckey (cited in Smith, 2011) revealed a high proportion of skull fractures (around 50 per cent of 94 the skulls examined) among people from the Northern Territory and the south-eastern region of South Australia, most likely inflicted during conflict. (For further discussion about research and study methods, and social and emotional wellbeing, see Chapters 11, 12 and 13 respectively.)

Health systems pre-invasion

The pre-invasion Indigenous health practitioners and healthcare delivery systems have been framed by Western observers as 'traditional medicine' delivered by 'clever men and women', 'traditional healers' and 'men of high degree' (Berndt, 1943; Elkin, 1946). The delivery of healthcare and healing was often described as 'magic' and 'sorcery'. This framing of pre-invasion healthcare most likely occurred because traditional healers placed equal emphasis on the spiritual and the physiological in their explanation and treatment of illness. From the descriptions of several authors, it is clear that traditional healers, medicine men and women, clever men and women, and native doctors looked heavily to the spiritual and supernatural worlds to explain illness and disease (Berndt, 1943; Elkin, 1946). However, it is equally the case that traditional healers were inclined to describe illness and disease as physiological manifestations.

While the clever men and women carried a heavy responsibility for dealing with health issues, they also had a broad range of other responsibilities, such as rainmaking, appeasing spirits and deciding on punishments. Within their communities, they represented what we today describe as 'the health system'. Just as contemporary health professionals use physical and medicinal treatments, so did traditional healers. There is a wide variety of records concerning the traditional use of plants for medicinal purposes (Bates, 1985; Berndt, 1943; Elkin, 1946; Locher, Semple & Simpson, 2013; Packer et al., 2012; Pearn, 1993; Smith, 2011; Walton et al., 2004). There is also evidence that injuries such as broken bones were treated in the pre-contact period. The 'healers' and 'native doctors' were predominantly male. Their knowledge was passed through the patrilineal line from father to son (Elkin, 1946). According to Berndt (1943), there are some documented accounts of women being responsible for these roles.

CASE STUDY

Pre-invasion pharmacopoeia and treatment of injury

Prior to invasion, Aboriginal and Torres Strait Islander people had a substantial knowledge of drug-making for curative and treatment purposes. There are substantial accounts of different tribal groups' knowledge of how to use plants and animal extracts for treatment. This summary of pre-invasion treatments is drawn from Locher, Semple & Simpson (2013), Packer et al. (2012) and Pearn (1993, 2005).

The most common treatments were used across many different tribal groups. This knowledge was usually the domain of the 'native doctor'. For example, a universal treatment for rheumatism involved crushing eucalyptus leaves and rubbing them over the affected area. A common treatment for headache also involved eucalyptus leaves, which were either crushed and steamed (with the steam inhaled) or boiled (with the resin ingested). There are accounts of infected wounds being treated with leeches to remove the infection. Wounds were treated (and infections prevented) through the application of an antiseptic rub from eucalyptus leaves mixed with mud or ochre.

(cont.)

Treatment of fractures appears to have been common and diverse. Accounts from Western Australia describe wrapping leg bones in possum or kangaroo skin and then applying straight tree branches to either side of the leg as a brace. Twine made from possum fur was used to hold the brace together. Other accounts from New South Wales and Queensland describe the use of possum fur mixed with clay to form a cast around a fractured limb. For compound fractures, eucalyptus leaf extracts in the form of paste would be applied to the wound before a clay cast was applied, a method similar to contemporary practices.

A guide to traditional bush medicines was published by the Northern Territory Health Department in 1988. In it, many treatments were identified as having recognised therapeutic properties (Aboriginal Communities of the Northern Territory, 1988).

Examination of traditional medicines continues today. For example, one substance obtained from a type of tree found in Central Australia and already identified as an antiseptic is also an effective treatment for rheumatism (Saggers & Gray, 1991). Scabies can be treated with tea tree oil (Walton et al., 2004), and antibiotics and antifungals with low toxicity are being developed from the Currant Bush (also known as the Maroon Bush) (Pearn, 1993). Plants and extracts that make up traditional pharmacopoeia continue to represent an area of research interest in an age of antibiotic resistance and advances in medical technology.

QUESTIONS FOR REFLECTION

- Who 'owns' this traditional knowledge of healing? Who should benefit when traditional pharmacopoeias are incorporated into current treatment approaches?
- If an Aboriginal and Torres Strait Islander client has a strong spiritual illness or wants to be treated by a traditional healer, how might traditional approaches be received by nursing staff in the hospital system today?
- How can traditional healing practices be incorporated into the care of Aboriginal and Torres Strait Islander clients in combination with Western medicine?

There are many accounts of other roles played by women in traditional healthcare. The most prominent was in the birthing process, in the role of midwife (discussed in detail in Chapters 7 and 8). While the care of women during birthing varied according to region, some similarities did exist (Bates, 1985; Hamilton, 1981). In many communities, when it was time to give birth the pregnant woman would leave the main camp and be attended by female relatives (often her mother or mother-in-law). Typically, men's attendance was forbidden during birthing. Another common feature was the seclusion of the mother for a period after the birth.

Aboriginal and Torres Strait Islander preventative healthcare pre-invasion

Treatment of disease and illness were common in pre-colonial Australia. There is also some evidence that preventative healthcare measures were practised by Aboriginal and Torres Strait Islander people in this era. For Aboriginal and Torres Strait Islander people, preventative healthcare does not just stop diseases or illnesses, but also enables holistic care and results in living a good life.

There is a lack of a comprehensive knowledge base about Aboriginal and Torres Strait Islander healthcare that can be attributed to the 'inherent deficiency caused by the omission of Indigenous knowledge' from the onset of colonisation (Blyton, 2009, p. 119). However, despite limited literature on preventative healthcare measures in the pre-colonial era, two examples show how Aboriginal and Torres Strait Islander people stayed healthy: caring for Elders and eating native bush foods.

Caring for Elders and old people is an integral part of Aboriginal and Torres Strait Islander cultures. Many early reports of Aboriginal and Torres Strait Islander people falsely claimed that the population only lived until around 40 years old. Instead, impressionist observations are of Elders and old people who were very healthy and likely living into their eighties, with the First Fleet's surgeon Worgan recounting numerous run-ins with old people, and stating, 'They seemingly enjoy uninterrupted Health, and live to a great Age' (Worgan, 1788). Cultural concepts of caring for old people, providing social support and delivering medicinal remedies are all factors of a preventative healthcare system that helped Aboriginal and Torres Strait Islander Elders and old people counter illness and live long, healthy lives (Blyton, 2009).

Another way that Aboriginal and Torres Strait Islander people maintained their health and prevented illness was through their diets. Aboriginal and Torres Strait Islander people traditionally ate 'native bush foods': seasonally and geographically dependent meat, fruits, vegetables, nuts, seeds and insects (Watarrka Foundation Limited, 2019). Native bush foods varied between differing Aboriginal nations and clans, depending on their geographic location. In Brisbane, for example, coastal mobs undertook traditional hunting and marine harvesting of dugong, turtle, fish and crustaceans, while mobs living inland traditionally ate kangaroo, emu, witchetty grubs and plants like yams, wild fig and grapes (Stuart-Fox, 2000).

Hunting, gathering, preparing and eating native bush foods were a communal feat (Blyton, 2009). This helped with knowledge sharing and a holistic approach to diets and health that is intrinsically linked to culture and caring for Country (Watarrka Foundation Limited, 2019). Varied and well-balanced diets, and the shared role of food preparation in communities, contributed to pre-colonial preventative healthcare of Aboriginal and Torres Strait Islander peoples.

The period of initial contact, separation and protection (1788–1940s)

Health status and health provision

This devastating era of health decline for Aboriginal and Torres Strait Islander people began immediately after the period of first contact and invasion. Between 1788 and the 1940s, the health of Aboriginal and Torres Strait Islander people fundamentally changed. People moved from the pre-invasion era of mostly good health to the very poor health status that we recognise today.

When Australia was established as a convict colony by the British, their first interactions with the Aboriginal and Torres Strait Islander population were meant to be peaceful (Saggers & Gray, 1991; Smith, 1980). However, from the outset, Aboriginal and Torres Strait Islander people were excluded from the economy (only convict labour was used in the early years), and other exclusionary practices ensured that conflicts arose. Most notably, land was taken through pastoral expansion from the early 1800s. Aboriginal and Torres Strait Islander people were pushed to the margins in the new economy and were separated from their traditional lands. Pastoral expansion began at a rapid rate, initiating a period of conflict between pastoralists and local mobs. The result was often the massacre of entire family groups or the movement of people to separate camps, settlements and stations on the fringes of towns and cities. The decline in Aboriginal and Torres Strait Islander health and the decline in population numbers both stem from this time. Policy decisions and societal factors from this period continue to have a lasting legacy.

During the early colonial period, many fundamental changes occurred in the lives of most Aboriginal and Torres Strait Islander people. Dietary habits were transformed. Tobacco was introduced, as were white flour, white sugar and high fat meats. People encountered introduced infectious diseases to which they had limited immunity. And they were forcibly moved: instead of living as small, highly mobile groups, they began to live in large, sedentary and mixed (tribal and family) groups. Together, these factors had a significant effect on morbidity and mortality.

The population figures presented in Table 2.1 illustrate the story of the destruction of Aboriginal and Torres Strait Islander communities. While the pre-contact population shown is contested (Butlin, 1982), there is no doubt that the health and wellbeing of Aboriginal and Torres Strait Islander people were significantly and negatively affected by colonisation, with estimates that two-thirds of the population did not survive.

Table 2.1 Estimated population, pre-invasion, and lowest estimated population

State	Estimated pre-contact population	Estimated lowest population	Year	Percentage of pre-contact population
NSW	48,000	7,434	1901	15.5
Vic	15,000	850	1901	5.7
Qld	120,000	22,500	1927	18.8
SA	15,000	4,598	1921	30.7
WA	62,000	17,500	1933	28.2
Tas	4,500	18	1861	0.4
NT	50,000	15,386	1933	30.8

Sources: Saggers & Gray (1991); Smith (1980).

The large-scale movement of Aboriginal and Torres Strait Islander people into reserves and settlements had a profound effect on their health, particularly in terms of infectious diseases. While records are scant, Abbie (1969) compiled a list of the most common diseases introduced at the time: malaria, hookworm, filariasis, leprosy, smallpox, influenza, pneumonia, typhoid, measles, chickenpox, whooping cough, mumps, scarlet fever, diphtheria, tuberculosis, gonorrhoea and syphilis. Aboriginal and Torres Strait Islander people did not have immunity to these diseases, as they did not exist in Australia prior to colonisation (Abbie, 1969). The severe impact of what was probably smallpox is evident from accounts of Governor Phillip about the Port Jackson area; he noted that the disease had killed half of the Aboriginal population and also appeared to spread inland and along the coast (Saggers & Gray, 1991; Stone, 1974). The explorer Charles Sturt also noticed the results of smallpox: on an inland journey into the Bourke region of New South Wales, he noted evidence of smallpox scars prevalent among the local Aboriginal population (Saggers & Gray, 1991).

Sexually transmissible diseases and infections, then known as 'venereal disease', also became a common cause of mortality, with reports of between half to two-thirds of the Aboriginal population in Port Phillip dying due to syphilis (Saggers & Gray, 1991). Venereal diseases were introduced by the English and were often transmitted as result of sexual abuse of Aboriginal women. Similar accounts were reported in parts of Western Australia and Queensland (Parsons, 2008). The concern about venereal diseases became so great that authorities soon devised measures of isolation for those suspected of having venereal disease, leading to the creation of the infamous **lock hospital** systems.

lock hospitals Remote hospitals where supposedly ill Aboriginal and Torres Strait Islander people were locked away, given little health treatment and left to die.

CASE STUDY

Lock hospitals in Queensland

In the early twentieth century, Queensland had two different systems for the control of venereal disease: one for the non-Indigenous population and another for the Aboriginal and Torres Strait Islander population.

The Department of Public Health was responsible for the non-Indigenous population, and focused on the reporting of venereal disease by general practitioners (GPs). This involved provision of free medical treatment and public health awareness and education programs. Sex workers who were infected could be detained forcibly at the Brisbane Venereal Disease Hospital. Once clear of infection, they were free to leave the hospital and return to the community.

For Aboriginal and Torres Strait Islander people, the responsibility fell to the Chief Protector of Aborigines, whose primary approach involved quarantine. Almost no attention was given to developing awareness and education. The Chief Protector established quarantine stations, such as the Fantome Island lock hospital. Similar quarantine stations were established across the country (Saggers & Gray, 1991).

In Queensland from 1928 until 1945, Aboriginal and Torres Strait Islander people who were suspected of having venereal disease were removed from communities and transported to the Fantome Island lock hospital. The island is 70 kilometres from Townsville and part of the Palm Islands group. The lock hospital was established on the (contested) basis that venereal disease was rampant among the Aboriginal

(cont.)

population and that the only solution was to separate those who were infected from the rest of the population.

Aboriginal people from Palm Island were sent to build the Fantome Island lock hospital in 1926. The hospital had an operating theatre, dispensary, treatment room and hospital ward. It also had an obstetric room, irrigation blocks, office, communal kitchen and barrack wards. Men and boys lived in the barrack wards – open-aired huts with a roof but no walls, which could accommodate up to 30 patients. Women were housed closer to the hospital in ward accommodation. The hospital was staffed by up to six Aboriginal and Torres Strait Islander people, a charge attendant and a visiting medical officer who was supposed to attend twice weekly.

When transported to the hospital, men were placed in neck chains, while women and children were placed in handcuffs. Once on the island, their treatment regimen, while consistent with medical knowledge of the day, was risky and often led to side-effects such as swelling, unconsciousness and toxic poisoning. The treatment included injections of arsenic, bismuth and occasionally even mercury.

The system for diagnosing disease differed for Aboriginal and non-Indigenous people. From 1930 onwards, bacteriological testing was available and incorporated into the clinical diagnosis for non-Indigenous people. This testing was not available to the patients at Fantome Island.

During the two years from 1940, five separate reports by inspectors at both Palm Island and Fantome Island described the widespread mismanagement of the lock hospital system. The inspectors recommended that the facility at Fantome Island be removed and reorganised to Palm Island, along with a significant improvement in facilities and treatment. When the patient profiles were reviewed, the inspectors discovered to their surprise that 146 of the 192 people at the facility were disease-free. In addition, there were no signs of infection – old or new. Despite these findings, the Department of Native Affairs was reluctant to release any disease-free patients and ensured that discharged people were relocated to reserves at Palm Island, Woorabinda or Cherbourg.

Source: Parsons (2008).

QUESTIONS FOR REFLECTION

- What do you think was behind the decision to create places like Fantome Island?
- If you were asked to administer medication that is not recommended for a specific treatment (and is not best practice), how would you manage this?

Health systems

In 1837, largely as a result of an inquiry by the British House of Commons that highlighted the appalling state of Aboriginal and Torres Strait Islander health, a new system of separation and 'protection' from the excesses of the European settlers was advocated. The colonial office was to retain responsibility for Aboriginal and Torres Strait Islander people, and the states were required to finance protection. Each state had a 'Protector of Aborigines' who would look after the interests of Aboriginal and Torres Strait Islander people.

This policy change saw the establishment of reserves and missions for Aboriginal and Torres Strait Islander people. Some people moved voluntarily, though many were forcibly relocated. At the time, there was a crude health system in the colony solely for the treatment of illness (Smith, 2011); minimal public health and primary healthcare were available. Only those Aboriginal and Torres Strait Islander people who were employed under contract or those retained under the *Aborigines Protection Act* were eligible to receive treatment. Fees were applied for treatment and had to be paid to the hospital from the Protector's office.

Magistrates had the power to dispense medication or send impoverished Aboriginal and Torres Strait Islander people to hospital. When people were referred to hospital, their treatment left much to be desired. Nurses were the primary caregivers during this period. The standard protocol for treating Aboriginal and Torres Strait Islander people was for treatment to be given outside in the yard or on the veranda, not in the hospital itself (Saggers & Gray, 1991). In some hospitals (for example, at Kempsey Hospital), Aboriginal and Torres Strait Islander people were admitted to separate wards. In some areas, this practice of separation continued into the 1950s (Smith, 2011). Anecdotal reports indicate that segregation wards and treatment of Aboriginal and Torres Strait Islander people on the verandas of hospitals continued into the 1970s (Forsyth, 2007).

One purpose of the reserve and mission system was to 'civilise' Aboriginal and Torres Strait Islander people and bring them into modern education, employment, religion and living standards (Pollard, 1988). From 1880, many Aboriginal and Torres Strait Islander children were forcibly removed from their communities without their parents' consent. Although not a violation of Australian law at the time, this practice was a violation of human rights and international law. The ways in which children were removed varied greatly. Sometimes it was achieved by deception, with parents being tricked into letting their children go with the government officials. Sometimes brutal force was used. It was not uncommon for Aboriginal and Torres Strait Islander mothers to be forced to sign forms giving consent for their children to be taken by the authorities without understanding the implications of the document being signed. It has been estimated that 13 per cent of the Aboriginal and Torres Strait Islander population were removed from their families (Stolen Generations). In addition, 31 per cent of the population had relatives who were part of the Stolen Generations, amounting to an estimated 44 per cent of the Aboriginal and Torres Strait Islander population being exposed to familial removal. People belonging to the Stolen Generations are significantly more likely to experience poorer health, and socioeconomic outcomes compared with Aboriginal and Torres Strait Islander people who were not removed from their families. These impacts include increased contact with the justice system (including incarceration), higher levels of violence, poorer self-assessed health, and lower household income. The effects of the Stolen Generations are also intergenerational: descendants of the Stolen Generation are more likely to experience adverse health, cultural and socioeconomic outcomes (AIHW, 2018).

Most of the children who were removed from their homes were between the ages of two and four years. There are accounts of newborn infants being taken from their mothers while at the hospital, with nurses sometimes involved in this process (HREOC, 1997). The justification for removing a child could be vague. Between 1915 and 1939, a reserve manager or police officer could remove a child on moral or spiritual welfare grounds, due to 'negligence' or even on the belief that it was 'necessary'.

From about 1900, health services slowly began to be established on the reserves and missions in an attempt to deal with the pressing health issues of the time. In Cherbourg (Queensland), a hospital was built eight years after the Barambah Aboriginal settlement was established (under the *Aboriginals Protection and Restriction of the Sale of Opium Act 1897)* (Cox, 2007). Similar arrangements were seen at reserves and missions across the country. The hospitals (sometimes called dormitories) were usually staffed by a non-Indigenous matron. Medical treatment was normally undertaken by visiting doctors on a rotational and sometimes irregular basis.

Although Aboriginal and Torres Strait Islander people were not allowed to participate in formal nursing education programs until much later, many (mainly females) were trained in basic nursing skills to look after patients in the reserve hospitals. They worked alongside the hospital matrons as nursing assistants. However, some Aboriginal and Torres Strait Islander women did undertake formal nursing training in the early 1900s, including May Yarrowick (Best & Howey, 2013). A letter dated 28 May 1906 from the Matron of Crown Street Women's Hospital to the board, accepting May Yarrowick, stated that 'the fact of her being a half caste was not a valid ground in refusing her to train as a nurse. A separate room would, however, be provided for her.' In the 1940s, Woorabinda mission began to offer a two-year nursing training program for 'native girls.' Cherbourg and Palm Island missions introduced similar training programs, with mixed success (Best, 2013).

The reserve and mission systems could have been an opportunity to create the systems and workforce required for effective healthcare provision, utilising local people during this period. Sadly, this was not the case, with only minimal education and training of Aboriginal and Torres Strait Islander people to become healthcare workers (including hospital and nursing aides) or nurses on those missions and reserves. The exception to this was the 'Native Nurses' training scheme that operated in Woorabinda, Cherbourg and Palm Island (Best, 2015). This scheme appears to be the only one of its kind across the country. It operated for about a decade, and Aboriginal and Torres Strait Islander women were trained in the local mission hospital achieving 'high results' (Director of Native Affairs (Queensland), 1948).

The widespread movement of people onto reserves and missions had an enormous effect on their health. Traditional approaches to health and wellbeing were compromised in many ways. Many people moved great distances from their traditional lands and now had limited access to plants that previously had been available for treatment. Western approaches to disease treatment took precedence, and 'native doctors' were discouraged and often prevented from practising. Much of the knowledge about traditional pharmacopoeias, relevant to specific regions of Australia, was lost. Traditional practices such as 'birthing on Country' were also severely compromised.

QUESTIONS FOR REFLECTION

- Many Aboriginal and Torres Strait Islander children were forcibly removed from their families. What are some of the ongoing health impacts that may be experienced by children who were removed? Consider social and emotional wellbeing health impacts, including the effects of being disconnected from family and culture.
- Nurses were sometimes involved in the removal of Aboriginal and Torres Strait Islander children. Reflect on your role as an incoming nurse or midwife in an industry with this history. What can be done in the future to ensure these histories are *acknowledged* but not *repeated*?

The period of assimilation

The assimilation period began in the 1940s, around the end of World War II. At this time, the dominant thinking changed from the idea that Aboriginal and Torres Strait Islander people would 'die out' because the population was in fact increasing. Assimilation policies emerged, with the aim of ensuring that Aboriginal and Torres Strait Islander people could become indistinguishable from non-Indigenous Australians. For this, Aboriginal and Torres Strait Islander people were transferred into 'training' programs to ensure that they became part of broader society. While the intention of the policy was to merge Aboriginal and Torres Strait Islander people into the rest of Australia, its implementation left much to be desired.

Much of the training focused on pastoral duties (farm labour and production) for males and domestic duties for females. This training often involved segregated programs and provided only basic education. Any Aboriginal or Torres Strait Islander person who wanted to move into a semi-professional or professional occupation (such as nursing) would face systemic racism. This was clearly described in the *Bringing Them Home* report:

> I wanted to be a nurse, only to be told that I was nothing but an immoral black lubra, and I was only fit to work on cattle and sheep properties ... I strived every year from Grade 5 up until Grade 8 to get that perfect 100% mark in my exams at the end of each year, which I did succeed in, only to be knocked back by saying that I wasn't fit to do these things ... Our education was really to train us to be domestics and to take orders.
>
> (HREOC, 1997)

During this period, the health status of Aboriginal and Torres Strait Islander people continued to be poor. The policy and treatment approaches remained essentially the same as during the segregation era. Aboriginal and Torres Strait Islander people were still unable to readily access the care they needed and were often refused the care they requested. Segregated treatment also continued (Saggers & Gray, 1991).

The most significant change during the assimilation period was the recognition of the appalling state of Aboriginal and Torres Strait Islander people's health. Information about their health status became more widely available. It was also during this period that infectious diseases began to be replaced by non-communicable diseases as a major cause of morbidity and mortality among Aboriginal and Torres Strait Islander people (Thomson, 1984). However, the assimilation era did see an upswing of Aboriginal and Torres Strait Islander women entering into registered nurse and midwifery training across the country.

The rise of self-determination and community controlled health services

From the early 1960s, both Aboriginal and Torres Strait Islander and non-Indigenous people who were concerned about health became increasingly frustrated with the lack of change in health outcomes of Aboriginal and Torres Strait Islander people. Advocates became organised, and a rights-based movement began the journey towards **self-determination**.

self-determination The 'ongoing process of choice'. Refers to the right of people to freely determine their own social, cultural, economic and political stances and development.

Health advocates increasingly recognised that the underlying causes of physical and emotional ill-health included the history of dispossession and alienation. Historical causes also contributed to the lack of involvement by Aboriginal and Torres Strait Islander people in the country's social, political and economic systems. The determination of those in the Aboriginal community to establish their own services led to the development of the **Aboriginal community controlled health services (ACCHSs)**, which are now a major part of Australia's health system.

Aboriginal community controlled health services (ACCHSs) Aboriginal primary healthcare services run by and for local communities. Also called Aboriginal Medical Services or Aboriginal community controlled health organisations (ACCHOs). ACCHSs are discussed in Chapter 6.

The ACCHSs were a response to concerns that health services were not available, and that where there were services, these were not meeting the needs of Aboriginal and Torres Strait Islander people. ACCHSs were also a recognition that existing health services represented significant geographical, financial and cultural barriers to appropriate health service provision. Many mainstream health services were clearly unwelcoming or openly discriminatory. The first ACCHS was established in Redfern (Sydney) in 1972 and the second by the Central Australian Aboriginal Congress in 1973. Importantly, when Redfern opened its doors for service it was Torres Strait Islander registered nurse and midwife Dulcie Flower who did so with a young doctor named Fred Hollows.

CASE STUDY

The development of the Central Australian Aboriginal Congress

The Central Australian Aboriginal Congress (CAAC) was established in 1973, largely as a political voice for the Aboriginal people living in Central Australia. It has since become the leading provider of comprehensive primary healthcare in the region.

CAAC's development stemmed from the 1967 Australian referendum that gave the federal government the right to make laws affecting Aboriginal and Torres Strait Islander people and saw them included in the population census. In the lead-up to the referendum, a number of important events occurred. Tensions came to the fore in the land rights movement, caused by the proposal to mine bauxite at Yirrkala in the Northern Territory. At the same time, there was a walk-off of Aboriginal people from the Wave Hill station over poor wages and poor working conditions. Around the same time, activists from Central Australia (in particular, Kumantjayi Perkins) who attended the University of Sydney became politically active. In 1965, Perkins launched the Freedom Rides that travelled throughout northern and central New South Wales to highlight racism and segregation in rural communities. Activists advocated for a move away from the desire for equal rights to self-determination. This was initially expressed through land rights campaigns, and then through legal aid and health organisations such as CAAC and the Redfern Aboriginal Medical Service.

On 9 June 1973, more than a hundred people from Alice Springs and surrounding towns came together to begin the process of establishing a legal entity (CAAC). They elected office bearers and prioritised the establishment of the Congress's legal services. In the early days, CAAC's activities covered a broad range of issues, including a program of temporary accommodation for people affected by the very wet season of 1975 and a program of arranging water, firewood and food drop-offs.

From its beginning, CAAC placed a strong emphasis on a comprehensive approach to health development for the community. CAAC sent a submission to the federal Minister for Aboriginal Affairs, highlighting the shortcomings of existing approaches to Aboriginal health. Another submission to the same minister requested that the Congress be supported to open a health service that would provide 'both a preventative and curative approach' to service delivery for Aboriginal and Torres Strait Islander people. The submission requested training for Aboriginal health workers (see Chapter 10) and suggested that the service include both traditional healers and interpreters. Dr Trevor Cutter, from Melbourne, assessed the situation in Alice Springs in 1974. He remained in Alice Springs and began to visit the town camps. In 1975, two female Aboriginal health workers were employed by CAAC, and the organisation moved into a converted house.

In its first year, CAAC provided around 4000 health consultations. By 1976, this had grown to almost 10,000 consultations. A dental service and welfare services were also added that year. By 1980, demands on the service were greater than the ability to meet them. In 1985, more than 28,000 medical consultations, 1500 dental consultations and 25,000 welfare consultations were conducted – equating to about 190 people being seen each day. In 1988, purpose-built premises were completed, which are still in operation today. CAAC continues to grow and currently operates a range of services, including housing, alcohol and drug treatment, family support, child care, health worker training and health promotion, from a number of different sites in Alice Springs.

Source: Rosewarne et al. (2007).

(cont.)

QUESTIONS FOR REFLECTION

- What do you think services such as CAAC contribute to the Australian healthcare system?
- What would be the effects today on hospitals and other services if CAAC did not exist?
- How might your nursing practice change if you were working in an ACCHS?

In 1973, the federal government proposed to assume full responsibility for Aboriginal and Torres Strait Islander policy and planning from the states and territories. All jurisdictions except Queensland accepted the proposal, and negotiations began for the transfer of responsibility for Aboriginal and Torres Strait Islander policy, planning and coordination. The Department of Aboriginal Affairs (DAA) was created in 1972 and was given central authority for policy administration. DAA began making direct allocations of funding to community organisations, including ACCHSs.

Local community control of health services is essential to Aboriginal and Torres Strait Islander peoples' definition of health and wellbeing. Each community needs to determine its own affairs, protocols and procedures. The National Aboriginal Community Controlled Health Organisation (NACCHO), the peak body representing community controlled health services at the national level and formerly called the National Aboriginal and Islander Health Organisation, was formed in 1974 to represent local Aboriginal and Torres Strait Islander community controlled services at the national level. NACCHO provides a 'coordinated response from the community sector, advocating for culturally respectful and needs-based approaches to improving health and wellbeing outcomes through ACCHSs' (NACCHO, 2020).

The ACCHSs continue to contribute significantly to the prevention and management of health issues for Aboriginal and Torres Strait Islander people. More recently, there has been a substantial and positive transformation in the broader Australian primary and tertiary health sector regarding access by, and treatment for, Aboriginal and Torres Strait Islander people.

Contemporary healthcare and systems

Closing the Gap

The contemporary policy setting in Australia relevant to the health of Aboriginal and Torres Strait Islander people is Closing the Gap. This is a national initiative that aims to eliminate the differences in health outcomes that currently exist between Aboriginal and Torres Strait Islander people and other Australians. The first Closing the Gap Report was released in 2009.

Target progress

There are six Closing the Gap targets, relating to life expectancy, child mortality, education and employment (DPMC, 2020). Each year, the Prime Minister provides the

Australian people with an update on each of the targets. Two Closing the Gap targets relate to health: reducing mortality of children under five years of age, and closing the life-expectancy gap.

The mortality rate for Aboriginal and Torres Strait Islander children under five years of age is currently twice the rate of other Australian children. In 2008, the infant mortality rate for Aboriginal and Torres Strait Islander children was 181 for every 100,000 children, compared with 104 per 100,000 for non-Indigenous children. There have been improvements in infant mortality rates between 2008 and 2016, although the Aboriginal and Torres Strait Islander infant mortality rate has consistently remained over twice the rate of the non-Indigenous child mortality rate (DPMC, 2020) (see Figure 2.1).

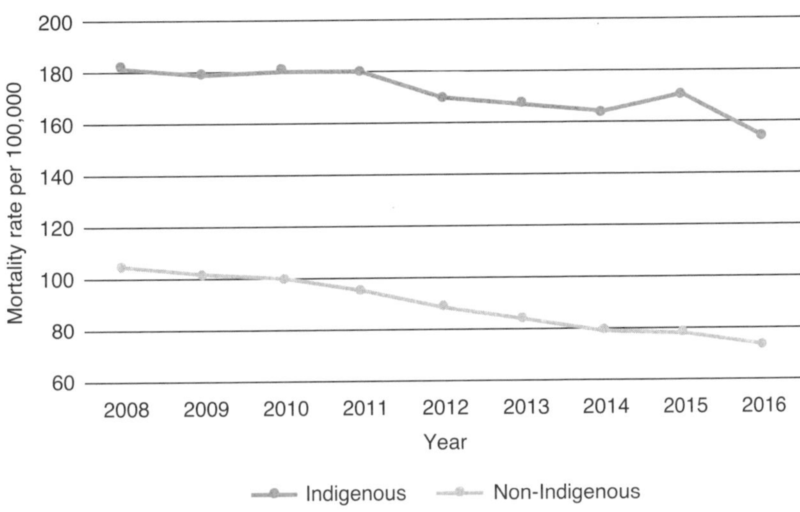

Figure 2.1 Under-five infant mortality rates by Indigenous status 2008–16

Source: Based on data from DPMC (2020).

The life-expectancy gap between Aboriginal and Torres Strait Islander people and other Australians is significant. Life expectancy is reported in three-year cycles. In 2015–17, Aboriginal and Torres Strait Islander life expectancy was estimated to be 75.6 years for females and 71.6 years for males, a lower life expectancy of 7.8 years for females and 8.6 years for males. Between 2010–12 and 2015–17, there was a small, non-significant reduction in the difference of 1.9 years for females and 2.5 years for males (DPMC, 2020) (see Figure 2.2).

These health outcomes are an indication of a person's or group's position within society. They reflect the access to education, employment and power and influence within society experienced by Aboriginal and Torres Strait Islander people. The poor health outcomes experienced by Aboriginal and Torres Strait Islander people reflect the importance of the social and **cultural determinants of health**. Social determinants of health, including education, income and social inclusion, account for at least 34 per cent of the health difference between Aboriginal and Torres Strait Islander people and non-Indigenous Australians (DPMC, 2020). Two other Closing the Gap goals are

cultural determinants of health A 'strength based perspective, acknowledging that stronger connections to culture and country build stronger individual and collective identities, a sense of self-esteem, [and] resilience' (Brown, n.d., cited in Lowitja Institute, 2014, p. 2). The cultural determinants of health 'are enabled, supported and protected through cultural practice, kinship, connection to land and Country, art, song and ceremony, dance, healing, spirituality, empowerment, ancestry, belonging and self-determination' (Department of Health, 2017, p. 7).

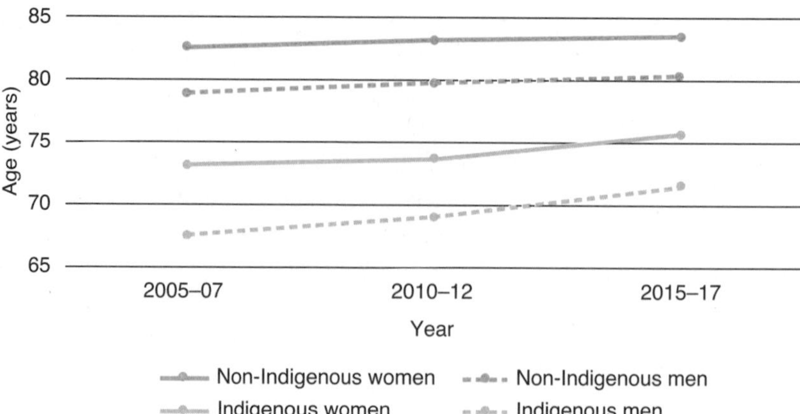

Figure 2.2 Life expectancy by Indigenous status and gender 2005–17

Note: Life expectancy data are reported in three-year cycles.

Sources: Based on data from DPMC (2019, 2020).

worth mentioning here. They show that significant resources continue to be required to achieve equality of outcomes between Aboriginal and Torres Strait Islander people and other Australians.

There remains a significant difference in Year 12 school attainment, but progress is being made. In 2018, just 66 per cent of Aboriginal and Torres Strait Islander people aged 20–24 years had completed Year 12, compared with 90 per cent of other Australians. However, between 2006 and 2016. the difference in Year 12 attainment was reduced by 24 per cent (DPMC, 2020) (see Figure 2.3).

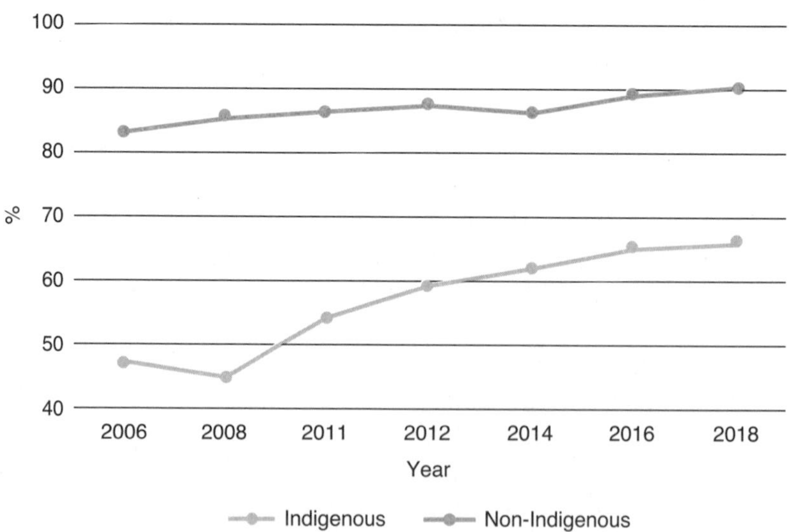

Figure 2.3 Year 12 attainment by Indigenous status 2006–19

Note: Data unavailable for 2010; data from 2011 are presented here instead.

Sources: Based on data from AIHW (2019) and DPMC (2016, 2017, 2019, 2020).

Compared with 2006, in 2018–19 there was in increase in Indigenous employment by 7 per cent (from 42 to 49 per cent); however, between 2006 and 2019 the difference between employment of Indigenous and other Australians remained at around 30 per cent (ABS, 2016; DPMC, 2020) (see Figure 2.4).

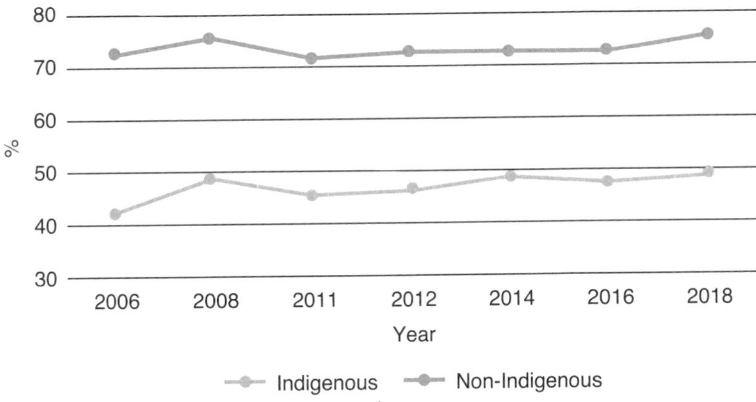

Figure 2.4 Employment by Indigenous status 2006–2019

Note: Data unavailable for 2010; data from 2011 are presented here instead.

Sources: Based on data from DPMC (2016, 2017, 2019, 2020).

Closing the Gap refresh

In 2018, the Council of Australian Governments (COAG) released the Closing the Gap Refresh statement (COAG, 2018). The refresh aimed to reset the relationship between governments and Aboriginal and Torres Strait Islander communities and to facilitate a shared 'ownership of and responsibility for' the Closing the Gap agenda (COAG, 2018). The approach seeks to increase ownership of the Closing the Gap targets by Aboriginal and Torres Strait Islander communities, use a strengths-based and community-led approach, and allow for empowerment and self-determination of Aboriginal and Torres Strait Islander people to assist in closing the gap.

Concerns about the Closing the Gap Refresh, including the epidemiological approach have been raised by Aboriginal and Torres Strait Islander people (Bond & Singh, 2020). The concerns are twofold. The first issue is a failure of the Closing the Gap policy to incorporate factors that contribute to inequality such as exposure to racism, socioeconomic and political exclusion and the causes of poor environmental and living conditions. Second, the Closing the Gap discourse, including the reporting framework, leads people to conclude that inequality results from the poor behaviour by Aboriginal and Torres Strait Islander people themselves, otherwise known as blaming the victim.

Bond & Singh (2020) call for a greater consideration and understanding of the underlying socioeconomic, political, environmental and racial factors that result in Aboriginal and Torres Strait Islander health inequalities, and would change the dominant school of thought – that Aboriginal and Torres Strait Islander individuals are a 'risk factor' for health inequality – and put the onus back onto socioeconomic, political and racist systems that are at the heart of health inequality.

QUESTIONS FOR REFLECTION

- How would Australian history, including the significant decline in Aboriginal and Torres Strait Islander health during the initial contact and assimilation periods, affect current Closing the Gap targets?
- Describe three examples of social determinants of health. How might these affect current Aboriginal and Torres Strait Islander health outcomes?
- What role do nurses and midwives play in helping to close the gap?

Contemporary Aboriginal community controlled health services

Today, Aboriginal and Torres Strait Islander communities operate 143 ACCHSs in urban, regional and remote Australia (NACCHO, 2020). ACCHSs can vary from large, multifunctional services with several medical practitioners that provide a wide range of services, to smaller services reliant on Aboriginal health workers and/or nurses to provide primary care. The smaller services often have a preventive, health education focus. The services form a network, but each remains autonomous and independent of one another and the government (NACCHO, 2020).

ACCHSs are local employment hubs for Aboriginal and Torres Strait Islander people and for other Australians, and their workforce might consist of Aboriginal health workers, Aboriginal and Torres Strait Islander nurses and midwives, doctors (some of whom are Aboriginal and/or Torres Strait Islander) and a range of other health professionals. ACCHSs also employ administrative staff and other ancillary staff such as cleaners and transport drivers. They are able to offer training and career advancement to staff. Some services also conduct research or have a dedicated research unit. The ACCHS model, therefore, does not just provide health and wellbeing services, but also helps to improve health and wellbeing through employment and community development. Through their research activity, the ACCHs are also able to contribute to knowledge about what programs and services work.

Holistic health: Aboriginal and Torres Strait Islander models of healthcare

Holistic healthcare

Aboriginal and Torres Strait Islander people view health as holistic, recognising that health is not merely the absence of disease, but rather the physical, social, emotional, cultural and spiritual wellbeing of individuals, families and communities (Dudgeon, Milroy & Walker, 2014). The cultural, political, historical and social determinants of health are important in holistic approaches to health. These can include access to housing, employment and education, interactions with the justice system, and colonisation (Harfield et al., 2018).

A holistic health approach helps us to understand other areas outside of health that can be addressed to help improve health outcomes for Aboriginal and Torres Strait Islander people:

> You can't fix the health gap in the doctor's surgery alone. And that's what everyone thinks. You can't fix it in the health system alone. All these other things, education, housing, environmental infrastructure, waste disposal … you need all those things in place to compliment the work that the health system does.
>
> (Gooda, 2013, cited in Neumayer, 2013, p. 43)

Emerging services are also acknowledging that the model of healthcare delivery developed by Aboriginal and Torres Strait Islander people is suitable for all Australians. Aboriginal and Torres Strait Islander people and non-Indigenous people alike benefit from a holistic approach to healthcare (Neumayer, 2013).

Culturally safe health service delivery

Since the late 1980s, the primary and tertiary health sectors have attempted to incorporate elements of cultural safety and culturally safe practice in their delivery of health services to Aboriginal and Torres Strait Islander people. This typically involves training that incorporates issues relevant to Aboriginal and Torres Strait Islander health, case scenarios involving Aboriginal and Torres Strait Islander clients and discussions about cultural safety (Newman, 1993). This is discussed in-depth in Chapter 3 and adheres to the fully theorised model of care by Māori nurse and scholar Irihapiti Ramsden.

Today, there is increasing support for 'birthing on Country' practices to be available to Aboriginal and Torres Strait Islander women and families. This model of care promotes culturally safe, holistic birthing practices that can include traditional birthing practices. Birthing on Country can provide an opportunity for the best start in life for Aboriginal and Torres Strait Islander babies and families (Kildea et al., 2013) and has been advocated to help improve both maternal and infant health outcomes (Kildea & Van Wagner, 2012). The basis of this model of care ensures that Aboriginal and Torres Strait Islander women are at the forefront in the design, delivery, development and evaluation of the services. Birthing on Country practices promote connection to land and country, place and belonging. They are community based and governed, and incorporate culturally safe nursing and midwifery practices, using a holistic approach to healthcare delivery. They provide Aboriginal and Torres Strait Islander women with the opportunity to include traditional practices in the birthing of their child and enrich connections with land and Country (CATSINaM, 2016). Importantly, the birthing on Country model of care can be delivered in any setting in Australia. The principles of birthing on Country enable Aboriginal and Torres Strait Islander women to have access to any relevant cultural aspects they wish to include in their birthing, irrespective of their location and birth setting (hospital, birthing centre).

There is an increasing focus on providing culturally safe nursing and midwifery services (NSW Health, 2013). The most common employment sector for Aboriginal and Torres Strait Islander people is in healthcare and social assistance, at 14 per cent

(ABS, 2018). Nurses make up the largest number of health professionals in community-based and tertiary health services in Australia. Approximately 330,000 nurses and midwives were registered in Australia in 2018 (Department of Health, 2019).

Government initiatives have aimed to increase the number of Aboriginal and Torres Strait Islander nurses, midwives and allied health professionals. Hospitals now commonly employ Aboriginal Health Workers and Liaison Officers (AHWLOs) (discussed in depth in Chapter 10), who help and advocate for Aboriginal and Torres Strait Islander clients and aim to break down cultural barriers to health service delivery (Mackean et al., 2020).

A 2020 review of AHWLOs in the acute care setting found limited literature on AHWLOs and their effects on quality care indicators. However, other information sources, including local and state health organisations, indicate that AHWLOs are a crucial component of holistic and culturally safe Aboriginal and Torres Strait Islander healthcare (Mackean et al., 2020).

NSW Health (NSW Ministry of Health, 2018), for example, states that AHWLOs play a 'key role in combating the high burden of disease and mortality rates in Aboriginal communities of NSW'. The Aboriginal Health Council of South Australia (AHCSA, 2020) similarly states that AHWLOs are 'crucial to improving health outcomes of Aboriginal and Torres Strait Islander people'.

Perhaps the greatest gains in health are made when organisations that are led and run by Aboriginal and Torres Strait Islander people provide an extensive range of health services to the wider community. The Maari Ma Aboriginal Corporation is an example of this approach.

CASE STUDY

Maari Ma Aboriginal Corporation

In the mid-1990s, a new model of Aboriginal primary healthcare service provision began in the far west of New South Wales. The model developed in response to continuing concerns about ill-health and the need for better primary healthcare for the region's Aboriginal population. The local community established an independent Aboriginal organisation to deal with 'health business'. Rather than set up a stand-alone Aboriginal Medical Service, the community decided to develop a model of primary healthcare delivery integrated with the health services provided in the region by the Greater Western Area Health Service (which was funded by the state and federal governments). The Maari Ma Aboriginal Corporation was established to provide broad-based health services.

Maari Ma took an optimistic, solutions-focused approach to healthcare provision. Richard Weston, CEO of Maari Ma at the time, noted that 'the leadership did not focus on the all the wrongs done to our people by the whitefellas. They chose instead to engage with white leadership and have dialogue. They did not dwell in the past, they got on with building the future' (Weston, 2013).

A recent evaluation identified the success of Maari Ma and led to increased funding for Aboriginal primary healthcare and greater primary healthcare activity. Many health indicators for the region show some improvement, including improved access to antenatal care in the first 20 weeks of pregnancy, reduced vaccine-preventable hospitalisations, reduced rates of premature birth and low birth weight and reduced rates of acute preventable hospitalisations.

Several factors identified in the evaluation contribute to the success of Maari Ma, including increased investment by federal and state governments into primary healthcare, Indigenous management of 'mainstream' health service delivery and significant employment of Aboriginal staff (including Aboriginal health workers). Other factors include the engagement of Aboriginal community leaders in mainstream health system development and the use of data and evidence-based programs to improve the service's response to key health priorities. Maari Ma particularly focuses on maternal and child health, the prevention and management of chronic disease and working with other sectors to address the social determinants of health.

Source: Grew & Houston (2007).

QUESTIONS FOR REFLECTION

- How do you think the establishment of Maari Ma would translate to an urban setting?
- What challenges would you expect to face as a student nurse placed in a Maari Ma service?

Conclusion

This chapter has shown how historical thinking and actions have informed Aboriginal and Torres Strait Islander health policy and practice. It also shows how historical mistakes such as segregation, isolation and protection contributed to devastating outcomes for the health of Aboriginal and Torres Strait Islander people. Current progress owes much to those who advocated, argued and rationalised for a better approach.

Despite recent positive changes in approach, we continue to see the legacy of historical policies and actions. The Closing the Gap targets demonstrate that we need to remain vigilant about improving the health of Aboriginal and Torres Strait Islander people. Improving the health of Aboriginal and Torres Strait Islander people means taking an approach that goes beyond traditional healthcare and considers the social and cultural determinants of health – including education, housing, employment and position in society.

Nurses and midwives are a significant force in healthcare delivery and systems for Aboriginal and Torres Strait Islander people. Appropriate education of nurses and midwives – including the education of both Aboriginal and Torres Strait Islander and non-Indigenous nurses and midwives – is the key to improving health services and delivery to Aboriginal and Torres Strait Islander people in Australia.

Learning activities

1. Research the missions and reserves that were established near where you were born or raised. (To start your search, visit the Aboriginal/reserve/mission map available at http://oa.anu.edu.au/entity/14540?eid=14581.)
2. Research an ACCHSs in your area. What services do they provide? (To start your search, visit www.naccho.org.au.)
3. Research the Aboriginal health policy and plans of your local health service. (To start your search, visit your state or territory Department of Health.)

FURTHER READING

ABS (2018). *Census of Population and Housing: Characteristics of Aboriginal and Torres Strait Islander Australians, 2016.* Canberra: ABS.

DPMC (2020). *Closing the Gap: Prime Minister's Report 2020.* Canberra: DPMC.

Saggers, S. & Gray, D. (1991). *Aboriginal Health and Society: The Traditional and Contemporary Aboriginal Struggle for Better Health.* Sydney: Allen & Unwin.

Thomson, N. (1984). Australian Aboriginal health and health-care. *Social Science & Medicine,* 18(11), 939–48.

Visit the companion website at www.cambridge.org/highereducation/isbn/9781108794695/resources to see further online resources.

REFERENCES

Abbie, A.A. (1969). *The Original Australians.* London: Muller.

Aboriginal Communities of the Northern Territory (1988). *Traditional Bush Medicines: An Aboriginal Pharmacopoeia.* Melbourne: Greenhouse Publications.

ABS (2016). *National Aboriginal and Torres Strait Islander Social Survey, 2014–15,* Canberra: ABS.

ABS (2018). *Census of Population and Housing: Characteristics of Aboriginal and Torres Strait Islander Australians, 2016.* Canberra: ABS.

AHCSA (2020). *Aboriginal Health Worker Role.* Adelaide: Aboriginal Health Council of South Australia.

AIHW (2018). *Aboriginal and Torres Strait Islander Stolen Generations and Descendants: Numbers, Demographic Characteristics and Selected Outcomes.* Canberra: AIHW.

AIHW (2019). *Indigenous Education and Skills.* Canberra: AIHW. Retrieved from www.aihw.gov.au/reports/australias-welfare/indigenous-education-and-skills.

Bates, D. (ed.) (1985). *The Native Tribes of Western Australia.* Canberra: National Library of Australia.

Berndt, R.M. (1943). *Wuradjeri Magic and 'Clever Men'.* Canberra: AIATSIS.

Best, O. (2013). The Native Nurses of Queensland: 1940s. Paper presented at the Australian Institute of Aboriginal and Torres Strait Islander Studies Nursing and Midwifery Seminar Series, Semester 1, Canberra.

Best, O. (2015). Training the 'natives' as nurses in Australia: So what went wrong? In H. Sweet & S.Hawkins (eds), *Colonial Caring: A History of Colonial and Post-colonial Nursing.* Manchester: Manchester University Press, pp. 104–25.

Best, O. & Howey, K. (2013). Finding May Yarrowick: Is she the first? Paper presented at the Aboriginal Institute of Aboriginal and Torres Strait Islander Studies Nursing and Midwifery Seminar Series, Semester 1, Canberra.

Blyton, G. (2009). Reflections, memories, and sources: Healthier times? Revisiting Indigenous Australian health history. *Australian and New Zealand Society of the History of Medicine, Inc. Health and History,* 11(2), 116–35.

Bond, C. & Singh, D. (2020). More than a refresh required for closing the gap of Indigenous health inequality. *Medical Journal of Australia,* 212(5), 198–9.

Butlin, N. (1982). *Close encounters of the worst kind: Modelling Aboriginal depopulation and resource competition 1788–1850.* Canberra: Australian National University Press.

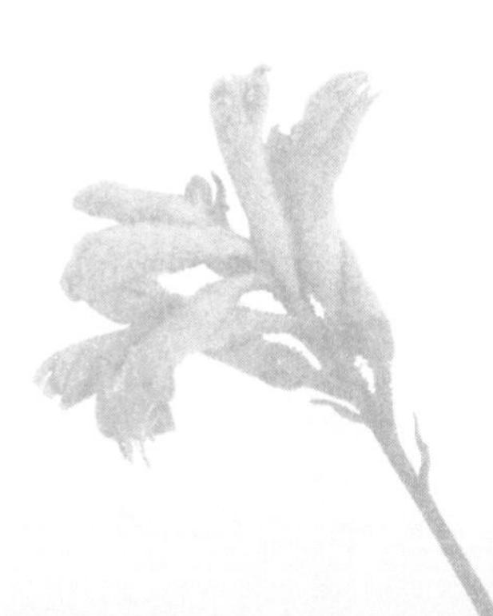

CATSINaM (2016). Birthing on Country position statement. *Congress of Aboriginal and Torres Strait Islander Nurses and Midwives*. Retrieved from www.catsinam.org.au/static/uploads/files/birthing-on-country-position-statement-endorsed-march-2016-wfaxpyhvmxrw.pdf

Clark, M. (1966). *Sources of Australian History*. London: Oxford University Press.

Cleland, J.B. (1928). Disease among the Australian Aborigines. *Journal of Tropical Medicine and Hygiene*, 31, 53–70.

COAG (2018). *COAG Statement on the Closing the Gap Refresh, 12 December 2018*. Canberra: COAG. Retrieved from www.coag.gov.au/sites/default/files/communique/coag-statement-closing-the-gap-refresh.pdf

Cox, L. (2007). Fear, trust and Aborigines: The historical experience of state institutions and current encounters in the health system. *Health and History: Journal of the Australian and New Zealand Society for the History of Medicine*, 9(2), 70–92.

Department of Health (2017). *My Life My Lead: Opportunities for Strengthening Approaches to the Social Determinants and Cultural Determinants of Indigenous Heaalth: Report on the National Consultations, December 2017*. Canberra: Department of Health. Retrieved from www1.health.gov.au/internet/main/publishing.nsf/Content/D2F6B905F3F667DACA2580D400014BF1/$File/My%20Life%20My%20Lead%20Consultation%20Report.pdf

Department of Health (2019). *Summary Statistics: Health Workforce Summaries. Health Workforce Data*. Available at: https://hwd.health.gov.au/summary.html

DPMC (2016). *Closing the Gap: Prime Minister's Report*. Canberra: DPMC.

DPMC (2017). *Closing the Gap: Prime Minister's Report 2017*. Canberra: DPMC.

DPMC (2019). *Closing the Gap: Prime Minister's Report 2019*. Canberra: DPMC.

DPMC (2020). *Closing the Gap: Prime Minister's Report 2020*. Canberra: DPMC.

Director of Native Affairs (Queensland) (1948). *Annual Report of the Director of Native Affairs for the Year Ending 30 June 1948*.

Dudgeon, P., Milroy, H. & Walker, R. (eds) (2014). *Working Together: Aboriginal and Torres Strait Islander Mental Health and Wellbeing Principles and Practice*. Canberra: Commonwealth of Australia.

Elkin, A.P. (1946). *Wuradjuri Magic: Aboriginal Men of High Degree*. Canberra: AIATSIS.

Forsyth, S. (2007). Telling stories: Nurses, politics and Aboriginal Australians, circa 1900–1980s. *Contemporary Nurse*, 24(1), 33–44.

Grew, R. & Houston, S. (2007). Review of the Management Agreement Between Maari Ma Health Aboriginal Corporation and Greater Western Area Health Service. Unpublished report by the Greater Western Area Health Service.

Hamilton, A. (1981). *Nature and Nurture: Aboriginal Child-rearing in North-Central Arnhem Land*. Canberra: AIATSIS.

Harfield, S.G., Davy, C., McArthur, A., Munn, Z., Brown, A. & Brown, N. (2018). Characteristics of Indigenous primary health care service delivery models: A systematic scoping review. *Globalization and Health*, 14(12). Retrieved from https://globalizationandhealth.biomedcentral.com/articles/10.1186/s12992-018-0332-2

HREOC (1997). *Bringing Them Home: Report of the National Inquiry into the Separation of Aboriginal and Torres Strait Islander Children from Their Families*. Sydney: HREOC.

Kildea, S., Magick Dennis, F. & Stapleton, H. (2013). *Birthing on Country Workshop Report, Alice Springs, 4 July 2012*. Australian Catholic University and Mater

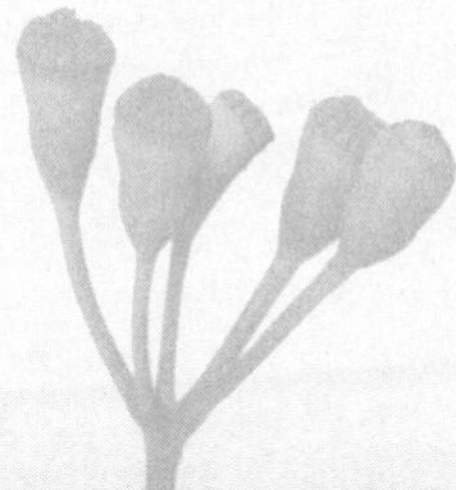

Medical Research Unit on behalf of the Maternity Services Interjurisdictional Committee for the Australian Health Ministers' Advisory Council.Sydney: AHMAC.

Kildea, S. & Van Wagner, V. (2012). *'Birthing on Country' Maternity Service Delivery Models: A Review of the Literature*. An Evidence Check rapid review brokered by the Sax Institute on behalf of the Maternity Services Inter-Jurisdictional Committee for the Australian Health Ministers Advisory Council. Sydney: AHMAC.

Locher, C., Semple, S.J. & Simpson, B.S. (2013). Traditional Australian Aboriginal medicinal plants: An untapped resource for novel therapeutic compounds? *Future Medicinal Chemistry*, 5(7), 733–6.

Lowitja Institute (2014). *Cultural Determinants Roundtable 2014: Background Paper*. Melbourne: Lowitja Institute. Retrieved from www.lowitja.org.au/content/Document/PDF/Cultural-Determinants-Roundtable-Background-Paper.pdf

Mackean, T., Withall, E., Dwyer, J. & Wilson, A. (2020). Role of Aboriginal Health Workers and Liaison Officers in quality care in the Australian acute care setting: a systematic review. *Australian Health Review*. Retrieved from www.publish.csiro.au/ah/pdf/AH19101

NACCHO (2020). About NACCHO. Retrieved from www.naccho.org.au/about

Neumayer, H. (2013). *Changing the Conversation: Strengthening a Rights-based Holistic Approach to Aboriginal and Torres Strait Islander Health and Wellbeing*. Canberra: Indigenous Allied Health Australia.

Newman, B. (1993). Nurses … bridging the gap: Australian Aboriginals and primary health care. *Journal of the Royal Society of Health*, 113(2), 87–90.

NSW Health (2013). *NSW Aboriginal Nursing and Midwifery Strategy*. Sydney: NSW Health. Retrieved from www.health.nsw.gov.au/nursing/aboriginal-strategy/Pages/default.aspx

NSW Ministry of Health (2018). *Aboriginal Health Worker Guidelines for NSW Health*. Sydney: NSW Ministry of Health.

Packer, J., Brouwer, N., Harrington, D., Gaikwad, J., Heron, R., Yaegl Community Elders … Jamie, J. (2012). An ethnobotanical study of medicinal plants used by the Yaegl Aboriginal community in northern New South Wales, Australia. *Journal of Ethnopharmacology*, 139(1), 244–55.

Parsons, M. (2008). Fantome Island lock hospital and Aboriginal venereal disease sufferers 1928–45. *Health and History*, 10(1), 41–62.

Pearn, J. (1993). Acacias and aesculapius. Australian native wattles and the doctors they commemorate. *Medical Journal of Australia*, 159(11–12), 729–38.

Pearn, J. (2005). The world's longest surviving paediatric practices: Some themes of Aboriginal medical ethnobotany in Australia. *Journal of Paediatrics and Child Health*, 41(5–6), 284–90.

Pollard, D. (1988). *Give and Take: The Losing Partnership in Aboriginal Poverty*. Sydney: Hale and Iremonger.

Rosewarne, C., Vaarzon-Morel, P., Bell, S., Carter, E., Liddle, M. & Liddle, J. (2007). The historical context of developing an Aboriginal community controlled health service: A social history of the first ten years of the Central Australian Aboriginal Congress. *Health & History*, 9(2), 114–43.

Saggers, S. & Gray, D. (1991). *Aboriginal Health and Society: The Traditional and Contemporary Aboriginal Struggle for Better Health*. Sydney: Allen & Unwin.

Smith, F.B. (2011). *Illness in Colonial Australia*. Melbourne: Australian Scholarly Publishing.

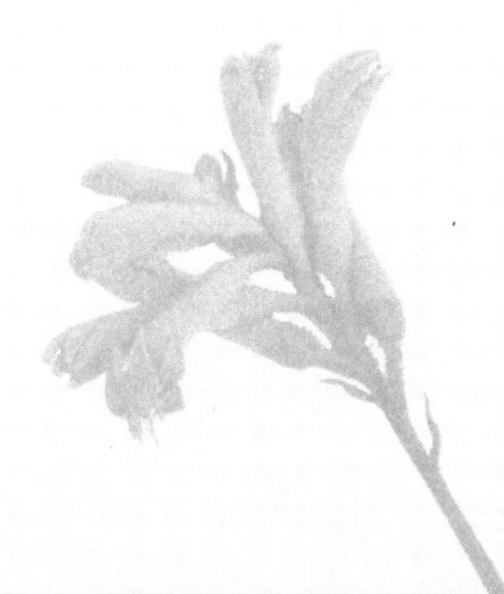

Smith, L. (1980). *The Aboriginal Population of Australia.* Canberra: Australian National University Press.

Solar, O. & Irwin, A. (2010). *A Conceptual Framework for Action on the Social Determinants of Health. Social Determinants of Health.* Geneva: WHO.

Stone, S. (ed.) (1974). *Aborigines in White Australia: A Documentary History of the Attitudes Affecting Official Policy and the Australian Aborigine, 1697–1973.* Melbourne: Heinemann.

Stuart-Fox, E. (2000). Survey on traditional and bush foods in the Aboriginal and Torres Strait Islander community in Brisbane. *Aboriginal and Islander Health Worker Journal*, 24(5), n.p.

Thomson, N. (1984). Australian Aboriginal health and health-care. *Social Science & Medicine*, 18(11), 939–48.

Walton, S.F., McKinnon, M., Pizzutto, S., Dougall, A., Williams, E. & Currie, B.J. (2004). Acaricidal activity of Melaleuca alternifolia (tea tree) oil: In vitro sensitivity of Sarcoptes scabiei var hominis to terpinen-4-ol. *Archives of Dermatology*, 140(5), 563–6.

Watarrka Foundation Limited (2019). *Traditional Aboriginal Foods.* Alice Springs: Watarrka Foundation. Retrieved from www.watarrkafoundation.org.au/blog/traditional-aboriginal-foods#:~:text=A%20large%20part%20of%20the,mulga%20seeds%20and%20wattle%20seeds.

Weston, R. (2013). *Early Steps of a New Aboriginal Health Service.* Broken Hill, NSW: Maari Ma Health Aboriginal Corporation.

WHO (2020). *Social Determinants of Health.* Geneva: WHO. Retrieved from www.who.int/gender-equity-rights/understanding/sdh-definition/en/#:~:text=Social%20determinants%20of%20health%E2%80%93The,global%2C%20national%20and%20local%20levels

Worgan, G. (1788). *Journal of a First Fleet Surgeon.* Prepared from the print edition published by Library Council of New South Wales; Library of Australian History Sydney 1978. Retrieved from http://adc.library.usyd.edu.au/data-2/worjour.pdf

LEGISLATION CITED

Aboriginals Protection and Restriction of the Sale of Opium Act 1897 (Qld)
Aborigines Protection Act 1909 (NSW)

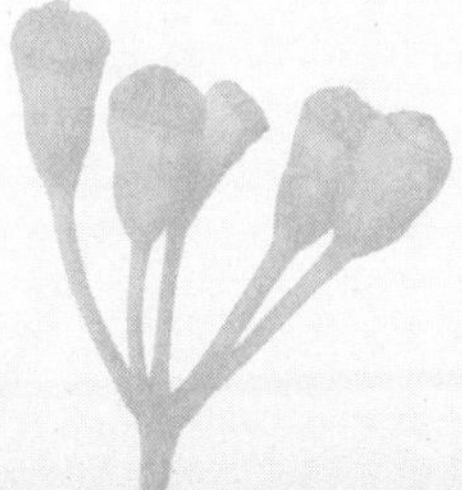

The cultural safety journey: An Aboriginal Australian nursing and midwifery context

Odette Best

> You people talk about legal safety, ethical safety, safety in clinical practice and a safe knowledge base, but what about Cultural Safety?
>
> (Ramsden, 2002, p. 1)

LEARNING OBJECTIVES

This chapter will help you to understand and examine:

- The effects of Australian colonial nursing history on Aboriginal and Torres Strait Islander people
- Your own beliefs, values and attitudes, and the influence these may have on your work with Aboriginal and Torres Strait Islander Australians
- Nursing and midwifery practice that respects the differences of clients
- The journey from cultural awareness to cultural safety

KEY WORDS

beliefs, values and attitudes
colonisation
cultural safety

Introduction

cultural safety The effective nursing of a person or family from another culture, determined by that person or family. Culture includes but is not restricted to age or generation; gender; sexual orientation; occupation; and socioeconomic status; ethnic origin or migrant experience; religious or spiritual belief and disability. The nurse delivering the service will have undertaken a process of reflection on [their] own cultural identity and will recognise the impact that [their] personal culture has on [their] professional practice. Unsafe cultural practice is any action which diminishes, demeans or disempowers the cultural identity and well-being of an individual. (NCNZ, 2011, p. 7)

This chapter explores the framework of **cultural safety** within nursing and midwifery practice. It discusses cultural safety from the perspective of an Aboriginal Registered Nurse with the focus on how cultural safety is relevant for Indigenous Australian people.

In 2019, the Australian Nursing and Midwifery Accreditation Council (ANMAC) released the updated Registered Nurse Accreditation Standards. The new standards mandated that cultural safety for all people be included in programs of study. Within Australia, across a range of health-related documents, we are bombarded with terms such as 'cultural competency', 'cultural humility', 'cultural responsibility' and 'cultural awareness'. There has been much confusion and foggy thinking about the meaning of cultural safety within Australia. The author of this chapter is a cultural safety purist as defined by Māori Registered Nurse Irihapeti Ramsden and her colleagues. There is no need to define nor redefine cultural safety in Australia. It is an already existing nursing framework developed by an Indigenous nurse, and was developed for the professions of nursing and midwifery for *all* nurses and midwives.

The chapter outlines the development of cultural safety framework by Irihapeti Ramsden. Cultural safety is placed within an historical context and is defined as a journey that all nurses and midwives need to undertake. Nursing and midwifery students are encouraged to consider the potential influence of their own cultures on their nursing and midwifery practice. This chapter uses an historical lens to explore the establishment of nursing in Australia and therefore the 'whiteness' of nursing, and its impacts on Indigenous Australian peoples and our health

Further, understanding cultural safety involves considering the different ways in which cultures define health. Within Australia, the biomedical model of health dominates; however, this is a relatively new model and is not the only one available or practised. This chapter provides an Indigenous Australian definition of health, and compares it with the World Health Organization's (WHO) definition to highlight the legitimate differences in defining health. The chapter explores how to cultivate cultural safety and embed it within nursing and midwifery practice.

Developing the theory of cultural safety

Māori nurse Irihapeti Ramsden developed the nursing framework of cultural safety. In her doctoral thesis, she stated 'that the dream of *Cultural Safety* was about helping people in nursing education, teachers and students, to become aware of their social conditioning and how it has affected them and therefore their practice' (Ramsden, 2002, p. 2). She argued that the framework for cultural safety was designed to demystify colonial history and prevent its impact on widespread attitudes and beliefs about Indigenous peoples.

colonisation The process of taking over land for the colonisers' use and establishing control over the Indigenous people. Colonisation typically involves taking political control of a country, occupying it with settlers and exploiting the country's resources.

Ramsden's work in cultural safety emerged from her own journey as a Māori student nurse and nursing graduate, and her response to the educational process, which 'was so obviously designed for student nurses who did not, and could not share the experience of the **colonisation** of my land and people and history' (Ramsden, 2002, p. 2).

For Ramsden, cultural safety requires an understanding of culture, which she defines as:

> The accumulated socially acquired result of shared geography, time, ideas and human experience. Culture may or may not involve kinship, but meanings and understandings are collectively held by group members. Culture is dynamic and mobile and changes according to time, individuals and groups.
>
> (Ramsden, 2002, p. 111)

It is important to note that *the concept of cultural safety does not anchor culture only to ethnicity*; instead, culture is expanded to incorporate many aspects that can make up an individual's culture. While ethnicity can often be an important aspect of one's culture, it is not the only aspect, and is not the only aspect of care that can have culturally unsafe care provided. Culturally unsafe care has been rampant throughout 'modern' nursing and midwifery care and histories that are not anchored to ethnicity. An example of such unsafe care is examined in the seminal work of English nurse scholar Dr Tommy Dickinson (2015). This work outlines the barbaric treatments and care provided to gay men and women within psychiatric hospitals where, until the 1980s, homosexuality was deemed a deviancy and an offence punishable by law. 'Curing' homosexuality was undertaken by admittance into psychiatric hospitals, where treatments such as chemical castration, electroconvulsive therapy and aversion therapies were utilised (Dickinson, 2015). Interestingly, in August 2020 Queensland became the first Australian state to outlaw gay conversion therapy and to make associated practices illegal. A further example of culturally unsafe care is demonstrated by Benedict and Shields (2014), who outline the horrendous involvement of nurses and midwives in the euthanasia programs against the Jews in Nazi Germany. While the above examples seem extreme, they are still a part of nursing and midwifery histories that demonstrate culturally unsafe care not necessarily anchored to ethnicity.

However, this chapter is focused on how culturally unsafe care has played a major role in the care of Indigenous Australians and has impacted upon the health status of Indigenous Australians.

Ramsden's definition of culture accepts that individuals may belong to multiple cultures at any one time. Within Australia's Aboriginal and Torres Strait Islander communities, culture can be determined by our ethnicity, link to land or Country, gender, profession, spirituality or sexuality. In this sense, Aboriginal and Torres Strait Islander Australians are no different from other Australians.

Within the context of Aboriginal and Torres Strait Islander peoples and their health, it is essential for nurses and midwives to recognise the immense diversity within the Indigenous Australian community. Aboriginal and Torres Strait Islander people hold a wide variety of beliefs, values and attitudes. There is just as much diversity within the Indigenous community as there is within the non-Indigenous community. Multiple cultures exist within the Indigenous community, quite apart from ethnicity.

Ramsden (2002, pp. 5–6) states that:

> Cultural Safety has been expanded to include all people encountered by nurses who differ in any way from the nurse. Whatever the difference, whether it is gender, sexuality, social class, occupational group, generation, ethnicity or a grand combination of variables, difference is acknowledged as legitimate and the nurse is seen as having the

primary responsibility to establish trust. Cultural Safety is therefore about the nurse rather than the patient. That is, the enactment of Cultural Safety is about the nurse while, for the consumer, Cultural Safety is the mechanism which allows the recipient of care to say whether or not the service is safe for them to approach and use. Safety is a subjective word deliberately chosen to give the power to the consumer.

As a newly graduated nurse, Ramsden was constantly expected to look after only Māori clients and their families. She reported that, at times, she would watch inappropriate care being given to Māori patients and recognise the distress of these clients. She would add to her own client load by helping or explaining things to the client that the *pakeha* (white) nurse had instructed them to do. One outcome of this extra work was that Māori patients would ask to be looked after by Ramsden; the *pakeha* nurses would shrug their shoulders, look at Ramsden and walk away (Ramsden, 2002). She explained that 'this meant dealing with such social mechanisms as personal and institutional racism in the context of a violent colonial history and coming to terms with the inherent power relations, both historical and contemporary' (Ramsden, 2002, p. 3). The experience described by Ramsden is common among Indigenous Australian nurses (Best & Bunda, 2020; Best & Gorman, 2016; Best & Nielsen, 2005; Nielsen, 2010;

Ramsden questioned the outcomes of inappropriate nursing care for Māori clients:

> Consciously or unconsciously such power reinforced by unsafe, prejudicial demeaning attitudes and wielded inappropriately by health workers, could cause people to distrust and avoid the health services. Nurses need to understand this process and become very skilled at the interpretation of the level of distrust experienced by many Indigenous people when interacting with the health service which has its roots in the colonial administration.
>
> (Ramsden, 2002, p. 3)

Ramsden's thinking about culture therefore began to focus on the power imbalance between the nurse and the client. This greatly informed her theory of cultural safety (Figure 3.1). She argued that 'cultural safety became concerned with social justice and quickly came to be about nurses, power, prejudice and attitude rather than the ethnicity or cultures of Māori or other patients' (Ramsden, 2002, p. 5). Just as Ramsden utilised the broadest definition of culture, the defining of 'cultural safety' also expanded to reflect this.

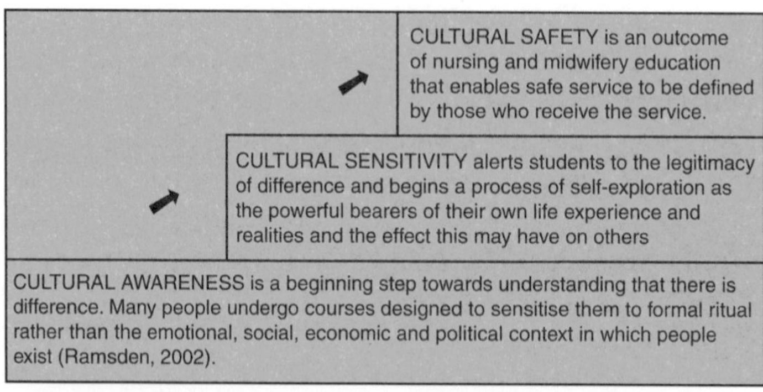

Figure 3.1 Ramsden's process of cultural safety in nursing and midwifery practice

Source: Reproduced from Ramsden (2002, p. 117).

Ramsden defines three steps for nurses and midwives to move through in order to become culturally safe practitioners and argues that work on cultural safety needs to be continuous. She proposes that nurses need to move from cultural awareness and through cultural sensitivity, before becoming culturally safe. (Ramsden, 2002, p. 117). Each step is individualised in its intent and the steps are not interchangeable.

Developing cultural awareness: Me, myself and I

Ramsden (2002, p. 117) identifies cultural awareness as the first phase on the journey to culturally safe practice. It is a 'beginning step towards understanding that there is a difference [between peoples and their lived experiences and political and social positionings]. Many people undergo courses designed to sensitise them to formal ritual rather than the emotional, social, economic and political context in which people exist.' This beginning step is one of self-reflection. It is essential for the nurse/midwife to understand their own cultures and the potential impact of these cultures on their clients/patients.

Cultural awareness training is common in Australian healthcare settings. Interestingly, most cultural training focuses on learning about Indigenous Australians. Little, if any, cultural awareness training encourages nurses to think about their own cultures, such as their ethnicity, or the nursing and midwifery cultures of the professions, or sexuality culture or gendered culture. Colonial nursing and midwifery practice and its impacts on nursing and midwifery care and Indigenous Australians are rarely discussed. McGibbon et al. (2013, p. 5) note that cultural awareness training that includes 'a focus on knowledge about cultural practices of diet, dancing and dress has taken us even further away from confronting colonialism in nursing.'

By and large, many non-Indigenous Australians have little sense of their own ethnicities. They often dismiss ethnicity as a culture by saying, 'I'm just Australian.' But what does that mean? Being Australian is not an ethnicity unless you are Indigenous. Non-Indigenous Australians do have many and varied ethnicities, but these ethnicities deemed Australian culture' are rarely examined. The author of this chapter argues that this is *an imagined sense of being acultural – meaning without culture*. This means that people with recognisable cultures (usually physically obvious ethnicities) are seen only by their ethnicity and are positioned as the ones who have culture.

QUESTION FOR REFLECTION

- Make a list of cultures with which you identify, including ethnicity. How and why do you identify with these cultures?

Understanding our own individual beliefs, values and attitudes

beliefs, values and attitudes The *Concise Oxford Dictionary* defines beliefs, values and attitudes in this way:

- **beliefs:** an acceptance that something exists or is true, especially without proof; firmly held opinions or convictions.
- **values:** principles or standards of behaviour.
- **attitudes:** a settled way of thinking or feeling.

Nurses and midwives must undertake a process of self-reflection to explore their *own* **beliefs, values and attitudes**, and must consider the potential impacts of these on recipients of their care.

Many misconceptions continue to inform widespread beliefs, values and attitudes about Indigenous Australians. These beliefs, values and attitudes are formed in early childhood and can be influenced by family, class, ethnicity, religion, schooling and social media. Arguably, this is due in part to Indigenous Australians being excluded from, or shown in negative ways in, mainstream media representations, and it is also because Indigenous Australians are rarely included in popular culture.

Cultural safety recognises that beliefs, values and attitudes are constructed through our social environments and will depend upon our childhood experiences. Cox and Taua (2013, p. 321) argue that cultural safety is underpinned by a philosophical commitment to social constructivism that 'refers to the socially constructed nature of reality, where humans come to know the world through experience and together construct reality by negotiating meanings through communication and power relationships'.

This approach to cultural safety makes it clear that nurses enter the profession with well-defined beliefs, values and attitudes about a whole range of issues. Accepted beliefs, values and attitudes will vary between nurses, midwives and their clients. Many nursing theorists and academics recognise that before nurses can move towards practising cultural safety, they must understand their own beliefs, values and attitudes, and the social structures in which they operate (Cox & Taua, 2017; Nielsen, 2010; Ramsden, 2002; Sherwood, 2013). The challenge is then for each individual nurse and midwife to understand that there are differences between people who may share at least one or more cultures. Part of the cultural safety journey is the development of nurses' and midwives' awareness of themselves and recognition that they do not necessarily know or understand the clients in their care. Nurses and midwives need to recognise how their personal beliefs, values and attitudes may influence their care of clients.

Nurses and midwives who do not reflect on their beliefs, values and attitudes, and how they were formed, may have nothing more than stereotyped, misleading myths to guide them in their attitudes and potential care of Indigenous Australians.

QUESTIONS FOR REFLECTION

- What are your own beliefs, values and attitudes about Aboriginal and Torres Strait Islander people? Where did you gain them from? How were they formed? Have you ever questioned whether they are valid or true?
- What are some of the commonly held beliefs about Indigenous Australians?

Who defines health?

Each person's beliefs, values and attitudes contribute to their understanding of what is meant by 'health'. The biomedical definition of health can be quite different from the definition of health advocated by Indigenous Australian communities. One of the most widely accepted definitions of health is outlined by the WHO (1946) as 'a state of complete physical, mental and social well-being and not merely the absence of disease or infirmity'. This definition has not been amended since 1946.

In contrast, the National Aboriginal Health Strategy (National Aboriginal Health Strategy Working Party, 1989, p. x) states that health is 'not just the physical well-being of the individual but the social, emotional and cultural well-being of the whole community. This is a whole of life view and it also includes the cyclical concept of life-death-life'. Swan and Raphael (1995, p. 19) extended the definition with this statement:

> The Aboriginal concept of health is holistic, encompassing mental health, physical, cultural and spiritual health. The holistic concept does not refer to the whole body but is in fact steeped in harmonised inter relations which constitute cultural well-being. These interrelating factors can be categorised largely into spiritual, environmental, ideological, political, social, economic, mental and physical. Crucially, it must be understood that when the harmony of these inter relations is disrupted, Aboriginal ill health will persist.

These definitions have some notable differences from the WHO definition. The Indigenous definition of health includes the community and the distinct interconnectedness of all elements. The Indigenous definition also outlines the continuation of health by including spirituality as the continuing cycle of 'life–death–life'. Every aspect of a person is regarded equally, including biological, psychological, sociological, spiritual and communal dimensions; today, this would be seen as 'holistic' health. In contrast, the WHO's definition operates from an individualist perspective and does not reflect community or spirituality. This definition of health is the one that dominates health discourses globally, and it is entrenched in biomedical dominance.

It is important to note that comparing and contrasting these definitions of health is not about trying to identify which is right or wrong. Instead, it is about recognising that an Indigenous definition of health may be different from the dominant Australian (Western) paradigm. Differences in defining health are valid and need to be acknowledged. The implication for nursing and midwifery practice is that different clients may hold different beliefs about what health means.

QUESTIONS FOR REFLECTION

- What is your personal definition of health?
- How have your beliefs, values and attitudes informed your definition of health?

Developing professional cultural awareness of the Australian nursing and midwifery professions

This section describes the development of the nursing profession in Australia. Understanding the history of nursing is an important aspect of your profession's culture. It positions nursing and midwifery within Australia's colonial history and helps to explain the evolution of the nursing profession (and therefore its 'whiteness'), the nursing profession's attitudes towards Indigenous Australians and the history that underpins the longstanding suspicion of nursing and midwifery held by many Indigenous people.

An important aspect of developing cultural awareness is to remember *not* to accept that 'the culture of nursing is normal to patients' (Ramsden, 2002, p. 110). While Ramsden wrote from a Māori perspective, this applies differently but equally to Indigenous Australians. Nursing and midwifery have their own cultures, with their own practices and language that can seem very strange to clients.

An historical understanding of Indigenous Australians' interface with health systems further explains the cultural distance between Indigenous clients and many nurses and midwives. Western approaches to nurse training in Australia began in 1838, with the first Sisters of Charity nurses arriving in Sydney (Francis, 2001). Australia's nurse training was influenced by the work of Florence Nightingale, who had established a nursing school in London by 1860; however, this was by no means the beginning of 'nursing' as a profession. In 1863, the widow of the NSW Chief Justice wrote to Nightingale, asking her to send trained nurses to Australia. This plea initially fell on deaf ears, but in 1864 doctors in Sydney requested of the Board of the Sydney Infirmary that it employ a small number of trained sisters from the Council of the Nightingale Fund. They argued that the 'doctors at the Sydney Infirmary were sure that nurses were the key to any effective cure' (Godden, 2006, p. 40). Six nurses trained by Nightingale arrived in Sydney in 1868 (Francis, 2001). By the 1890s, many hospitals across Australia had become 'nurse training institutions' (Madsen, 2007, p. 14).

In the early days of the Australian colony, little was done for the health of Indigenous people. However, the introduction of diseases such as whooping cough and sexually transmissible infections had devastating impacts on Indigenous people. These diseases were unknown prior to invasion, and Indigenous health practices had no experience in treating them. Initially, there was little interest from the colonisers in either the prevention or the treatment of the health of Aboriginal people. Interestingly, though, Nightingale had conducted research on the health of Aboriginal Australians before her nurses started their work in Australia. Her interest in the health of Aboriginal people had begun after a meeting with Sir George Grey, 'who had discussed with her the apparent deterioration and gradual disappearance of native races after contact with white civilisation' (Seaman, 1992, p. 90). Nightingale applied to the Colonial Office for aid to carry out an inquiry 'to ascertain, if possible the precise influence which school training exercised on the health of native children' (Nightingale, 1863, p. 3). She successfully obtained funding and devised a 'simple school form' that was sent to the native schools in the colonies. She received responses from Western Australia and South Australia, and presented her research in York (England) in 1864 (Nightingale, 1865).

The responses from Australia that described Aboriginal people were highly racist and showed gross ignorance. Aboriginal people were described as 'savages', 'uncivilised' and in urgent need of being brought into a state of civilisation. Throughout this period, the 'civilising' of Aboriginal people involved conversion to Christian beliefs. Aboriginal spirituality was not acknowledged, and people's spiritual beliefs were not regarded as essential to their health and identity.

However, within Nightingale's writings, there is no acknowledgement of the efficacy of Aboriginal health and healing practices, such as caring for the sick, using traditional medicines, child-bearing practices, healing the injured and caring for the frail aged and very young. One person who responded to Nightingale's study hinted at the use of traditional medicines. Bishop Salvadore wrote:

> A native belonging to the institution became ill with spitting of blood; a sure mark of fatal disease, if the patient is treated in the usual way. The patient begged to be allowed to go into the bush; and after days hunting of horses, he returned sufficiently recovered to resume his occupations.
>
> (Nightingale, 1865, p. 4)

Nightingale was scathing about the effects of colonisation on the health of Aboriginal Australians. She outlined what she believed were the root causes of their health decline:

1. the introduction to the natives of intoxicating liquor
2. the use of native women as prostitutes
3. hunger, as a result of deprivation of traditional hunting grounds
4. attempts to 'civilise' the natives by interfering with their traditional habits and customs
5. poor sanitary conditions as the result of natives being brought into schools or buildings under more confined conditions than had been their custom
6. cruelty and ill-treatment.

(Nightingale, 1863, cited in Seaman, 1992).

Nightingale's work is filled with contradictory views that were common at the time. She identified alcohol as a problem, but gave little attention to the fact that alcohol was often used as payment and bribes. Nightingale believed that aspects of Aboriginal people's declining health were due to attempts to civilise Indigenous people and the interruptions to their traditional lifestyles, but she argued that there was a strong need to educate them into the Christian belief system. She identified education as essential for civilising Aboriginal people, but did not take into account the deeply entrenched health practices of Aboriginal people, which were based on responsibility for land, understanding of the seasons, migration patterns across Country to gather resources and the making and utilisation of traditional medicine.

The overarching belief that Aboriginal Australians needed 'civilising' was evident in all of Nightingale's work and underpinned much of her analysis. Of course, this belief was not only held by Nightingale: it was also very much part of the colonial project. Nightingale's beliefs, values and attitudes also influenced her decisions about which women were 'appropriate' to be trained as nurses. The Nightingale scheme of nurse training 'emphasized good moral character as a qualification for nursing education and to reinforce this, trainees were to be resident at the hospital under the vigilant eye of home sisters' (Gregory & Brasil, 1993, p. viii). At this time, there was no thought of training Aboriginal nurses or teaching Aboriginal health to nurses and midwives. One response to Nightingale, from a Mrs Camfield from Western Australia, stated:

> There is not in nature, I think, a more filthy, loathsome, revolting creature than a native woman in her wild state. Every animal has something to recommend it; but a native woman is all together unlovable.
>
> (Nightingale, 1865, p. 7)

Nightingale's research provides a context for the emergence of the nursing profession in Australia. Her system of nursing was introduced into Australia as a way to improve the health of the new colonists. Nursing and midwifery began to gain legitimacy as professions, with nursing and midwifery training programs introduced across the country in the 1890s. This training had little or no regard for Indigenous Australian women. Further, there are no documented records of what these early trainee nurses and midwives were being taught about Australian 'natives' and their 'uncivilised' ways. Indeed, it would take well over a century for an Australian nursing authority to mandate the inclusion of Indigenous health to be taught within Schools of Nursing and Midwifery. This certainly was not the case in hospital-based training programs.

However, within the jurisdiction of hospital-based training programs, the growing nursing and midwifery professions gave little regard to the possibility of training Aboriginal and Torres Strait Islander nurses and midwives. Interestingly, an inquiry and subsequent report was undertaken in England in 1945, when the Colonial Office on Command of His Majesty presented to Parliament the *Report of the Committee on the Training of Nurses for the Colonies* (Colonial Office, 1945). Following a preliminary survey examining the state of nursing and midwifery services in colonial territories, two subcommittees were formed to consider retrospectively:

- the training of nurses in the United Kingdom and its Dominions for service in the colonial territories
- the training given in the colonies to Indigenous nurses.

When the report was released, it clearly noted that:

> At first the only trained nurses were those who were recruited in the United Kingdom and the Dominions or from nursing sisterhoods in Europe, but it was speedily recognized that no great extension of medical services could take place unless the greater part of the nursing staff was drawn from the local populations.
>
> (Colonial Office, 1945, p. 3)

The first recommendation of the Colonial Office Report gave a comprehensive overview of the training needs and requirements of nurses, midwives and mental health nurses across the colonies. However, the second recommendation – the training of Indigenous nurses – was largely ignored in Australia. The overall policy environment relating to the segregation and treatment of Aboriginal people in principle was in conflict with the second recommendation. It is no surprise that the recommendation was ignored (Best, 2015).

This section has outlined the culture of the nursing and midwifery professions within Australia as burgeoning professions. It aimed to highlight how Indigenous peoples were positioned within research undertaken by the mother of 'modern' nursing and how exclusionary practices of not teaching Indigenous health or training Indigenous nurses and midwives are grounded within the early culture of nursing and midwifery. The section has demonstrated a history of culturally unsafe practices in the professions and systems with regard to Indigenous Australians. Developing cultural awareness requires a recognition of the culture that underpins nursing and midwifery in Australia.

While the above has outlined an historical context of the professions developing in Australia, it is essential to understand that their development still informs the culture of contemporary practice. There is a great need to be aware of the impacts of historic practice on the professions in terms of their ongoing legacy for Indigenous Australians.

QUESTION FOR REFLECTION

- How did Florence Nightingale's beliefs, values and attitudes determine the status of Aboriginal Australians in the nursing profession?

Cultural sensitivity: Understanding the legitimacy of difference

According to Ramsden (2002), cultural sensitivity is the second phase in the journey towards becoming a culturally safe practitioner. She defines cultural sensitivity as 'alerting the student to the legitimacy of difference' that 'begins a process of self-exploration as the powerful bearers of their own life experiences and realities and the impact this may have on others' (Ramsden, 2002). In order to move from cultural awareness (of one's self and the professions) to cultural sensitivity (understanding the legitimacy of difference), it is the responsibility of each nurse and midwife to engage with colonial histories that alert you to the legitimacy of difference between Indigenous and non-Indigenous Australians. Some obvious examples of the legitimacy of difference outside of nursing and midwifery are the exclusion of Indigenous Australians in the Constitution and the establishment of missions and reserves, which were set up only for Indigenous Australians.

Missions and reserves were established through Acts of Parliament, and were used to segregate people. Entire communities were incarcerated, and traditional medical practices began to fracture as the use of traditional medicine was seen as 'witchcraft' and forbidden on the missions and reserves. (For an in-depth explanation of missions and reserves, see Chapters 1 and 2.)

Cox (2007) describes the trauma and the legacy experienced by many Aboriginal people from the system of missions and reserves. Forde (1990) describes the role of nurses on missions and reserves. At Woorabinda Mission in Queensland in the 1940s, Johnson (a visiting medical officer) stated that

> the appalling conditions and high death rates of Woorabinda were in part due to the staff and is made up of three officers of the Department who are too fond of drinking, a mentally unstable Matron and a professionally negligent Medical Officer.
>
> (Johnson, cited in Forde, 1990, p. 48)

The 'whiteness' of nursing

The Australian healthcare system is inherently 'white', and nursing is no exception. Cox and Taua (2017, p. 271) state that 'members of the white (or mainstream) culture are inheritors of unearned, unexamined and unacknowledged privilege'.

Aboriginal Doctor Anne-Maree Nielsen practised as a Registered Nurse for over a decade prior to going into medicine. In her Honours work, Nielsen articulated

> the structural and systematic white dominance of this profession which pervades all areas from colleague interactions to the provision of client care. As a predominantly Westernised system within this country, the field of healthcare is permeated by the social norms and expectations defined by white culture.
>
> (Nielsen, 2010, p. 23).

Aboriginal Distinguished Professor Moreton-Robinson explains:

> Whiteness in its contemporary form in Australian society is culturally based. It controls institutions, which are extensions of white Australian culture and is governed by the values, beliefs and assumptions of that culture and its history. Australian culture is less white than it used to be, but whiteness forms the centre and is commonly referred to in public discourse as the 'mainstream' or 'middle ground.'
>
> (Moreton-Robinson, 1999, p. 28)

Puzan (2003, p. 3), a white American nurse, offers some insights into experiences of nursing in the United States: 'Evidence of the entrenchment of whiteness within nursing can be found not only in practice, but even more fundamentally, in the locations where the formative giving and receiving of nursing education takes place.'

In Australia, the nursing profession is clearly entrenched within the Western biomedical model. As Cox and Taua (2017) argue, for many Australians this is taken by default to be the most legitimate system – both socially and politically. The biomedical model has excluded Indigenous health knowledges, and throughout much of colonial history it also involved the active exclusion of Indigenous peoples from nursing and midwifery education.

Currently, there is little research being conducted in Australia on the 'whiteness of nursing'. In her research, Nielsen (2010) explored Aboriginal nurses' experiences of the cultural challenges involved in working in mainstream healthcare. Nielsen's research involved interviews with Indigenous nurses to explore their experiences. She identified four major themes that influence the practice of contemporary Indigenous nurses:

1. discrimination
2. the whiteness of nursing
3. cultural clashes within nursing
4. cultural vitality (Nielsen, 2010, p. 12).

However, Nielsen argues that 'the dominance of whiteness within nursing is an ever present and saturating force and one that is keenly felt by Indigenous nurses and therefore the broader Indigenous community' (Nielsen, 2010, p. 20).

A culturally sensitive approach means that the nurse recognises and legitimises the differences between them and the client. When caring for Indigenous

Australians, it is necessary to understand the history and the colonial authorities that controlled Indigenous Australians since invasion, as this has a profound effect on the Indigenous client. It is also important to understand that the nursing profession has 'power' and 'whiteness' that impacts on clients. In a healthcare setting, nurses and midwives are typically in a position of power over clients. The Nursing Council of New Zealand (NCSZ, 1996, p. 8) states that 'when one group uses its position of power to impose its own values upon another a state of serious imbalance occurs. This threatens the identity, security and ease of the other cultural group creating a state of dis-ease.'

An historical lens helps us to understand the legitimacy of difference and why some Indigenous women are reluctant to visit hospitals for antenatal care. They are influenced by the recent memory of generations of children being stolen from their Aboriginal mothers while they were hospitalised to give birth. Historical practices have created a great deal of distrust among Indigenous peoples towards hospitals, due to segregated wards, forced sterilisation of Aboriginal women and the stealing of babies in our recent history (Forsyth, 2007). Nurses and midwives have certainly been used as government agents for popular administrative policies enforced upon Aboriginal people, particularly women. Yet rarely are these abuses of power and racism acknowledged or discussed as the barriers for Aboriginal people not wanting to or continuing to utilise health services. Within nursing and midwifery, the language of non-compliance is therefore often utilised in describing this behaviour in place of understanding the legitimacy of difference for Indigenous peoples.

To understand the legitimacy of difference is to acknowledge the racism that is inherent within the healthcare system and its impacts upon Indigenous Australians. Racism has been discussed and documented by many Indigenous Australian nurses over many decades, and can be experienced from their peers, patients and educators (Best, 2011, 2015; Best & Bunda 2020; Best and Gorman, 2016).

QUESTIONS FOR REFLECTION

- Identify how the 'whiteness of nursing' may affect care provided to Indigenous people in Australia.
- Provide two examples of past practices towards Indigenous peoples that legitimise difference between the treatment of Indigenous and non-Indigenous Australians in a healthcare context.

Becoming a culturally safe practitioner

Cultural safety requires nurses and midwives to understand their own cultures (including their own ethnicity), acknowledge the power imbalance inherent within nursing and midwifery practice (their own professional culture), have an understanding of colonial histories and their impact on Indigenous Australians, and have the ability to question biomedical dominance.

For Ramsden (2002, p. 117) cultural safety is an ongoing journey that allows clients to define their own care:

> Cultural safety is an outcome of nursing and midwifery education that enables safe service to be defined by those that receive the service and is achieved when the recipients of care deem the care to be meeting their cultural needs.

As nurses and midwives, we often work in a system that is resource and time poor. Within these systems, care is often dictated by the service provider and not the recipients of the care. However, the undeniable legacy of culturally unsafe care of Indigenous people is ever so obvious and reflected in the outstanding life differentials that remain between Indigenous and non-Indigenous Australians. The journey towards becoming a culturally safe practitioner is one of continual learning and self-reflection, which can be difficult to the time poor nurse and at times can seem overwhelming. The interface of Indigenous peoples and Australian healthcare systems is littered with examples of culturally unsafe care and the need for student nurses and midwives to learn to be culturally safe practitioners is an imperative to change this.

Ramsden noticed that her experiences as a Māori nurse and the experiences of *pakeha* (white) nurses were in stark contrast. She found that her *pakeha* nursing peers had little understanding of the brutal colonial and racist history of New Zealand:

> The omission of the colonial history of New Zealand in the basic state education system had led to a serious deficit in the knowledge of citizens as to the cause and effect outcomes of colonialism. Without a sound knowledge base it seemed to me that those citizens who became nurses and midwives had little information of substance on which to build their practice among this seriously at risk group.
>
> (Ramsden, 2002, p. 3)

It is the responsibility of *all* nurses and midwives to become culturally safe practitioners and activists for social justice for all. It is a continuous journey that will ultimately provide culturally safe care for Indigenous Australians. Progressing through the cultural safety journey is understanding *your own cultures* and their impacts on the care you provide, and understanding that there is a significant legitimacy of difference for Indigenous Australians accessing the healthcare system. Understanding *your own values, beliefs and attitudes* is an imperative of your journey and their impact on care you provide. While it may appear overwhelming to do this, there are small but significant actions that you can take. An example of this is understanding the power of nurses in determining who is Aboriginal. For example, as a young student nurse I was constantly challenged about my Aboriginality due to being urban born and raised. I was not considered a 'real Aborigine' due to not living in the outback, where the 'real ones' lived. I was often asked, 'But you're only part Aborigine aren't you?'

The Australian Indigenous community is eclectic – just like the broader Australian population. Overwhelmingly in the Aboriginal community, Aboriginality is not determined by skin colour. The underlying common myth that the darker a person's skin colour the more Aboriginal they are does not typically apply within Indigenous communities. This means that comments from nurses, such as, 'Oh, but you don't look Aboriginal' or, 'But you are only part Aboriginal', are demeaning for many Aboriginal people. It also means that we need to ask all our patients whether they are Indigenous to collect true data and not just leave this to our own assumptions about what Indigenous Australians look like. Aboriginal people do not determine Aboriginality by skin colour; using language relating to skin colour or suggesting blood quantum is highly offensive. While undertaking your admission assessments, it is vitally important that you ask whether your clients are Indigenous. It is not culturally safe practice to assume that someone is not Indigenous on the basis of their appearance.

To become culturally safe practitioners is a call to action for all student nurses and midwives. As nurses and midwives, we are often the front line in service provision for Indigenous peoples, so there is a need to be culturally aware of yourself and your profession, and particularly the potential impacts on Indigenous Australians. We need to be culturally sensitive in understanding the legitimacy of difference in the lived experiences of Indigenous lives that has had such profound impacts on the Indigenous community. A deep understanding of these prepares us well to answer the call of action of being culturally safe practitioners (Geia et al., 2020).

CASE STUDY

My experience as a patient

While I was working as a nursing director, I was admitted to a large tertiary hospital as a patient. I was diagnosed with a double ear infection, which required hospitalisation for intensive intravenous (IV) antibiotic treatment and pain management. I had a cannula inserted to receive IV antibiotics in the emergency department and was administered fentanyl subcutaneously. I was prescribed Endone for pain relief. When I was admitted to the ward, I was not asked whether I identified as Aboriginal, nor was I asked about my occupation.

Four hours after being admitted to the ward, my pain began to escalate. I requested Endone from the Registered Nurse (who had not introduced himself at the beginning of his shift). He looked at my medication chart and went to get the pain relief. He returned and offered me two Panadol. I questioned him about what medication I was being offered, and he explained that 'these are Panadol'. I stated that the doctor in the emergency department had written me up to receive Endone. The nurse replied that 'We don't give Endone out *willy nilly* and Panadol should hold your pain.' My pain soon escalated severely and I became highly agitated. The nurse avoided me.

Shortly after this encounter, the Aboriginal hospital liaison officer arrived. I asked how she knew that I had been admitted, and she explained, 'You identified within the emergency department and the box had been ticked.'

I rang a friend who worked as an anaesthetist at the hospital. In my highly distressed state, I asked him to come and see me. Simon (the anaesthetist) took my chart and read through my notes to ascertain my clinical history and the reason for my admission. He then took my chart to the nurses' station and asked why I was not receiving adequate pain relief, as written up. Within a few moments, the nurse appeared with the prescribed dose of Endone. The Registered Nurse in charge of the shift also arrived and apologised for the error. I then asked not to be looked after by my designated nurse for the rest of the shift.

(cont.)

QUESTIONS FOR REFLECTION

- Reflect on your own practice:
  - Considering the practice of the Registered Nurse in the above scenario, what areas of his practice should he reflect on and why?
  - What potentially were the beliefs, values and attitudes that influenced his culturally unsafe nursing practice?
- Seek to minimise the power differentials:
  - Describe one example of how the nurse used power differentials in his caregiving.
  - Describe an example of how the nurse could have minimised power differentials.
- Ensure that you do not diminish, demean or disempower others through your actions:
  - Name the actions of the nurse that were diminishing, demeaning and disempowering.

Reflecting on your answers to these questions, think about where you would place the care provided by this nurse along the defined journey of cultural safety and why?

Conclusion

This chapter has focused on the concept of cultural safety from the perspective of an Aboriginal Registered Nurse. Through a discussion about the history of nursing and the power of the nursing profession, the chapter encourages today's nurses to undertake their own journey towards becoming culturally safe practitioners. Nurses and midwives need to understand the history of healthcare for Aboriginal and Torres Strait Islander people and understand the legacy that remains from colonisation. Through examining your own beliefs, values and attitudes and how these impact on patient care, as nurses and midwives you will be able to understand what it is to be culturally aware. This becomes a very powerful tool in your practice coupled with an understanding of the 'whiteness' of nursing and midwifery. Examining colonial practices through an historical lens allows you to grasp what is meant by cultural sensitivity through understanding the legitimacy of difference. It allows you, as a nurse and/or midwife, to understand the legitimacy of difference for Indigenous Australians is real and has lasting impact on life differentials for Indigenous Australians. Cultural safety allows you to work in and towards culturally safe practices through understanding your own privileges and the legitimacy of differences between Indigenous and non-Indigenous Australians. Nurses and midwives are in a unique position to promote health for Indigenous Australians, particularly if they consciously reflect on their own practice.

Nurses and midwives are engaged in culturally safe practice when their care is determined to be safe by the recipients of that care. The capacity for reflective practice should become second nature for nurses and midwives who are culturally safe practitioners.

Learning activities

1. Define where you would position yourself on the cultural safety journey.
2. Identify what you need to do to progress along the cultural safety journey.
3. Outline the significance of teaching cultural safety in the Australian healthcare education setting for Aboriginal and Indigenous Australians.

FURTHER READING

Cox, L. & Taua, C. (2013). Socio-cultural considerations and nursing practice. In J. Crisp, C. Taylor, C. Douglas & G. Rebeiro (eds), *Fundamentals of Nursing* (4th edn). Sydney: Elsevier, pp. 320–40.

Forsyth, S. (2007). Telling stories: Nurses, politics and Aboriginal Australians, c. 1900–1980. *Contemporary Nurse*, 24(1), 33–44.

Happell, B., Cowin, L, Roper, C, Lakeman, R. & Cox, L. (2013a). Cultural safety. In B. Happell, L. Cowin, C. Roper, R. Lakeman & L. Cox (eds), *Introducing Mental Health Nursing: A Service User-oriented Approach* (2nd edn). Sydney: Allen & Unwin, pp. 347–64.

Happell, B., Cowin, L., Roper, C., Lakeman, R. & Cox, L. (2013b). Sociological understandings of mental health and Indigenous social and emotional well-being. In B. Happell, L. Cowin, C. Roper, R. Lakeman & L. Cox (eds), *Introducing Mental Health Nursing: A Service User-oriented Approach* (2nd edn). Sydney: Allen & Unwin, pp. 183–212.

McCubbin, L. (2006). Indigenous values, cultural safety and improving health care: The case of Native Hawaiians. *Contemporary Nurse*, 22(2), 214–17.

Stout, M. & Downey, B. (2006). Nursing, Indigenous peoples and cultural safety: So what? Now what? *Contemporary Nurse*, 22(2), 327–32.

Visit the companion website at www.cambridge.org/highereducation/isbn/9781108794695/resources to see further online resources.

REFERENCES

ANMAC (2019). *Registered Nurse Accreditation Standards*. Canberra: ANMC.

Benedict, S. & Shields, L. (2014). *Nurses and Midwives in Nazi Germany: The 'Euthanasia Programs'*. London: Routledge.

Best, O. (2011). Yatdjuligin: The stories of Aboriginal Queensland nurses 1950s–2005. Unpublished PhD thesis, University of Southern Queensland.

Best, O. (2015). Training the 'natives' as nurses in Australia: So what went wrong? In H. Sweet & S. Hawkins (eds), *Colonial Caring: A History of Colonial and Post-colonial Nursing*. Manchester: Manchester University Press.

Best, O. & Bunda, T. (2020). Disrupting dominant discourse: Indigenous women as trained nurses and midwives 1900s–1950s. *Collegian*, 10 October. Retrieved from www.collegianjournal.com/article/S1322-7696(20)30109-8/fulltext

Best, O. & Gorman, D. (2016). 'Some of us pushed forward and let the world see what could be done': Aboriginal Australian Nurses and Midwives, 1900–2005. *Labour History*, 111, 149–64.

Best, O. & Nielsen, A.M. (2005). *Indigenous Graduates' Experience of Their University Nursing Education: Report to the Queensland Nursing Council Research Committee*. Brisbane: Queensland Nursing Council Research Committee.

Colonial Office (1945). *Report of the Committee on the Training of Nurses for the Colonies*. London: His Majesty's Stationary Office.

Cox, L. (2007). Fear, trust and Aborigines: The historical experience of state institutions and current encounters in the health system. *Health and History: Journal of the Australian and New Zealand Society for the History of Medicine*, 9(2), 70–92.

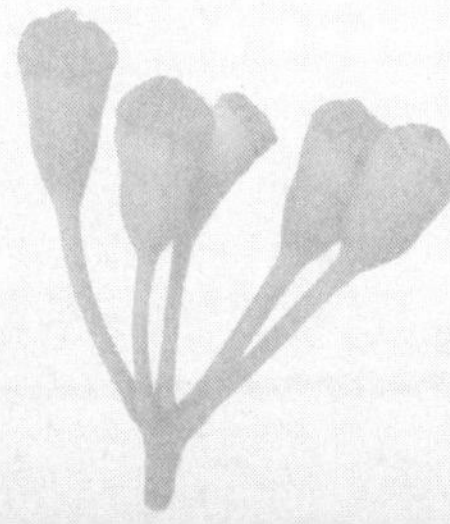

Cox, L. & Taua, C. (2013). Sociocultural considerations and nursing practice. In J. Crisp, C. Taylor, C. Douglas & G. Rebero (eds), *Potter and Perry's Fundamentals of Nursing*. Sydney: Mosby, pp. 320–45.

Cox, L. & Taua, C. (2017). Understanding and applying cultural safety: Philosophy and practice of a social determinants approach. In J. Crisp, C. Taylor, C. Douglas & G. Rebero (eds), *Potter and Perry's Fundamentals of Nursing* (5th edn). Sydney: Mosby, pp. 260–88.

Dickinson, T. (2015). *'Curing Queers': Mental Nurses and Their Patients, 1935–1974*. Manchester: Manchester University Press.

Forde, T. (1990). Confinement and control: A History of Woorabinda Aboriginal community 1927–1990. Unpublished Honours thesis, University of Queensland.

Forsyth, S. (2007). Telling stories: Nurses, politics and Aboriginal Australians, circa 1900–1980s. *Contemporary Nurse*, 24(1), 33–44

Francis, K. (2001). Service to the poor: The foundations of community nursing in England, Ireland and New South Wales. *International Journal of Nursing Practice*, 7, 169–76.

Geia, L., Baird, K., Bail, K., … & Wynne, R. (2020). A unified call to action from Australian nursing and midwifery leaders: Ensuring that Black lives matter. *Contemporary Nurse*. doi:10.1080/10376178.2020.1809107.

Godden, J. (2006). *Lucy Osbourne, a Lady Displaced*. Sydney: Sydney University Press.

Gregory, H. & Brasil, C. (1993). *Bearers of the Tradition, Nurses of the Royal Brisbane Hospital 1888–1993*. Brisbane: Boolarong Press.

Madsen, W. (2007). *Nursing History: Foundations of a Profession*. Sydney:Pearson.

McGibbon, E., Mulaudzi, F., Didham, P., Barton, S. & Sochan, A. (2013). Towards decolonizing nursing: The colonization of nursing and strategies for increasing the counter-narrative. *Nursing Inquiry*, 21(3), 179–91

Moreton-Robinson, A. (1999). Unmasking whiteness: A Goori Jondal's look at some Duggai business. In B. McKay (ed.), *Unmasking Whiteness: Race Relations and Reconciliation*. Brisbane: Griffith University, pp. 28–37.

National Aboriginal Health Strategy Working Party (1989). *A National Aboriginal Health Strategy*. Canberra: Australian Government. Retrieved from www.health.gov.au/internet/main/publishing.nsf/Content/health-oatsih-pubs-NAHS1998

Nielsen, A.-M. (2010). What are Aboriginal registered nurses' experiences of the cultural challenges, if any, involved in working in mainstream healthcare? Unpublished MA(Hons) thesis, University of Southern Queensland.

Nightingale, F. (1863). *Sanitary Statistics: Native Colonial Schools and Hospitals*. London: George E. Eyre & William Spottiswoode. Retrieved from http://archive.org/details/sanitarystatisti00byunigh

Nightingale, F. (1865). *Note on the Aboriginal Races of Australia. Presented to the Annual Meeting of the National Association for the Promotion of Social Science, 1864, at York (England)*. London: Emily Faithfull. Retrieved from http://archive.org/details/noteonaboriginal00nigh

NCNZ (1996). *Guidelines For Cultural Safety in Nursing And Midwifery*. Wellington: NCNZ.

NCNZ (2011). *Guidelines For Cultural Safety, the Treaty of Waitangi and Maori Health in Nursing Education and Practice*. Wellington: NCNZ. Retrieved from www.nursingcouncil.org.nz.

Puzan, E. (2003). The unbearable whiteness of being (in nursing). *Nursing Enquiry*, 10(3), 193–200.

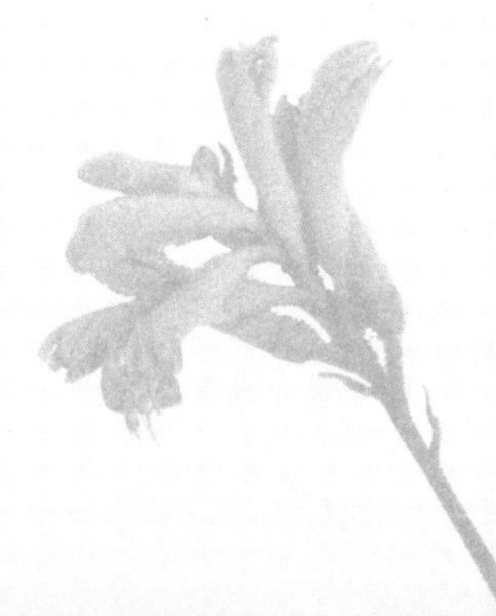

Ramsden, I.M. (2002). Cultural safety and nursing education in Aotearoa and Te Waipounamu. Unpublished PhD thesis, Victoria University of Wellington.

Seaman, K. (1992). Florence Nightingale and the Australian Aborigines. *Journal of the Historical Society of South Australia*, 20, 90–6.

Sherwood, J. (2013). Colonisation – it's bad for your health: The context of Aboriginal health. *Contemporary Nurse*, 46(1), 28–40.

Swan, P. & Raphael, B. (1995). *Ways Forward: National Aboriginal and Torres Strait Islander Mental Health Policy National Consultancy Report*. Canberra: Australian Government Publishing Service. Retrieved from www.health.gov.au/internet/publications/publishing.nsf/Content/mental-pubs-w-wayforw-toc~mental-pubs-w-wayforw-pro

WHO (1946). *Constitution*. New York: World Health Organization. Retrieved from https://apps.who.int/gb/bd/PDF/bd47/EN/constitution-en.pdf?ua=1

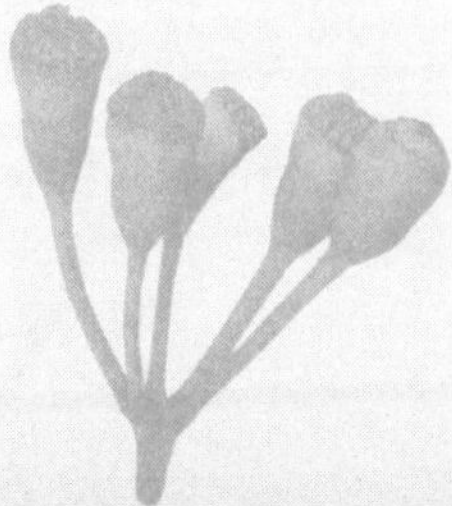

Torres Strait Islander health and wellbeing

Ali Drummond, Yoko Mills, Sam Mills and Francis Nona

4

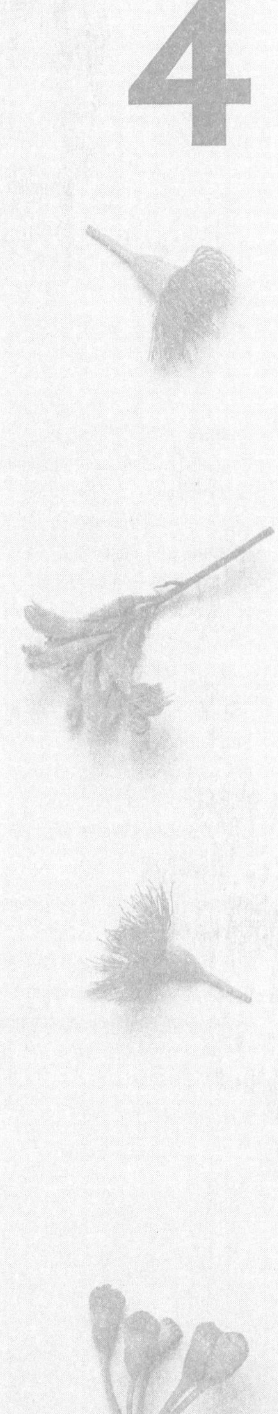

LEARNING OBJECTIVES

This chapter will help you to understand:

- The location and pre-colonisation history of Zenadth Kes and Islanders
- Islander identity and belonging, the colonial imaginations of these and their implications for health and wellbeing
- Islander perspectives of health and wellbeing, and the changes throughout colonial history
- Islander approaches to healthcare and wellbeing
- The impact of climate change on Islanders

KEY WORDS

autonomy
climate change
Country
Ged
Lag
Sea Country
self-determination

Introduction

Australia's First Nations peoples are a collection of multiple language groups; they are the sovereign peoples of the lands and waterways of their countries, which are now confined within the boundaries of the modern-day colonial nation-state of Australia. Torres Strait Islanders (Islanders) are a collection of First Nations peoples from the region commonly known as the Torres Straits, which for Islanders is increasingly being reclaimed and reknown as Zenadth Kes. The assertion of using the local name instead of the colonial name is an exercise of sovereignty. The reclaiming of places through knowing their local name is an important part of truth-telling and decolonising Country. Thus, this chapter predominantly refers to the Torres Strait Islands as Zenadth Kes. The Islanders have called the region home since time immemorial.

This chapter invites you to learn more about Zenadth Kes and the people who belong to it. Specifically, in keeping with cultural safety, this chapter aims to highlight the limitations of the colonial perceptions of Islanders. These imaginations of Islanders have historically informed what opportunities were afforded them. This includes equitable access to health inclusive of social determinants of health, compared with non-Indigenous Australians.

Today, Islanders reside all over Australia. Despite the distance, the belongingness to our **Country** (both Land and **Sea Country**) and kin remains strong.

Country Specific geographical location associated with Islanders' belonging and ownership. This ownership is different from Western understanding of ownership, as it is less about possession and exploitation, and more about connectivity to kin, present and past, and Country itself.

Sea Country Islander knowing of Country extends beyond land, unlike Western understanding of land ownership, to seas and sea-beds.

autonomy The right to self-govern. In the context of the Zenadth Kes, the right to engage with the globalised world as sovereign people, uninhibited by the colonial rule and aspirations of the Australian nation-state.

This chapter will look at the transformation of health and health service delivery to the people of Zenadth Kes, the significance of empowerment of the people, and the aspiration of **autonomy** or self-determination. Briefly, we look at the promise of this through the Torres Strait Model for Primary Health Care. Finally, the chapter explores how global warming and resulting rising sea levels are impacting the health and wellbeing of the Islanders of Zenadth Kes. The destruction of Country has real implications for the social, emotional and cultural health of Islanders – both individuals and the community.

Cultural safety is an essential part of contemporary practice. In the context of healthcare delivery to Islanders, this chapter will uncover how by exercising cultural safety as individuals, and members of health disciplines and health services, you can support the empowerment of Islanders, their families and communities. This will realise culturally safe care, which privileges Islanders' individual, family and community wellbeing.

Zenadth Kes, its peoples and their health and wellbeing

From the beginning of the engagement between Islanders and outsiders, Islanders have been framed as different things – cannibals, lost souls, noble savages, to name just a few. Nakata (2014) asserts that this was common for scientists and missionaries who came to document, research, change and save Islanders, because this was believed to be in the best interests of Islanders:

> To missionaries and scientists alike, Islanders were a people from the past. The position of Islanders has been framed, pre-conditioned and subsequently described, explained and understood – disciplined – by a scientific community of scholars.
>
> (Nakata, 2014, p. 30)

Islanders were rarely asked, or enabled to identify what was best for them, let alone enabled to fulfil this.

This first section celebrates the diversity of Islanders, and their connection to Country and kin. Relationality is significant to wellbeing, as through relationality Islanders fulfil roles and responsibilities to each other, caring for individuals and the community. We are humans, with different ways of knowing, being and doing – ways that are as valuable as those of other peoples. This was something historical figures of colonisation could neither comprehend nor accept.

Further, this section explores the failures of historical approaches of colonising Islanders. It looks at the diminishing, demeaning and disempowering violence of colonisation in its ambition for domination and control of Zenadth Kes, and thus Islanders as well. Understanding the failures of the past is essential, as this should inform contemporary knowledge and skills. Critiquing the past also provides an opportunity for Islanders to regain power, including their humanity, which is essential for culturally safe care.

Ged and *Lag:* Home

Zenadth Kes is home to Islanders; it is where Islanders belong in the universe, their centre within its vastness. Islanders have a long tradition of astronomy and have generations of experience of using knowledge of the stars to know time and direction. Our family has belonged here since time immemorial. Our family yet to come has deep roots within Zenadth Kes. The role of each generation since colonisation has been to maintain this connection to ***Ged*** or ***Lag***, which translates to 'home' in Meriam Mir and Kalaw Lagaw Ya, the two main dialects of Zenadth Kes.

Ged Meriam Mir language for home – home beyond the colonial understanding of home, incorporating Country and kin.

Lag Kala Lagaw Ya for home – home beyond the colonial understanding of home, incorporating Country and kin.

Zenadth Kes includes Land and Sea Country that lies between the tip of Cape York Peninsula, Australia and Papua New Guinea (PNG) (Figure 4.1). It lies within the borders of the Australian nation-state, having been annexed by Queensland in 1879. This specific part of the border is co-managed to ensure that Islanders and local Papua New Guinea (PNG) citizens can share the fisheries resources. This is enabled through the Torres Strait Treaty. Additional allowances include the ability for some Islanders and PNG citizens from thirteen PNG villages to move freely across the border for traditional activities. This allowance recognises the historical relationship between Islanders and PNG peoples of the region (DFAT, 1985).

There are over 200 islands in the region and seventeen of these have established communities. The Islanders have a number of language groups and island groups, and tribe or clan groups. Language groups correlate with island groups, and tribal groups are smaller communities of each island.

The two main language groups are Meriam Mir and Kala Lagaw Ya, and the latter includes a number of dialects. Miriam Mir is spoken in the Eastern Island group of Zenadth Kes, specifically by the Islanders of Mer, Erub and Ugar. The dialects of Kala Lagaw Ya are spoken in the Central Island group (Masig, Iama, Poruma and Warraber), Top Western Island group (Boigu, Dauan and Saibai), Western Island group (Mabuaig, Badu, and Kubin and St Paul villages of Moa) and Inner Islands group (Waiben, Ngurupai, Muralag and Kirriri [or Keriri]) (Lawrence & Lawrence, 2004; SLQ, 2020) (Figure 4.1).

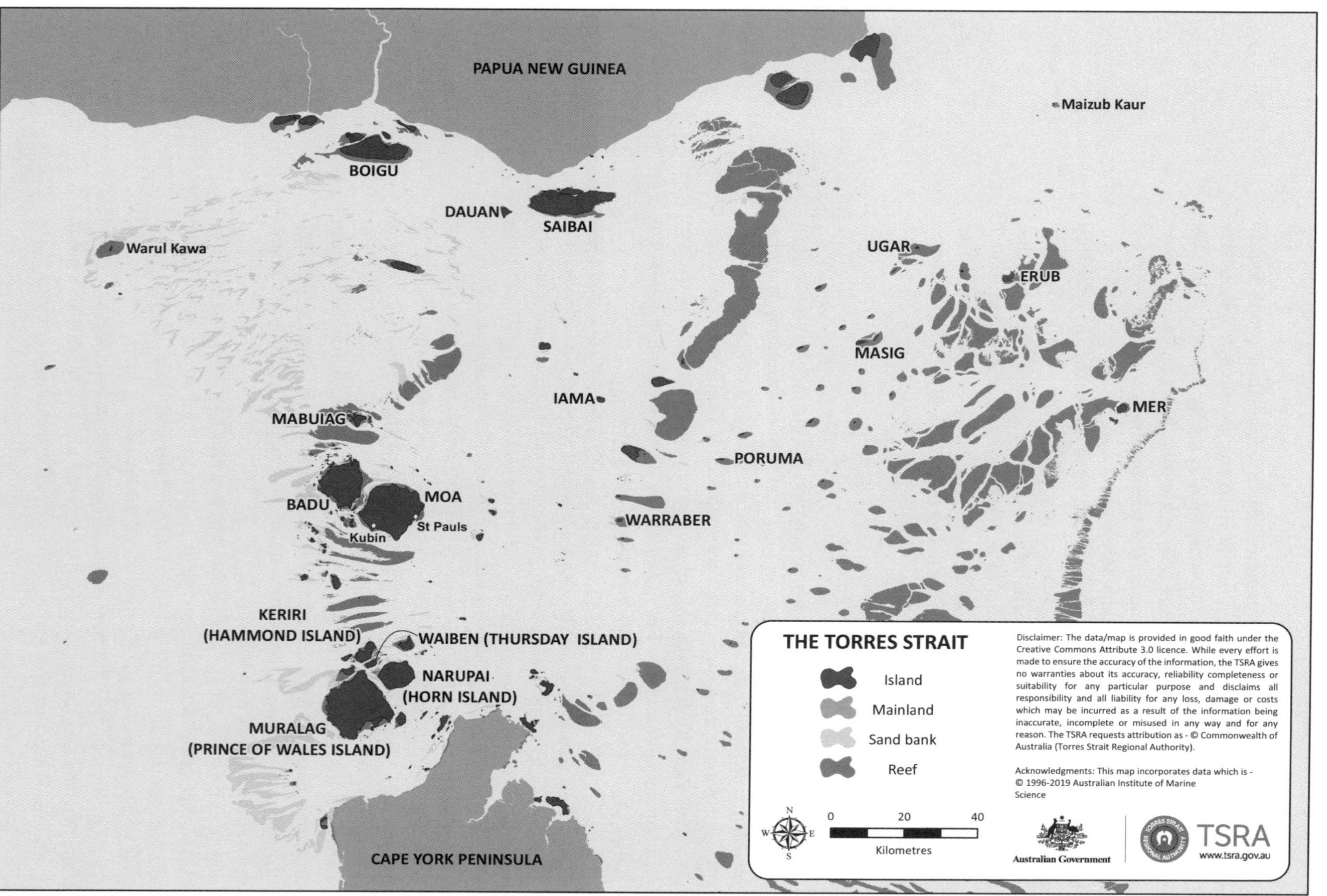

Figure 4.1 Map of Zenadth Kes

Source: Torres Strait Regional Authority, cited in ANAO (2013, p. 14).

Islanders also speak Torres Strait Kriol, a Creole or *lingua franca* that was initially spoken by Islander crew on pearling luggers, and by children so that Islanders from different language groups could communicate. It is a common language that is spoken in the region, and in Islander communities on mainland Australia (Lawrence & Lawrence, 2004).

Of the 10 per cent of Indigenous people who speak at least one of the 150 Indigenous languages still spoken, approximately 12 per cent speak one of the Torres Strait Islander languages. It should be noted that most Islanders are fluent English speakers as well (ABS, 2017).

Islander relationality and belonging

Most Islanders maintain a strong sense of belonging to their tribe or clan. Tribes and clans have associated totems, living things and seasonal elements, which are important parts of Islander belonging (Sharp, 2013).

The understanding of one's belonging is important: one's language group, Island group, tribe or clan group locates individuals within the broader family or kinship network, which expands beyond Western understanding of the nuclear family. These connections, or kinship relationships, define the roles and responsibilities that individuals will have towards each other.

As it is for Aboriginal people (Moreton-Robinson, 2016), relationality is an epistemological imperative for Islanders. That is to say, the relationships between Islanders, and between Islanders and their living earth (*Ged*, *Lag* or home), are essential knowledge. The more that is known, the greater the connection to Country and kin.

The knowledge and practice of these roles and responsibilities exemplify the dynamism of kinship networks. These networks are sensitive to contextual change – that is, any given context requires varying responses from members of the kinship network. These responses may be familiar to outsiders (e.g. teaching younger members of the family about fishing or gardening), while other responses may seem unorthodox (e.g. the role of family in-laws during significant occasions). These actions are often considered 'customary' or 'traditional' practice by outsiders, but are normal ways of being and doing for Islanders.

QUESTIONS FOR REFLECTION

- Reflect on the complexity of Islander belonging to language groups, island groups, tribe/clan groups, and the shifting roles and responsibilities within one's kinship network:
  - How does this relate to your understanding of family and the geographical location/s you associate with your childhood?
  - How does the exercise of relationality compare with the expectations and obligations that you have to your immediate and broader family?

Since time immemorial

Late Elder and respected Chief of the Wagadagam tribe of Mabuaig Athe Ephraim Bani was a linguist, and his work included the revitalisation of the Mabuaig language. A fluent language speaker, he developed the phonetic orthography for the Mabuaig language, which helps speakers to accurately annunciate words.

He also famously said that 'the past must exist, for a present, to create a future' (Gab Titui Cultural Centre, 2020). It speaks to the significance of Islander history, before colonisation with each other, with Country. Islanders come from generations of warriors, hunters, fishermen, gardeners, humans who harnessed knowledge of the region and surrounding water, sky and cosmos. This history remains within Islanders. It speaks to the significance of the present, to the imperative of immediate Islander leadership: asserting sovereignty. Islanders continue to be optimistic and opportunistic, changing tactics with new waves of colonialism. It speaks to Islander obligation to their future, one that they can imagine for themselves, their families and communities.

The peoples of Zenadth Kes proudly pronounce that they have been of their country 'since time immemorial', meaning since the beginning of their creation stories and before their gods arrived to establish their laws that are still in place today. These creation stories continue to be passed on, alongside Christian and Western scientific creation stories. Islanders' laws are also bequeathed to the next generation but remain superseded by laws of the Australian nation-state. Islander sense of belonging grows only stronger under colonial rule, as it is founded on knowing that Islanders have been in the region for many thousands of years.

Radiocarbon data suggest that Islanders have settled in the region for over 8000 years (Wright & Jacobsen, 2013). However, due to the changing environment since the end of the last ice age, and the limited available sites on which to conduct radiocarbon dating, the available data vary from island to island. For example, the data from the Western islands of Badu and Mabuaig suggest up to 7000–8000 years of settlement (Wright & Jacobsen, 2013, p. 79); data from Kirriri (or Keriri) suggest up to 2700 years of settlement (Brady & Ash, 2018, p. 98); and data from the Eastern Islands of Mer and Dauar show evidence of 2000 years of horticultural practices and up to 3000 years of a maritime subsistence economy (Carter et al., 2004). Radiocarbon dating from proximal areas of Australia and Papua New Guinea suggests up to 45,000 years of settlement (Wright & Jacobsen, 2013).

This demonstrates that Islanders have been in the region for a long time – certainly time immemorial for other current and previous civilisations. This emphasises our belongingness to Country and highlights the relatively short time that Australia has been colonised. Generations of Islanders have developed knowledge about the Country, its animals, plants, seasons, changes in the skies and cosmos, and of course the relationship between them (Sharp, 2013). Time has enabled Islanders to develop complex understandings of time associated with the patterns of these relationships.

This intimate relationship with Country and its entities meant that Islanders lived with Country, fishing and hunting, as well as gardening land and sea crops and creatures (Sharp, 2013). Islanders also traded goods with other Islanders, Papua New

Guineans and Aboriginal peoples. Of course, relationships existed between tribal groups, island groups and language groups of the region and the surrounding region of modern-day Australia and Papua New Guinea.

Perspectives of health and wellbeing

Invasion and colonisation: Sovereignty of land

In 1606, Spanish explorer and general Philomath Don Diego de Prado y Tovar, his second-in-command Luis Baez de Torres and their crew sailed to the islands of Zenadth Kes. They sought to be the first Europeans to locate the Australian mainland, but only got as far as the reefs and islands of Zenadth Kes (Windolf, 2010).

Prado's account of navigating the reefs includes descriptions of taking advantage of Islanders. He describes the killing of a number of Islander men who he portrays as strong and protective, apparently different from other black people he has seen in his 'adventures'. He also describes the kidnapping and rape of three Islander women (Windolf, 2010). The link between these crimes against the Islanders and Islander aggressive retaliation is not made by Prado.

Despite being second in command, it was Torres's letter to King Philip III of Spain that resulted in Torres's name being imposed upon the region (Windolf, 2010) – a 'gift' endowed despite Torres's obvious lack of connection to and his seeming disinterest in the region.

The next assault on the Islanders' sovereignty to the Country came with British explorer Commander James Cook, a Lieutenant when he sailed the East-Coast of Australia. He completed his navigation of the Australian East coast by planting a flag on Bedanug, an island in the Country belonging to the Kaurareg of Zenadth Kes. Cook called it Possession Island, claiming the east coast of Australia for Britain and King George III (National Museum Australia, 2020). A plaque on Bedanug reads:

> Lieutenant James Cook R.N. of the 'Endeavour' landed on this island which he named Possession Island and in the name of His Majesty King George III took possession of the whole Eastern coast of Australia from the latitude of 38° South of this place August 22nd 1770.
>
> (Royal Historical Society of Queensland, 2019)

These explorers were the initial assailants on the sovereignty of the Islanders of Zenadth Kes. Islanders' belongingness and sovereignty over their Country have been dismissed by Europeans since their earliest arrival in their region. The imagination and belief of Islanders as sub-humans, and the lack of relationship between Islanders and European Monarchies deemed Islanders, like other Indigenous peoples, unimaginable as landowners, let alone sovereign peoples of their Countries (Moreton-Robinson, 2015). Islanders were simple ornaments in the explorers' narratives about their conquest of imperialism.

Moreton-Robinson (2015), a Quandamooka women and eminent race scholar, unpacks the logic of possession and whiteness exercised by these European explorers. Moreton-Robinson (2015) sees the logic of possession as inherently a cultural element of Western civilisation, one that privileges the commodifying of raw material and labour as mere goods and services. In this view, land becomes a commodity that has a comparably decreased value compared with the relational value held by Indigenous peoples, including Islanders (Moreton-Robinson, 2015).

Pivotal to this logic is an acceptance of racial hierarchy, one that positions white people at the top, closer to God, and black people such as Indigenous peoples closer to animals. Herbert Spencer, nineteenth-century anthropologist and sociologist, used Charles Darwin's work on biological evolution to establish Social Darwinism, which asserted that Darwin's theory of the survival of the fittest supports the theory of racial hierarchy, and that certain human races – namely white Europeans – should inherit the world (Eckermann et al., 2010). Belief in racial hierarchy among humans makes it reasonable to take from others who are deemed not human enough – in other words, not worthy enough.

It is this possession that makes the relationship between Indigenous peoples, including Islanders, and the Country to which they belong invisible to Western outsiders (Moreton-Robinson, 2015). This is the logic that inspired the Spanish naming of the region after a Spanish second-in-command and Cook's claim of possession of the east coast of Australia. This is the racialised logic that legitimised the settlers' reasoning of Indigenous peoples as being less human than them and their Western monarchy and subjects (Moreton-Robinson, 2015).

QUESTIONS FOR REFLECTION

- Unfortunately, the dehumanising and racialised imaginations of Islanders still exist today. Knowing what we know about the vileness and inaccuracy of racism, how does this make you feel?
- Reflect on the image of Commander James Cook (he never earned the title of Captain), one that you may have learnt at school, at home with your family, and through the media and political stories about this explorer. How do these stories relate to the way Islanders would have felt about his visit to their Country?
- Can you list any popular imaginations about Indigenous peoples that were established from initial engagement between Indigenous peoples (including Islanders) and Western explorers and that still exist today?

Colonisation through Western empirical science: Sovereignty of our bodies

The aspirations of scientists who visited Zenadth Kes also aligned with this possessive logic. Most notable of all scientists is the late Cambridge Professor Alfred Haddon, who visited the region in 1888 while a Professor of Zoology, and later returned in 1898 as a budding anthropologist. In his second visit, Haddon was accompanied by fellow scientists on an expedition known as the Cambridge Anthropological Expedition of the Torres Straits (Nakata, 2014). Haddon and his colleagues were keen to capture the culture of Islanders before it was consumed by British colonisation. There was an expectation that this was an inevitable fate for Islanders, so their role was to capture the culture in their writings as much as possible, and not to stand in the way of colonisation.

Prominent Zenadth Kes education scholar Professor Martin Nakata highlights the functions of the possessive logic of these scientists. Their primary interest was to in further developing their science practice, which they asserted was unbiased. However, their science supported the theory of racial hierarchy and the presumed inferiority of Islanders. Their expedition to Zenadth Kes aimed to collect information that maintained the belief in racial inferiority (Nakata, 2014). Islander bodies were now seen as the subject of their colonising sciences. The 'noble savage' was conceptualised as 'mankind living in a primitive state of innocence in nature; their own nature as yet unspoiled by the depredation and contamination of civilisation' (Nakata, 2014, p. 21). This reflects the logic of Social Darwinism, specifically the proposed position of Australia's Indigenous peoples in the racial hierarchy: Islanders were not quite primitive savages, and they would never be deemed human, so they became 'noble savages'. Islanders were not the cannibals from popular colonial conceptions of Islanders; instead, Haddon found generous and hospitable peoples who shared what they had and did not want for anything (Nakata, 2014).

Colonisation through religion: Sovereignty of souls

In 1871, the London Missionary Society (LMS) arrived in Zenadth Kes to 'save the souls' of the peoples of Papua New Guinea. The LMS head missionary, Reverend Samuel Macfarlane thought the island of Erub was part of Papua New Guinea. This demonstrates that Macfarlane could not imagine that the land, water and skies as already known to the people that belonged there. Further, this ignores the established relationships between the peoples of the region. Islanders were merely natives who needed saving – from themselves and from the evil of British civilisation (Nakata, 2014).

Islanders were imagined to be barbaric and primitive, and the idea of the cannibal native was popularised. Thus, any retaliation from Islanders by trespassing outsiders was seen in this light. The remedy for this was colonisation through religion. The LMS was successful in its evangelising of the Zenadth Kes (Nakata, 2014). Stories of Christianity resonated with Islander creation stories. These commonalities were opportunistically mechanised to instil Christianity as a logical evolution of known religion of the region.

The contemporary privileging of Christianity within Islander families and communities is often considered a testament to the success of the LMS. However, this celebrates the civilising tool of Christianity while downplaying the agency of Islanders. While confined within colonial oppression, Islanders still exercise their spiritual agency.

Citizenships and power

In 1897, the Queensland government established the *Aboriginals Protection and Restriction of the Sale of Opium Act 1897* (Qld) (the Protection Act). The Protection Act was designed to legalise control over the Aboriginal peoples who lived within the borders of Queensland, as well as prohibit the sale of opium to Aboriginal peoples. This legislation created the roles of the local Protectors and Chief Protectors of Queensland, who held legal responsibility for Aboriginal people who became wards of the state through this Protection Act. The Islanders were not considered as Aboriginal peoples in this legislation. In 1903, amendments to the Protection Act resulted in Islanders being considered the same as Aboriginal peoples. This immediately placed Islanders as wards of the state under the care of the chief and local Protectors.

In 1939, the Queensland government passed the *Torres Strait Islanders Act 1939* (the TSI Act), which removed Islanders from the Protection Act. Under this Act, certain 'privileges' were awarded to Islanders that Aboriginal peoples under the Protection Act could not access. The most significant of these was the legal ability for Islanders to engage in the democratic process of voting to elect local Islander councils. While this was a great win for Islanders, the control that the Queensland government exercised over Islanders, specifically their subjection to power of local Protectors and the Director of Native Affairs, remained in place. The Islanders were empowered to have some control of local matters; however, their decisions remained subject to the appetite of the local Protector.

The TSI Act established a definition of Islanders that would distinguish them from Aboriginal peoples and other Australians. It asserted that a Torres Strait Islander was:

(a) one of the native race of the Torres Strait islands (sic),
(b) a descendent of the native race of the Torres Strait islands (sic) and is habitually associating with islanders ..., or:
(c) a person other than an islander ... who is living on a reserve with an islander as so defined as wife or husband or any such person other than an official or person authorised by the protector who habitually associates on a reserve with islanders as so defined.

Torres Strait Islanders Act 1939 (Qld) (pp. 17802–3)

This definition recognised heritage, the proximity to Zenadth Kes and Islanders as significant. This does not account for the significance of belonging experienced by Islanders living away from the region, supporting the incorrect assumption that Islanders lose their identity when they live away from the region (Watkin, 2009). This categorising of Islanders was a tool to apply control differently to Islanders and this definition was not interested in the relationality of Islanders.

Contemporary definitions of Australian Indigenous peoples' identity requires individuals to confirm the following three parts:

1. They are of Aboriginal and/or Torres Strait Islander descent.
2. They identify as Aboriginal and/or Torres Strait Islander persons.
3. They are accepted in the community with which they identify.

Like the definition within the TSI Act, this definition serves the purpose to identify individuals who may access 'privileges' designed for Indigenous peoples. However, these privileges remain limited to the appetite of Australian governments, and their departments.

The TSI Act was eventually succeeded by the *Aboriginal and Torres Strait Islander Affairs Act 1965* (Qld), then the *Aborigines Act 1971* (Qld) and finally the *Community Services (Aborigines) Act 1984* (Qld) (Daniels, 2017).

The invasion of Zenadth Kes and colonisation have constituted a devastating assault on Islanders, their ways of knowing, being and doing, and their health and wellbeing. However, their connections to Country and kin remain strong. Identity is a problematic concept, as it is superficial categorising that supports the continued control of Islanders. Australian history about how Islanders have been treated by successive British and Australian governments shows constant determination to diminish, demean and disempower Islanders. Externally imposed ideas of identity are part of that. Understanding Islander belonging is far more liberating, and is aligned with aspirations of **self-determination** and autonomy.

self-determination The right to freely determine political status, and freely pursue economic, social and cultural development appropriate for one's people. Within the context of the Zenadth Kes, this includes recognition of the historical and contemporary impact of colonisation and how this informs contemporary access to human rights.

CASE STUDY

Somebody now: Aunty Ellie Gaffney's story

Aunty Ellie was a Torres Strait Islander nurse and midwife who was born in the Torres Straits in 1932. She spent her childhood and young adulthood growing up in Zenadth Kes, at the Cowal Creek Mission on Cape York Peninsula, Cherbourg (a three-hour drive north-west of Brisbane) and in Brisbane.

Despite the challenges associated with entering and completing her nursing and midwifery training, Aunty Ellie persisted, successfully completed her general nursing training in 1954 at the Royal Brisbane Hospital, and her obstetric training soon after.

After completing her training, Aunty Ellie eventually returned home to be with family again, and to contribute to the health and wellbeing of her own people. While not surprising to her, Aunty Ellie recounts the normalised racism that was exercised by the non-Indigenous community on Thursday Island. Social groups such as the local tennis club and the local bowls club were covertly segregated. These same people exercised influence over the social norms of public institutions such as the local health services.

Aunty Ellie used her influence as a nurse and midwife to challenge the overt and covert personal racism she encountered, whether directed at her or other Islanders. She also used both professional and personal roles and relationships to effect change from an institutional level – for example, changing service delivery and the segregated dining areas. Her belongingness and established roles and responsibilities to the community who claimed her were the driving force. This is the strength of the Islander nurse working with her people.

Aunty Ellie eventually left the nursing profession and the health service to invest her time and energy into community programs, most of which still exist today. The Mura Kosker Sorority provides a range of health and social services aimed at addressing domestic violence. The Torres Strait Islander Media Association (TSIMA) continues to broadcast locally specific programs (and national ABC programs) to the

(cont.)

Zenadth Kes region. The Star of the Sea Home for the Aged continues to increase its capacity to care for more Islander older peoples and Elders. All of these community programs are based on Thursday Island.

Aunty Ellie Gaffney left a significant legacy for future Islander nurses and midwives. The authors pay their respect to her, and recognise our shared commitment to our Country and our kin.

Source: Gaffney (1989).

QUESTIONS FOR REFLECTION

- Aunty Ellie identified the normalised racism and whiteness of the health services and health workforce (including the nursing and midwifery workforce) on Thursday Island. Describe how the overt and covert actions of these non-Indigenous peoples resonate with the beliefs of the non-Indigenous explorers, missionaries and scientists that came before them.
- The normalised racism is historically evident in how Islanders were seen as inferior to non-Indigenous outsiders. Whiteness is exercised in the perpetuation of this myth, but also in how non-Indigenous culture continues to reimagine itself as superior and as saviours of Islanders. How does this relate to contemporary narratives about the role of the nurse and midwife as saviours?

Demographics

Islanders make up a small proportion of Australia's population. Thus, data on Islanders are usually included among data relating to Aboriginal peoples. Islander health status is therefore difficult to quantify, as data that are collected and presented by relevant national organisations often include both Aboriginal peoples and Islanders. This invisibilises Islanders in reporting by assuming similarities with Aboriginal peoples that may not be accurate. National Indigenous data are reliable, but it is currently not well known where there may be differences between Aboriginal peoples and Islanders.

Population

The 2016 census identified 649,200 people who identified as being Aboriginal and/or Torres Strait Islander people, which equates to approximately 2.8 per cent of the Australian population. Of this, 59,112 people identified as Torres Strait Islanders as well as identifying as both Aboriginal and Torres Strait Islanders. Islanders makes up 9.1 per cent of the Indigenous population and 0.25 per cent of Australia's population (ABS, 2017).

The ABS (2017) found a 18 per cent increase of people who identified as being an Aboriginal and/or Torres Strait Islander person between the 2011 and 2016 censuses. Islander-specific data indicate only a 10 per cent increase. The ABS found a similar increase between the 2006 and 2011 survey, and suggested that potential contributing factors could include improved census coverage and individuals who originally selected unknown Indigenous status now knowing and identifying as such, which may also be a result of an increased number of parents identifying their children as being Aboriginal and/or Torres Strait Islander (ABS, 2013).

Following World War II, the regulations on Islander movements were moderated to enable Islanders to leave Zenadth Kes for work and access more opportunities for themselves and their families (Lawrence & Lawrence, 2004). Islanders not abiding by the expectations of Queensland government and local Islander leadership were also forcibly removed and sent to government missions. Some Islanders were also forced to move due to changing environmental conditions that compromised the safety of living on their island homes (Watkin, 2009).

Today, Islanders reside all over Australia. The majority live in Queensland (37,547), followed by New South Wales (8919) and Victoria (3195). Islanders even call the colder parts of Australia home, with 2,008 Islanders living in Tasmania and 366 in the Australian Capital Territory (ABS, 2017) (Figure 4.2).

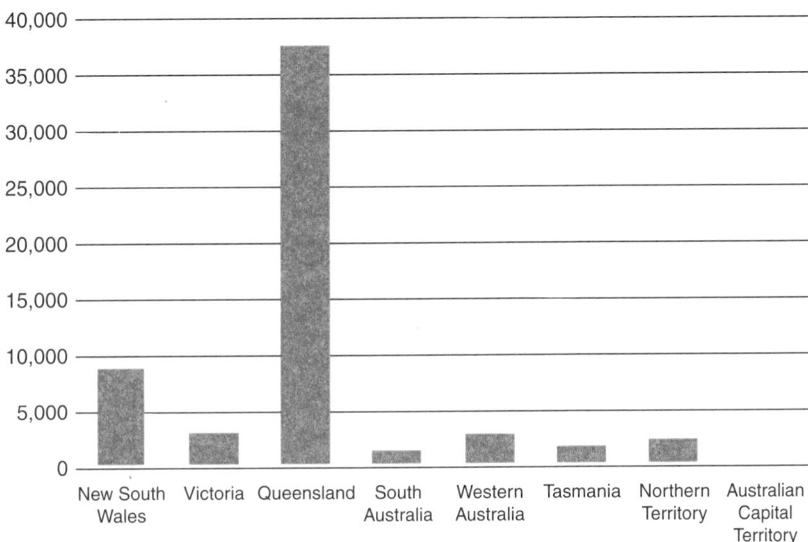

Figure 4.2 Distribution of the Torres Strait Islander population by Australian state/territory (2016 census data)

Source: Based on data from ABS (2017).

*Includes people who identified as Torres Strait Islander, as well as Aboriginal and Torres Strait Islander.

QUESTIONS FOR REFLECTION

It is common health practice to ask the people seeking healthcare about their Indigenous status – that is, if they identify as an Aboriginal person and/or a Torres Strait Islander. This information helps connect patients to Indigenous-specific support services, and also ensures that health services are being funded adequately to address the additional needs of Indigenous peoples.

However, asking about someone's Indigenous status has proven to be challenging for some clinicians. Uncertainty about why the question is being asked, and anxiety about what patients will think or say as a response, are a couple of examples of these challenges. Better informed clinicians are able to support patients and fellow staff with this important process (Scotney et al., 2010).

- How do you feel about asking all your patients about their Indigenous status?
- It is important to avoid *policing* someone's Indigenous status, as this is culturally unsafe. Policing may be exercised by comparing an Indigenous person to a static prescription of what an Indigenous person should look like or what they should be good at (e.g. assume that they should have dark skin and black curly hair, or be good at football). The information in this chapter is designed to support the development of your knowledge and confidence. As a culturally safe practitioner, how will you ensure that you don't use this knowledge to police Islanders' identity?

Health and wellbeing

Delivering culturally safe care to Islanders requires a critical understanding of how health services may perpetuate the colonial imaginations of Islanders. The dominance of the biomedical approach to health and wellbeing is inherently culturally unsafe. It discounts different understandings of health and wellbeing. This does not mean that the biomedical approach is wrong, but that its dominance limits the effectiveness of contemporary healthcare delivery, including nursing and midwifery care. It can only accept a particular way of knowing and practising health, and historically has diminished and demeaned other ways of knowing and practising health.

Definition of health and wellbeing

The National Aboriginal Health Strategy 1989 (NAHS) promotes the Aboriginal definition of health:

> Aboriginal health means not just the physical well-being of an individual but refers to the social, emotional and cultural well-being of the whole Community in which each individual is able to achieve their full potential as a human being thereby bringing about the total well-being of their Community. It is a whole of life view and includes the cyclical concept of life-death-life.
>
> (NACCHO, 1989)

This definition was established through consensus, which included the contribution of a number of Islanders. The lack of the mention of Islanders in this definition does not mean that it is not applicable to Islanders' understanding of health and wellbeing. On the contrary, the consensus acceptance of this definition persists.

Moreover, this definition is broader in its scope than the dominant biomedical understanding of health. It goes beyond the individual to consider the health of the community. Additionally, this definition of health promotes the need to focus on the physical as well as social, emotional and cultural wellbeing of the community. The significance of collective wellbeing is emphasised, highlighting the importance of recognising relationality, specifically how family members care for each other.

This definition also asserts Indigenous peoples' ownership and value of their knowledges. The cyclical concept of life–death–life highlights the significance of death as an important part of life, which is in contrast to a biomedical approach that positions death as bad. Belief in an afterlife is common; however, this definition brings to light a philosophical perspective that is not often considered an essential part of the biomedical understanding of health. This definition asserts Indigenous peoples' ownership and sovereignty over their bodies.

Health service provision in Zenadth Kes

Zenadth Kes is serviced by Queensland Health's Torres and Cape Hospital and Health Services (TCHHS). The TCHHS is responsible for delivering public healthcare to over 26,000 people in north Queensland; Indigenous peoples make up 70 per cent of this population.

The median age of death during the 2013–15 period was 59 years for Indigenous people and 67 years for non-Indigenous people (Queensland Health, 2018, p. 35). While this is not the same as life expectancy, these figures do tell us something about the health of the peoples in the TCHHS catchment area, and the effectiveness of the health service. What is also obvious is the gap between the median age of death of Indigenous people and that of non-Indigenous people in North Queensland.

In *The Health of Queenslanders 2018* (Queensland Health, 2018), Queensland Health's Chief Health Officer identified high levels of potentially preventable hospitalisation in the region (twice the rate of Queensland's average). This was mostly due to 'diabetes complications, cellulitis, and dental conditions', which accounted for 52 per cent of potentially preventable hospitalisation (Queensland Health, 2018, p. 44). This suggests that improvements can be made in preventing hospitalisation for these priority areas.

Torres Strait Model for Primary Health Care

Delivery of healthcare in the Torres Strait prior to 1997 was dominated by a biomedical approach in that it prioritised acute presentations, whereby the focus primarily was on 'What we do' as opposed to 'How we approach health' within the whole health system. To address the burden of ill-health among Islanders, a model for primary health care, commonly referred to as the Torres Strait Model for Primary Health Care (TSMPHC), was established in 1997. It aimed to strategically enable service-wide alignment to a population health approach that reflected the Indigenous definition of health. This would normalise a holistic approach based on social justice, equity, community participation, social acceptability, cultural safety and trust (Smith, 2016). Islander health leader Phillip Mills asserted that this approach aligned with the WHO-endorsed Alma Ata Declaration (P. Mills, personal communication, 1997).

The development of the TSMPHC encompassed three human rights principles, including clients/communities' rights to access healthcare that is affordable, accessible and appropriate (McMurray, 1999). Further to this, the TSMPHC also encapsulated the recommendations and aspirations of key health reports including the *Torres Strait Health Strategy 1993* and the *Implementation Plan for the Torres Strait Health Strategy 1996*.

In addressing the health priorities of the people Zenadth Kes the Torres Strait Health Strategy 1993 was developed by the community with local solutions. This strategy encompassed accessible services that were culturally safe and community controlled. Implementation plan for the Torres Strait Health Strategy 1996 was an important enabler of the former report. It came into fruition to achieve better outcomes for the people in the Torres Strait and Northern Peninsula Area. This entailed Indigenous management of service, better training for staff and a culturally accessible model for Primary Health Care

The goal of the TSMPHC was to optimise access of healthcare services outside the hospital, ensuring that these services were more client friendly and accessible to community members through a culturally safe model and community /client driven healthcare processes (Mills, 1997). The TSMPHC, which is still practised today, is driven by an Indigenous management structure that focuses on five core services: primary care; disease screening and prevention; education; health promotion; and community development. These core services are realised across all healthcare programs/services. Delivery of care for a client was, and continues to be, based on providing a holistic approach through being a one-stop-shop – that is, doing everything you can for the client when they engage the health service.

Traditional medicines practice and Torres Strait Islanders

As a clinician, it is important to understand that when a person seeks your services, the holistic needs of the person must be considered: 'Their relationships: their immediate health issues; their past issues; their lives. They're not just their illness, and they're not just their condition, or their reason for admission to hospital' (Queensland Health, 2014)

Prior to colonisation, traditional forms of healing, such as the use of traditional healers, were called upon to address not only the physical wellbeing of a person but their social, emotional and spiritual wellbeing. Although the impact of colonisation has removed and disconnected people from their Country and kin, many Aboriginal people and Islanders still use traditional medicine, food and remedies, including consultations with a traditional healer.

The use of traditional medicines by Islanders is not something that is openly discussed. These were practices that were deemed witchcraft by the missionaries, and Islanders faced harsh penalties if caught exercising Islander knowledge. Traditional healing practices include knowledge of traditional medicines, their preparation and use. This knowledge remains sacred knowledge and is not for the authors to share.

In practice, there are no or limited formal policies and procedures within hospitals and health services that support a safe and high-quality engagement with traditional Islander medicine. Traditional healing practices are exercised by many Indigenous communities and families. Indigenous peoples have been here a very long time and have developed a deep understanding of pharmacopeia of local plants and animal products. Additionally, knowledge about how these medicines work continues to be passed down in some communities. Therefore, it may not be unusual for an Indigenous person in hospital to be visited by large groups of immediate and extended family, and their own healers.

Health professionals should aspire to build therapeutic relationships with the patient and their family. Exercise culturally safe care so that if the patient or their family wishes to engage with a traditional healer, they will inform the health team. This is an opportunity to exercise flexibility with care provision and negotiate with the patient and their family about what is achievable in the context of hospital and health professional policy and regulation. Not all requests will be unimaginable; however, some may take some innovation to fulfil.

Environmental health: The wellbeing of our Country

The Islanders have a physical and spiritual connection to the Straits that go back at least 8000 years and potentially up to 45,000 years (Wright & Jacobsen, 2013). **Climate change** threatens to disrupt the spiritual and physical relationship between Islanders and their Country.

climate change Dramatic changes to global climate patterns since the mid- to late twentieth century as a result of increased levels of atmospheric carbon. Rising water levels is one outcome, a result of melting glaciers and ice sheets, and thermal expansion of sea water.

Zenadth Kes spans 48,000 kilometres of open sea. Within its borders are the northern reefs of the Great Barrier Reef and the shallow continental shelf that limits the energy and height of the waves that break across the islands (Duce et al., 2010; Green et al., 2010). In addition to the connection to islands, Islanders also assert a connection to this Sea Country that makes up approximately 90 per cent of the Zenadth Kes region and is an important part of Islander culture and spirituality. Practically, it also provides hunting and fishing food resources (O'Neill et al., 2012, p. 1104).

The five main island groups mentioned earlier also differ in their geological composition. The diversity includes low-lying sand-cay islands, continental islands, volcanic islands and reef islands. Low-lying sand cay islands are particularly vulnerable to weather extremes, as some islands are only 1 metre above sea level with communities that stretch to the edge of the beach (Duce et al., 2010, p. 31; Green et al., 2010).

According to the Torres Strait Regional Authority (TSRA, 2014), the main issues identified as result of climate change for Zenadth Kes are increasing air and sea temperatures, increasingly unpredictable and extreme weather events (including storm surges and inundations), a rise in sea level, rougher oceans making travel between islands more dangerous or inaccessible, and rising carbon dioxide levels increasing the ocean's acidity. The *TSRA Report* (TSRA 2014) states that these impacts are already evident and that increasing sea levels that are anticipated to get progressively worse will affect Zenadth Kes and its people, their exercise of their ways of knowing, being and doing on their Country, and their flora and fauna. A combination of even a small rise in sea levels and stronger winds is likely to cause more dangerous storm tides and increase the risk of inundation to the local environment and damage to infrastructure (Green & Ruddock, 2008). Of particular distress to Islanders is damage to infrastructure of cultural significance through loss of land to erosion, such as the cemetery on Saibai Island (O'Neill et al., 2012, p. 1107).

Duce et al (2010) state that global observations since the 2007 Intergovernmental Panel on Climate Change (IPCC) suggest that global sea levels have increased 80 per cent faster than predicted, indicating a global sea level rise of around 1 metre by the year 2100. This projected change in climate, sea level, ocean chemistry and water temperature will have major ecological impacts on the evidently vulnerable Zenadth Kes region. The existing socioeconomic disadvantage and the remoteness of the region will exacerbate the effects of climate change (Briggs, 2010; Green, 2006; Green et al. 2010).

The potential of damage to crops and diminished or lost marine ecology damaging traditional hunting and fishing will impact the nutritional status of Islanders. Already negative impacts on marine fisheries in the region are being reported (Johnson & Welch, 2015, p. 611). The warnings of potentially significant, negative disruption to marine micro-organisms should also be heeded (Cavicchioli et al., 2019).

Considering the Indigenous definition of health, and the impact of loss of island Country, the spiritual, social, emotional and physical wellbeing of entire communities will be compromised with the loss of island Countries – a real risk with increased sea levels associated with climate change.

Caring for Country for the Islanders is integral to the wellbeing of the community and the local environment (McNamara & Westoby, 2011a, p. 895; Scott & Mullrennan 1999). Western paradigms may not fully recognise the impact of the loss of connection with Country. Research indicates that

> whilst nostalgia – a feeling of melancholy or yearning when absent from one's home – is well known, similar negative emotions can be felt by people who experience distress because of environmental changes that harm their home environment, with resultant loss of solace.
>
> (McNamara & Westoby, 2011b, p. 233)

The potential impacts of climate change on the Zenadth Kes islands and Islanders are complex and often interconnected, in the same way the culture, health and spirituality of the people is tied to Country. The impacts are compounded as the people in the area already suffer socioeconomic disadvantage disproportionately in geographically remote locations compared with regional and urban parts of Australia. This has a real impact on all residents, with Indigenous peoples experiencing higher burdens. This makes adaptions to climate change even more difficult for individuals, but ever more important for governments, and for national and international leaders (Gutierrez & LePrevost, 2016, p. 1).

CASE STUDY

Climate change and dengue fever

You are the local nurse and midwife on Erub. It is November, so the monsoon season is approaching, which will bring very high tides and storms. Last monsoon season saw mass erosion of the beaches, and high tides that lapped close to people's homes – closer than the previous year. Governments had announced the building of a sea wall on the low beaches most susceptible to tidal flooding; however, despite the announcement, the wall has not yet been constructed.

Your immediate concern, however, is working with the visiting environmental health team from Thursday Island regarding dengue fever prevention. In 2020, the WHO identified dengue fever as the most prevalent viral infections globally. There were 96 million symptomatic dengue cases globally with 40,000 deaths (WHO, 2020). The Aedes aegypti mosquito is the vector for the dengue virus and it can be found in Zenadth Kes and other regions of Queensland.

The environmental health team is made up of a number of Torres Strait Islander health workers. They are on Erub for two days, delivering health promotion sessions to the community about dengue prevention. Community members are advised to use insect repellent and wear long-sleeved shirts and long pants at dawn and dusk. If their homes do not have insect screens, community members are encouraged to purchase mosquito nets and use mosquito coils.

The environmental health team also conducted inspections of people's homes and businesses, assessing yards for containers and other items that may pool water and create a reservoir for the dengue mosquito, tipping over containers with water and encouraging community members to store these undercover.

This broad approach to health and wellbeing is reflective of the Torres Strait Model for Primary Health Care.

QUESTIONS FOR REFLECTION

Dengue fever is a significant public health concern for the peoples of Zenadth Kes, one that is not realised by many other Australians. As a health professional working in Zenadth Kes, you are expected to work within the Torres Strait Model for Primary Health Care, which includes being involved in environmental health campaigns.

- To ensure a truly holistic approach, you will have to engage colleagues from the school, the local council and the local shops. What could their contribution be to dengue prevention?

Climate change-induced sea level rise is compromising the connection between Islanders and their Land and Sea Country.

- Thinking holistically, what may need to be considered in the healthcare plan for Islanders within Zenadth Kes?

Conclusion

Zenadth Kes is an ancient place, one that is sacred to Islanders. Appreciating the significance of connection between Islanders, Country and kin is essential to culturally safe care. Aspiring to establish and maintain an effective therapeutic relationship with Islander patients and their families is paramount to culturally safe care and resonates with the significance of relationality to Islanders.

As a culturally safe practitioner, it is important to endeavour to learn about the varying accounts of history and not just rely on single stories. Published work about Islander history has rarely been written by Islanders. These narratives betray the sophistication of Islander society, and intently frame them as noble savages or subhuman. This has permitted centuries of violent colonisation. Culturally safe practitioners understand how these beliefs can inform individual practice and the way institutions function.

Islanders now reside all across Australia. Their proximity to Country and kin remains important. A culturally safe practitioner will understand the history associated with control and freedom for Islanders, but will not use this to police the identity of Islanders. Identity is a shallow concept: the sense of belongingness for Islanders is within them.

There is so much to learn from Islanders, particularly their understanding and practice of health and wellbeing. More research is required to ensure that the dominant biomedical model can be sufficiently complemented with Islander-led approaches. Until then, culturally safe practitioners must be flexible in their service delivery, and advocate for change where they see that this is possible.

While Islanders continue to challenge the new waves of colonisation that continue to try to contain and control Islanders, they also face new challenges. Climate change is real for Islanders. Islands are washing away, and with them material possessions such as homes, but also irreplaceable things like sacred places. The Sea Country that Islanders have revered for generations is taking our islands as a result of climate change. A culturally safe practitioner appreciates the Indigenous definition of health and thus acknowledges the sorrow associated with this loss of Country.

Learning activities

1. What has been the most significant thing you have learnt about yourself while reading this chapter and completing the activities? Why was it so significant?
2. How has your understanding of caring for Indigenous people, particularly Torres Strait Islanders, changed since reading this book? What new knowledge have you gained? What do you still find confusing?
3. Describe your level of confidence of exercising culturally safe care to a Torres Strait Islander person and their family. What are your strengths? What are areas you need to continue to develop?
4. Visit the Torres and Cape Hospital and Health Services, Queensland Health website (www.health.qld.gov.au/torres-cape). Search for health professional job vacancies. Once you have found a position, learn more about the island where this position is located by visiting the Community Profiles page of the Torres Strait Regional Authority website (www.tsra.gov.au/the-torres-strait/community-profiles).

FURTHER READING

There are a number of books written on Zenadth Kes and Islanders. Below is a collection of books that privilege the voices and experiences of Islanders.

Faulkner, S. (2007). *Life B'long Ali Drummond: A Life in the Torres Strait*. Canberra: Aboriginal Studies Press.

Gibson, H.D. & Neuenfeldt, K. (2013). *Steady Steady: The Life and Music of Seaman Dan*. Canberra: Aboriginal Studies Press.

Nakata, M. (2014). *Disciplining the Savages, Savaging the Discipline*. Canberra: Aboriginal Studies Press.

Titasey, C. (2012). *Ina's Story: The Memoir of a Torres Strait Islander Woman*. Thursday Island: Catherine Titasey.

Visit the companion website at www.cambridge.org/highereducation/isbn/9781108794695/resources to see further online resources.

REFERENCES

ABS (2013). *Changing Propensity to Identify as Being of Aboriginal and Torres Strait Islander Origin Between Censuses*. Retrieved from www.abs.gov.au/ausstats/abs@.nsf/Lookup/2077.0main+features52006-2011

ABS (2017). *Aboriginal and Torres Strait Islander population – 2016 Census Data Summary*. Retrieved from www.abs.gov.au/ausstats/abs@.nsf/Lookup/by%20Subject/2071.0~2016~Main%20Features~Aboriginal%20and%20Torres%20Strait%20Islander%20Population%20Data%20Summary~10

ANAO (2013). *Torres Strait Regional Authority – Service Delivery*. Canberra: ANAO. Retrieved from www.anao.gov.au/sites/default/files/AuditReport_2013–2014_10.pdf

Brady, L.M. & Ash, J. (2018). New radiocarbon dates from Kirriri 4: extending the 2,500 BP signature for the onset of the Torres Strait Cultural Complex to South Western Torres Strait, Northeast Queensland, *Australian Archaeology*, 84(1), 98–104.

Briggs, G. (2010). *Strategic Analysis Paper: The Impact of Climate Change on the Torres Strait and Australia's Indian Ocean Territories*. Perth: Future Directions International. Retrieved from www.futuredirections.org.au/wp-content/uploads/2011/05/1269915280-FDI%20Strategic%20Analysis%20Paper%20-%2030%20March%202010.pdf

Carter, M., Barham, A.J., Veth, P., Bird, D.W., O'Connor, S. & Bird, R.B. (2004). The Murray Islands archaeological project: Excavations on Mer and Dauar, Eastern Torres Strait, *Memoirs of the Queensland Museum, Cultural Heritage Series*, 3(1), 163–82.

Cavicchioli, R., Ripple, W.J., Timmis, K.N. … Webster, N.S. (2019). Scientists' warning to humanity: Microorganisms and climate change. *Nature Reviews Microbiology*, 17(9), 569–86.

Daniels, E. (2017). *Community Services (Aborigines) Act 1984* September 2020. Retrieved from www.findandconnect.gov.au/ref/qld/biogs/QE01020b.htm

DFAT (1985). *The Torres Strait Treaty*. Retrieved from www.dfat.gov.au/geo/torres-strait/Pages/the-torres-strait-treaty

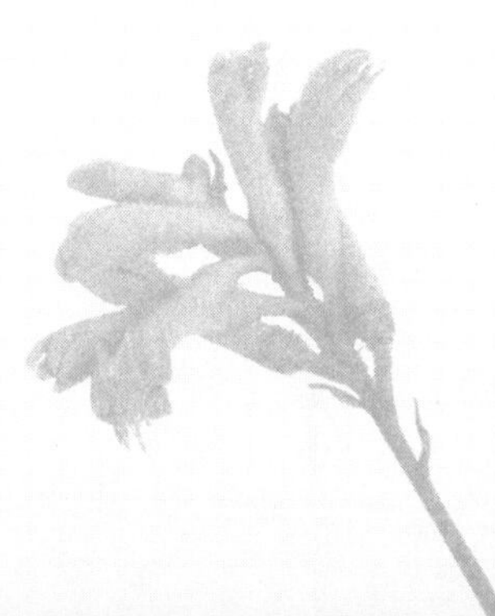

Duce, S.J., Parnell, K.E., Smithers, S.G. & McNamara, K.E. (2010). *A Synthesis of Climate Change and Coastal Science to Support Adaptation in the Communities of the Torres Strait.* Cairns: Reef & Rainforest Research Centre.

Eckermann, A.K., Dowd, T., Chong, E., Nixon, L., Gray, R. & Johnson, S. (2010). *Binan Goonj: Bridging Cultures in Aboriginal Health* (3rd ed.). Sydney: Elsevier.

Gab Titui Cultural Centre (2020). Ephraim Bani Gallery. Retrieved from www.tsra.gov.au/gabtitui/gab-titui/galleries/ephraim-bani-gallery

Gaffney, E. (1989). *The Autobiography of Ellie Gaffney, a Woman of Torres Strait.* Canberra: Aboriginal Studies Press.

Green, D. (2006). *How Might Climate Change Affect Island Culture in the Torres Strait?* Melbourne: CSIRO. Retrieved from www.cmar.csiro.au/e-print/open/greendl_2006a.pdf

Green, D., Alexander, L., McLnnes, K., Church, J., Nicholls, N. & White, N. (2010). An assessment of climate change impacts and adaptation for the Torres Strait Islands, Australia. *Climatic Change*, 102(3), 405–33.

Green, D. & Ruddock, K. (2008). Climate change impacts in the Torres Strait, Australia. *Indigenous Law Bulletin*, 7(8), 2–3,6.

Gutierrez, K.S. & LePrevost, C. (2016). Climate justice in rural southeastern United States: A review of climate change impacts and effects on human health. *International Journal of Environmental Research and Public Health*, 13(2), 189.

Johnson, J.E. & Welch, D.J. (2015). Climate change implications for Torres Strait fisheries: Assessing vulnerability to inform adaptation. *Climatic Change*, 135(3–4), 611–24.

Lawrence, D. & Lawrence, H.R. (2004). *Woven Histories, Dancing Lives: Torres Strait Islander Identity, Culture and History*. Canberra: Aboriginal Studies Press.

McMurray A. (1999). *Community Health & Wellness: Primary Health Care in Practice.* London: Churchill Livingstone.

McNamara, K.E. & Westoby, R. (2011a). Local knowledge and climate change adaptation on Erub Island, Torres Strait. *The International Journal of Justice and Sustainability*, 16(9), 887–901.

McNamara, K.E. & Westoby, R. (2011b). Solastalgia and the gendered nature of climate change: An example from Erub Island, Torres Strait. *Ecohealth*, 8(2), 233–36.

Mills, P. (1997). Personal communication.

Moreton-Robinson, A. (2015). *The White Possessive: Poverty, Power, and Indigenous Sovereignty*. Minneapolis, MN: University of Minnesota Press.

Moreton-Robinson, A. (2016). Relationality: A key presupposition of an Indigenous social research paradigm. In C. Andersen & J.M. O'Brien (eds), *Sources and Methods of Indigenous Studies*. London: Routledge, pp. 69–77.

Nakata, M. (2014). *Disciplining the Savages, Savaging the Discipline*. Canberra: Aboriginal Studies Press.

NACCHO (1989). *Definitions.* Canberra: NACCHO. Retrieved from www.naccho.org.au/about/aboriginal-health-history/definitions

National Museum Australia (2020). Cook claims Australia. Retrieved from www.nma.gov.au/defining-moments/resources/cook-claims-australia

O'Neill, C., Green, D. & Lui, W. (2012). How to make climate change research relevant for Indigenous communities in Torres Strait, Australia. *The International Journal of Justice and Sustainability*, 17(10), 1104–1120.

Queensland Health (2014). *Aboriginal and Torres Strait Islander Patient Care* Guideline. Retrieved from https://healthinfonet.ecu.edu.au/healthinfonet/getContent.php?

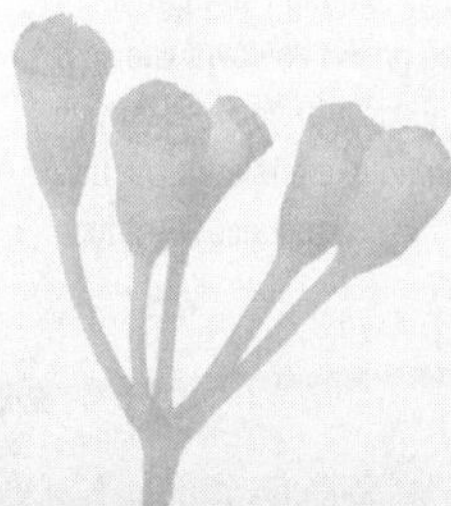

linkid=366304&title=Aboriginal+and+Torres+Strait+Islander+patient+care+guideline&contentid=30786_1

Queensland Health (2018). *The Health of Queenslanders 2018: Report of the Chief Health Officer Queensland*. Brisbane: Queensland Health. Retrieved from www.health.qld.gov.au/__data/assets/pdf_file/0032/732794/cho-report-2018-full.pdf

RHSQ (2019). From the archives: Possession Island. Retrieved from https://queenslandhistory.org/2019/08/from-the-archives-possession-island

Scotney, A., Guthrie, J.A. , Lokuge, K. & Kelly, P.M. (2010). 'Just ask!' Identifying as Indigenous in mainstream general practice setting: A consumer perspective. *Medical Journal of Australia*, 192(10), 609.

Scott, C. & Mullrennan, M. (1999). Land and sea tenure at Erub, Torres Strait: Property, sovereignty and the adjudication of cultural continuity. *Oceania*, 70(2), 146–76.

Sharp, N. (2013). *Stars of Tagai*. Canberra: Aboriginal Studies Press.

SLQ (2020). Information awareness – Torres Strait Islands. Retrieved from http://iaha.com.au/wp-content/uploads/2013/03/000210_informationawareness_tis.pdf

Smith, J.D. (2016). *Australia's Rural, Remote and Indigenous Health*. Sydney: Elsevier.

TSRA (2014). *Torres Strait Climate Change Strategy 2014–2018*. Retrieved from www.tsra.gov.au/__data/assets/pdf_file/0003/6393/TSRA-Climate-Change-Strategy-2014–2018-Upload.pdf

Watkin, F. (2009). My island home: a study of identity across different generations of Torres Strait Islanders living outside the Torres Strait. Unpublished PhD thesis, James Cook University.

WHO (2020). Vector-borne diseases. Retrieved from www.who.int/en/news-room/fact-sheets/detail/vector-borne-diseases

Windolf, J.F.P. (2010). With Torres on the search for Terra Australis: Don Diego de Prado y Tovar. *Queensland History Journal*, 21(2), 117–26.

Wright, D. & Jacobsen, G. (2013). Further radiocarbon dates from Dabangay, a mid-to late Holocene settlement site in western Torres Strait. *Australian Archaeology*, 76(1), 79–83.

LEGISLATION CITED

Aboriginal and Torres Strait Islander Affairs Act 1965 (Qld)
Aboriginals Protection and Restriction of the Sale of Opium Act 1897 (Qld)
Aborigines Act 1971 (Qld)
Community Services (Aborigines) Act 1984 (Qld)
Torres Strait Islanders Act 1939 (Qld)

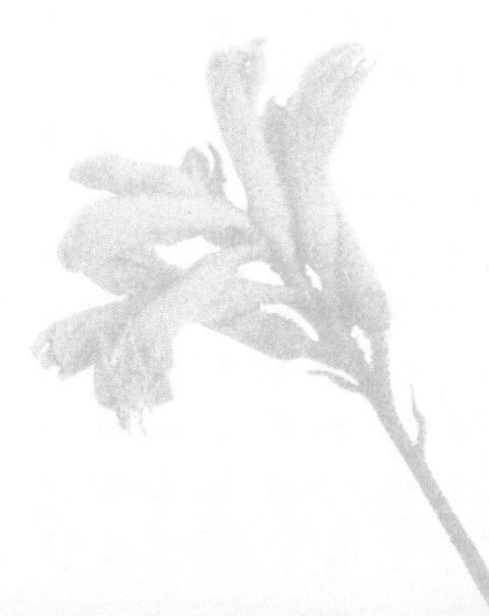

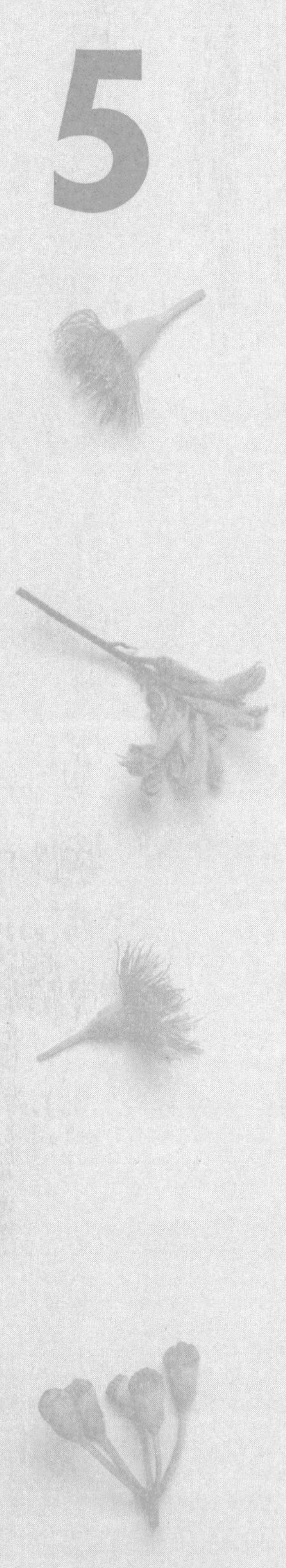

5 Indigenous gendered health perspectives

Bronwyn Fredericks, Mick Adams and Odette Best

LEARNING OBJECTIVES

This chapter will help you to understand:

- The gendered reality of Aboriginal men's and women's lives
- Gendered Indigenous health perspectives
- The differences between women's health and men's health
- Relevant policies and strategies and the role of nurses in gendered healthcare

KEY WORDS

gendered realities
men's business
women's business

Introduction

Historically, Aboriginal and Torres Strait Islander women and men held defined **gendered realities**. Within each clan group, the common ties of culture held people together, but gendered realities defined the specific roles of women and men. Women's business defined the knowledge and activities shared among women, which would not be shared with men. In turn, men's business defined the knowledge and activities that were shared among men and kept separate from women. Aboriginal and Torres Strait Islander men and women had processes for mediating and negotiating their shared responsibilities. Their communication was defined by their gendered realities, and occurred within the gendered cultural boundaries that were accepted by the group. Men and women held distinct, defined roles that were of vital importance to the balance of community.

gendered realities The life experiences that are available to individuals on the basis of their gender.

Even today, Aboriginal and Torres Strait Islander people maintain the separation of women's business and men's business. This separation is particularly relevant to discussions about the health status of Aboriginal and Torres Strait Islander people. It is also relevant to discussions about health interventions, as the gendered realities of women's business and men's business influence decisions about health promotion and the provision of healthcare. This chapter explores the gendered realities of the contemporary health experiences of Aboriginal and Torres Strait Islander people and examines gender issues that are relevant to nursing and midwifery practice.

Gender and Indigenous people

Gender is a widely discussed, debated and contested topic in Australia. Discussions about identity, gender and sexuality are conducted within many disciplines. In some disciplines, gender is defined in terms of biological sex characteristics; in others, gender is seen as a socialised condition that relies heavily upon cultural norms. Within the health sector, discussions about gender tend to focus on equality of access, the different health needs of women and men, and the different health outcomes experienced by women and men. In the broad context of Australian society, discussions about gender intersect with discussions about many other social issues, such as ethnicity, socioeconomic status and educational opportunity.

At first glance, discussions about gender within the context of Aboriginal and Torres Strait Islander people may appear to be associated primarily with sexual and reproductive issues. However, discussions about gender within Aboriginal and Torres Strait Islander communities are equally as complex as discussions about gender within the broader Australian community. While some Aboriginal communities have very clearly defined gender roles and expected gendered behaviours, there is also wide variation. For example, some Aboriginal and Torres Strait Islander communities readily accept varied gender roles (where, for example, a male dresses and behaves as a female and is described as a 'sistergirl'). Many communities have multiple ways of defining gender (in recognition of this, the Australian Passport Office now records three possible gender categories: F (female), M (male) and X (indeterminate/unspecified/intersex) (DFAT, 2013).

Through the processes of colonisation and the introduction of Christianity, Western understandings of gender identity and a system of patriarchy were introduced to Aboriginal and Torres Strait Islander communities. Traditional Aboriginal concepts and social understandings of gender and sexual identity were undermined, challenged and changed. Some communities today reflect a combination of gender concepts, with fragments of traditional gender roles sitting alongside Western understandings. For example, an Aboriginal woman might participate in Aboriginal **women's business** activities and be married in a Western-style ceremony conducted in a church or by a civil celebrant. Some may be married in the 'Aboriginal way'. Aboriginal men and women may use the terms 'ladies' and 'gentlemen' when referring to Aboriginal women and non-Indigenous women, and Aboriginal men and non-Indigenous men, respectively. While the terms 'ladies' and 'gentlemen' are embedded in Western notions of what 'ladies' or 'gentlemen' are supposed to be, they are at times used within Indigenous communities. We acknowledge these terms are used in some communities and may be more commonly used by older people. In these contemporary times, Aboriginal men may undertake **men's business** activities in the traditional way and also undertake to care for small infants and young children while their women partners are out shopping, or might be single fathers or be in other situations that are different from their traditional roles. Some communities, particularly those in which Aboriginal people have married non-Indigenous people, are dominated by Western understandings of gender.

women's business Customs, cultural practices and laws shared among women and taught to young women by their Elders, but not shared with men. Women's health issues are an important part of women's business.

men's business Customs, cultural practices and laws shared among men and taught to young men by their Elders, but not shared with women.

QUESTIONS FOR REFLECTION

Who are the women and men in your region?

Imagine that you have just accepted the position of Registered Nurse in a fairly isolated Aboriginal community.

- How might you develop your understanding of gender in that community?
- How is your understanding of yourself relevant to your work? What gender are you? How do you define your sexuality? What other aspects and factors do you use to define yourself? Where and how did you develop these defining characteristics?
- In thinking of your new role as a Registered Nurse, what are some of the day-to-day aspects that you might need to consider with respect to your gender? How will you manage your gender while working within an Aboriginal community that may have different understandings of gender from your own?

A gendered Indigenous perspective of health

The National Aboriginal Health Strategy (NAHSWP, 1989, p. ix) notes that, prior to colonisation, Aboriginal people 'were able to determine their "very-being", the nature of which ensured their psychological fulfilment and incorporated the cultural, social and spiritual sense'. This concept of 'very-being' relates to an individual's and community's core identity. It encompasses cultural traditions and practices that ensure people feel confident about and comfortable with who they are. This also includes being able to determine one's 'very-being' regarding gender.

As noted in the early chapters of this text, the processes of colonisation in Australia greatly affected the health status and wellbeing of Aboriginal women and men. We see its continuing effects today in the appalling health status of Aboriginal and Torres Strait Islander people.

The National Aboriginal and Torres Strait Islander Health Council report (NATSIHC, 2001, p. 5) states that

> the ill health of Aboriginal and Torres Strait Islander peoples exceeds that of any other sector of Australian society and the causes can be partly attributed to the impact of colonisation on the health of Aboriginal and Torres Strait Islander peoples.

As noted earlier in this text, the Aboriginal understanding of health is quite different from the standard definition broadly used throughout Australia. The National Aboriginal Health Strategy quotes John Newfong, who stated that, 'In Aboriginal society there was no word, term or expression for "health" as it is understood as in Western society' (NAHSWP, 1989, p. ix). Aboriginal people did not deconstruct or separate one element of a person's life as 'health'. Rather, health was traditionally the essence of everything about life; it encompassed all aspects of a person's life, including their land, environment, physical body, community, relationships and law. The word 'health', 'as it is used in Western society almost defies translation but the nearest translation in an Aboriginal context would probably be a term such as "life is health is life"' (NAHSWP, 1989, p. ix). For Aboriginal people, this means that health

> is a matter of determining all aspects of their life, including control over their physical environment, of dignity, of community self-esteem, and of justice. It is not merely a matter of the provision of doctors, hospitals, medicines or the absence of disease and incapacity.
>
> (NAHSWP, 1989, p. ix)

Many groups, agencies and organisations have since built on this statement. For example, in 1999 the Queensland Aboriginal and Islander Health Forum (QAIHF), now called the Queensland Aboriginal and Islander Health Council (QAIHC), issued its Corporate Plan, which stated:

> Health for Aboriginal peoples is cultural well-being. Cultural well-being is the integrity and harmony of physical, social, political, environmental, economic, ideological and emotional inter-relations which operate at the individual, family and community levels and constitute the essence of our Aboriginality.
>
> (QAIHF, 1999, p. 1)

The underlying concept is that, for Aboriginal and Torres Strait Islander peoples, health is linked to Aboriginality itself. Aboriginality underpins people's health and wellbeing. It is within this context that gender becomes relevant: for Aboriginal and

Torres Strait Islander people, gender must be explored within the overall framework of Aboriginality and a holistic view of health.

A chapter in the National Aboriginal Health Strategy addresses women's business (NAHSWP, 1989, pp. 179–90). It is considered a seminal document and was the first time an official document focused on Indigenous women's health issues, including health awareness, health education and promotion, family planning, birthing centres, antenatal and postnatal care, and cervical and breast cancer screening. The 'Women's Business' chapter acknowledges that 'health for Aboriginal women is not seen in the context of "white women's" issues or problems, but as part of their overall well-being, which is inextricably linked to that of their families and communities' (NAHSWP, 1989, p. 179). The chapter notes that women's business 'is not normally discussed openly or widely in a public forum; however, women's health issues need to be debated widely by Aboriginal women first before agreement can be reached on comprehensive, representative strategies' (NAHSWP, 1989, p. 179). Three gendered issues relevant to Aboriginal and Torres Strait Islander women are revealed in the 'Women's Business' chapter: the holistic view of health that is relevant for Aboriginal and Torres Strait Islander women; the difficulties that Aboriginal and Torres Strait Islander women often experience when accessing mainstream health services; and the reluctance of Aboriginal and Torres Strait Islander women to discuss their health issues – matters considered to be strictly women's business – within a public forum or one with mixed genders present.

The authors of the National Aboriginal Health Strategy (NAHSWP, 1989) advocated for separate conversations about men's business and women's business as integrally important to developing strategies for improving health. These separate conversations, which initially are based on culturally safe gender segregation, allow men and women to discuss their separate business before then coming together to make joint decisions. These separate conversations are not designed to promote gender division, but rather to recognise that women's business is most appropriately discussed by women, and men's business is most appropriately discussed by men. As the Strategy document stated, 'This is not to say that women's health issues can be isolated from general health issues affecting men, children, families and community at large' (NAHSWP, 1989, p. 179).

The National Aboriginal Health Strategy was a particularly important document for Aboriginal and Torres Strait Islander women, as it was the first time that any national policy published for broad circulation acknowledged Aboriginal women's ownership of Aboriginal women's issues. For the first time in public policy, the interests of Aboriginal women and their ownership of their interests was clearly articulated and supported. While Aboriginal people have always recognised the distinction between women's business, men's business and community business, it had not previously been articulated in public policy, nor has it been as articulated since this time in any comprehensive policy.

The National Aboriginal Health Strategy (NAHSWP, 1989) also recognised the interplay between traditional culture and contemporary approaches and acknowledged that the separation of women's business and men's business remains appropriate today. It stated that, 'while many Aboriginal people do not live traditionally, these traditional Aboriginal formats for discussion are the ones with which the majority of Aboriginal people feel most comfortable' (1989, p. 179). Although many urban Aboriginal and Torres Strait Islander people do not seem to live a 'traditional life', they may practise cultural traditions that remain relevant to them. The separation of women's business, men's business and community business is a common example of this.

CASE STUDY

Planning

Imagine you are a Registered Nurse working in a small health service in a rural community. Women have many different roles in the community and seem to be involved in the community's life in a variety of ways.

The local branch of the Country Women's Association (CWA) has asked you to be involved in planning a Ladies' Health Day. They know that you have a growing number of Aboriginal and Torres Strait Islander women clients and they want you to invite those women to be part of the Ladies' Health Day.

The CWA is hoping to invite a female general practitioner from the city to visit women in the community. They also plan to invite guest speakers from the larger regional town about 200 kilometres away.

QUESTIONS FOR REFLECTION

- What might you need to consider as you decide whether or not to be involved in the Ladies' Health Day?
- What might you suggest to the women from the CWA as they plan the event?
- Are there other guest speakers who might need to be asked?
- What factors might you need to consider in seeking involvement from Aboriginal women in your community?
- What effect might this have on your relationships with Aboriginal women and men in your community?

Health status and gender

As discussed elsewhere in this book, there are significant health disparities throughout Australia between Indigenous and non-Indigenous men and women. Indigenous men and women are the most socially and economically disadvantaged population group in Australia and have the poorest health outcomes (AIHW, 2015; Fredericks et al., 2017). Despite government initiatives, programs and strategies, the situation continues to be mostly unchanged. Of particular relevance to the discussion about gendered health perspectives are these statistics:

- Digestive organ cancers were each responsible for 20 per cent of deaths from cancer among Aboriginal and Torres Strait Islander females, and female genital cancers (mainly cervical cancer) for 17 per cent (ABS, 2007).

- Between 2011 and 2012, 38 per cent of Indigenous women aged 50–69 years participated in a BreastScreen program, compared with 54 per cent of non-Indigenous women (AIHW, 2015, p. 122).
- Indigenous Australians were 1.2 times as likely to report a cardiovascular disease when compared with the non-Indigenous population (with significantly higher rates of coronary heart diseases and rheumatic fever), with women more likely to have cardiovascular disease than men (14 per cent compared with 11 per cent) (AIHW, 2015, pp. 80; 89; AIHW, 2019a).
- Both Indigenous men and Indigenous women are reported as having higher rates of blood pressure than non-Indigenous people. Indigenous adults are 1.2 times as likely to have high blood pressure compared with non-Indigenous adults (AIHW, 2015).
- Indigenous men aged 15–34 years are three times more likely to die from external causes than non-Indigenous men, and Indigenous women four times as likely than non-Indigenous women (AIHW, 2015, p. 100).
- Indigenous women are fifteen times more likely and Indigenous men seven times more likely than non-Indigenous women and men respectively to experience hospitalisation as a result of chronic kidney disease (AIHW, 2015, p. 95).

Adams (2007) argues that Aboriginal and Torres Strait Islander men face two key issues in relation to poor overall health. First, the use of alcohol and other drugs and their exposure to violence place them at higher risk of harm and increase their likelihood of being isolated from their communities in prisons or detention centres compared with other Australians (AIHW, 2015). Indigenous men use illicit substances at higher rates than non-Indigenous men and also at higher rates than Indigenous women (AIHW, 2015), and in addition have higher rates of tobacco smoking, risky alcohol consumption, chronic disease (such as lung cancer, diabetes and kidney disease), along with health conditions (such as scabies, trachoma and acute rheumatic fever) that are uncommon in the general population (AIHW, 2015; Wenitong et al., 2014). Adding to this complexity is Aboriginal and Torres Strait Islander men's reluctance to speak about health issues and to seek assistance for their health problems. This is an important contributor to poor health outcomes for Aboriginal and Torres Strait Islander men. Since Aboriginal and Torres Strait Islander men have the poorest health outcomes and the lowest life expectancy of any group of men in Australia, this is an important issue for health professionals and policy-makers.

Aboriginal and Torres Strait Islander men and women are likely to present at clinics, health services and hospitals with diverse and complex health problems. Often, their health problems are exacerbated because the individual has delayed seeking medical attention for a variety of reasons, including fear of shame, concern about being unfairly judged, worries about inappropriate and discriminatory behaviour, or fear about medical procedures. They may worry that they will need to be transported to another town for treatment, and thereby will be separated from their communities. They may also be concerned that their cultural beliefs about gender-appropriate behaviour will be dismissed in the Westernised medical system. There are numerous articles, reports and papers documenting their concerns.

Gender-appropriate care

The 2006 Census of Population and Housing (ABS & AIHW, 2008) reported that approximately 4 per cent of Aboriginal and Torres Strait Islander respondents required assistance with the core activities of daily living. For example, they needed help with eating, bathing, dressing, general self-care, mobility and communication. Aboriginal and Torres Strait Islander people require this type of daily assistance at twice the rate of the non-Indigenous population (ABS & AIHW 2008, p. 55; AIHW, 2015).

Receiving care and support with the activities of daily living is a gendered experience for many Aboriginal and Torres Strait Islander people. It may not be appropriate for male carers to provide support for women, or for female carers to provide support for men. Ensuring appropriate access to male and female carers can be a vital part of ensuring positive health outcomes and a greater sense of wellbeing.

In the Aboriginal context, personal care needs do not remove the struggles that many people face daily, such as unstable housing situations, family relationship issues and the death of loved ones. Many Aboriginal and Torres Strait Islander families must cope with multiple family deaths each year. It is well understood that, in the older population, Aboriginal men and women represent only 4 per cent of people over the age of 65 years (compared with 16 per cent in the non-Indigenous population), which is the time when most of the general population are beginning to live on the old-age pension or their superannuation funds (AIHW, 2019b). The deaths of babies, young people and one's family members are a constant reminder of one's own mortality.

CASE STUDY

Culturally safe, gendered practice

Imagine you are working a late shift in a busy urban hospital and have been allocated a room of five male patients. During handover, you are informed that another admission is expected within the hour. The Registered Nurse conducting the handover tells you that the incoming patient has a hernia and will be admitted and prepared for theatre on the morning list.

The incoming patient has been identified as 'problematic' by staff in the accident and emergency department and is being considered for referral and a psychiatric evaluation. The incoming patient is an Aboriginal 'man' wearing a dress and identifying as a 'sistergirl' named Belinda. Belinda refuses to be admitted to a male ward and has threatened to discharge herself if this occurs.

QUESTIONS FOR REFLECTION

- Who would describe themselves as a 'sistergirl'? If you do not know, you need to seek out this information. What do you know about gender and sexuality in other cultures? How might you address your lack of knowledge about this if you do not know?

(cont.)

- What is culturally unsafe about the care Belinda has received in the accident and emergency department?
- Refer to Chapter 3, about cultural safety. Where along the cultural safety journey would you identify the actions and language of the nurse who provided the handover about Belinda?
- How might you provide culturally safe care for Belinda?
- Identify some possible support mechanisms that may be put in place for Belinda as she is admitted to the ward.

Changing the situation

Over the years, Australian agendas for women's health and men's health have varied in their ability to include the needs of Aboriginal and Torres Strait Islander men and women. Often, broad policy agendas generalise about men and women and minimise the differences between these broad groups. This can mean that the voices and needs of minority groups, such as Aboriginal and Torres Strait Islander people (or people from other ethnic backgrounds, or people living with disability) can be lost in the broader discussion about gendered health. For example, women's health centres and policy approaches that are designed specifically to meet the needs of men or women tend to generalise about the needs that are shared by all women and all men. Sometimes, the specific health needs of Indigenous men and women are overlooked. In contrast, approaches that have focused on the health needs of Aboriginal and Torres Strait Islander people generally have tended to minimise gender distinctions.

It is possible that more concrete gains would be made if Aboriginal and Torres Strait Islander health issues were discussed within a framework of gender. For example, if the men's health movement addressed as its core priority the significant discrepancies between Aboriginal men's health and the health of other men, we might see real gains in Aboriginal men's health status and wellbeing. In the same way, when the women's health movement speaks in broad terms about women's health, it tends to minimise the urgency of addressing the health status of Australia's Indigenous women. A focus on the health discrepancies between Aboriginal and Torres Strait Islander women and other Australian women could lead to concrete change.

Aboriginal and Torres Strait Islander men and women should not feel as though they have to make a choice between gender issues and Indigeneity when they are trying to gain access to services (Bessarab, 2006; Fredericks, 2007, 2009; Fredericks et al., 2017). They should not be asked to separate their gender from their culture. At the same time, they should never feel that they cannot have culture without gender (whether they opt for manhood, womanhood or some other kind of personhood). An individual's sense of being should not have to be measured against something else in order to gain access to basic healthcare. This suggests that mainstream providers of care need to address the ways in which Western medical culture dominates over others and affects the people who seek access to healthcare. Perhaps we need to question more closely whether current health categories (such as women's issues, men's issues,

Indigenous issues and so on) are applicable and helpful when seeking to meet the needs of individual clients.

Australia has experienced a revitalised interest in the different health issues that are experienced by men and women. In 2007, the then opposition leader, Kevin Rudd, made an election promise to develop a National Women's Health Policy. In response, the Department of Health and Ageing (DHA, 2009) released the *National Women's Health Policy: Consultation Discussion Paper*, which argued that the new health policy would 'recognise gender as a basic determinant of health, which gives rise to different health outcomes and different needs for women and men' (DHA, 2009, p. 1). In the introduction, the then Minister for Health and Ageing stated that the new policy would 'emphasise prevention, health inequalities and the social determinants of those inequalities' (DHA, 2009, p. iii). However, while the discussion paper foreshadowed promising developments in recognising the importance of gender within health policy, its implementation to date has been disappointing.

The consultations for the National Women's Health Policy received numerous submissions, including some from Aboriginal and Torres Strait Islander women. In 2009, the Australian Women's Health Network (AWHN) received approximately $100,000 from the Australian Department of Health and Ageing (Gender and Reproductive Health Branch) to consult with Aboriginal and Torres Strait Islander women and provide input into the submissions for the new National Women's Health Policy. The AWHN is not an Indigenous organisation, nor does it have a broad Indigenous membership. To implement the project, Indigenous women worked under the governance structure of the AWHN and established the Australian Women's Health Network Talking Circle (AWHN, 2009; Angus & AWHN-TC, 2009), which included Aboriginal and Torres Strait Islander women; the Talking Circle helped to develop the National Aboriginal and Torres Strait Islander Women's Health Strategy. The Strategy is available online, as is an article describing the project (see Fredericks, Adams & Angus, 2010; Fredericks et al., 2011).

The National Aboriginal and Torres Strait Islander Women's Health Strategy was launched at the AWHN National Conference held in 2010. The Strategy did not replace other documents, and needs to be seen as a document that supplements and complements other strategies. It was designed to build on work to improve the health and wellbeing of Indigenous women (e.g. see Best & Lucashenko, 1995; Daylight & Johnstone, 1986; Fredericks, 2003, 2008, 2010; Fredericks et al., 2010; Harrison, 1991; Huggins, 1994; Moreton-Robinson, 2000). The Strategy offers a platform for advocacy and current and future work inclusive of community-based programs (e.g. see Fredericks et al., 2016, 2017; McPhail-Bell et al., 2015) and cross-disciplinary Indigenous activism that raises issues for Indigenous women (e.g. see Baker et al., 2016). The National Women's Health Policy was launched in 2010 (DHA, 2010b). Some of the elements of the Strategy are also reflected in the National Aboriginal and Torres Strait Islander Health Plan 2013–2023 (NATSIHP), which provides the foundation for all state and territory Aboriginal Health Plans (Department of Health, 2013). NATSIHP provides a national overarching framework in partnership with a range of other plans and strategies, including some gender-specific plans and strategies to help Close the Gap in Indigenous health status and outcomes (Department of Health, 2013).

QUESTIONS FOR REFLECTION

Look up and read the National Aboriginal and Torres Strait Islander Women's Health Strategy (Fredericks et al., 2010).

- What do you notice about the document? What stands out? What can you draw upon for your studies? What can you learn about working with Indigenous women?
- See whether you can find a comparable Indigenous men's health strategy. Can you locate any specific Indigenous men's health strategies developed by state or territory governments? What have you found? What do you notice about the documents? What stands out?
- Look up the National Men's Health Policy (DHA, 2010a). How does it link to the other documents? What can you draw upon for your studies? What can you learn about working with Indigenous men?
- Look up the National Aboriginal and Torres Strait Islander Health Plan 2013–2023 (NATSIHP)(Department of Health, 2013). How and where are women's and men's health specifically addressed? How does your state or territory Aboriginal Health Plan relate to these documents?
- As a Registered Nurse, how might you implement a framework of culturally safe practices when caring for and treating Indigenous men and Indigenous women?

Rethinking Indigenous male health

Adams (2014) observes that there has been no systematic research about the relative disadvantages in reproductive and sexual health for Aboriginal and Torres Strait Islander males, and therefore there is very little information available, even at a basic descriptive level. Much of what we can learn in this area depends on self-reporting of symptoms and perceived sexual and interpersonal difficulties. Lawrence et al. (2004) also observed that there was very little research conducted on men who have sex with men (MSM), so they set out to gather data from MSM of Aboriginal and Torres Strait Islander background in Queensland, asking about their risk-taking behaviours, such as unprotected anal intercourse (UAI); understanding of and attitude towards HIV; interaction with Indigenous and gay communities; and ability to access relevant resources and services. There is limited research available for Indigenous people with regard to sexuality and sexual behaviours beyond reported sexually transmitted infections (STIs) (Adams, 2014).

While STIs such as gonorrhoea, chlamydia and syphilis are easily detected and curable with short courses of antibiotics, rates continue to be high among Aboriginal and Torres Strait Islander people, particularly in many remote communities of Australia (AIHW, 2018; Kirby Institute, 2017). Ward et al. (2013) state that there are few statistics about the incidence and prevalence of these diseases among Aboriginal people because of systemic issues associated with reporting of Aboriginal status in the notifiable diseases surveillance system.

Ward et al. (2013) explain that the remoteness of many Aboriginal communities, a lack of cultural and social acceptability of services, and the adequacy and effectiveness of local services in the development and delivery of programs can also act as barriers to access for young Aboriginal people. Little has changed for young people in remote communities since this time. Young Aboriginal and Torres Strait Islander people in urban communities face some of the same issues, although a growing number of Aboriginal and Torres Strait Islander community controlled services and programs are being implemented, targeted at young people. For example, the Brisbane Aboriginal and Torres Strait Islander Health Service (BATSIHS) has a young people's program, and there is increasing service uptake by services provided through the Institute for Urban Indigenous Health (IUIH) in Southeast Queensland.

There may also be sistergirls in the community – often males who identify as a girl being trapped in a boy's body. Depending on the community, being transgender might also mean observing strict cultural practices as defined by male and female gender roles (Clarke, 2015; Kerry, 2018). While there has seen significant progress on LGBTIQ issues over the years, sistergirls might still struggle with acceptance in their own communities and may choose to leave and live where they feel accepted and supported. In some communities, sistergirls may experience profound impacts on their health and wellbeing as a result of losses to their identity, sense of worth and spirituality, and having to act in ways that don't feel comfortable to them.

In a range of communities, transphobia may result in forms of punishment or what may be termed payback, through which retribution for social transgressions is brought down on community members. For example, Kerry (2018) offers an example from the Tiwi Islands on the north coast of Australia where for decades a sistergirl's family and community enacted payback because she advocated on behalf of sistergirls (and brotherboys). The payback included verbal harassment, physical assault and rape against the sistergirl herself, as well as immediate members of her family. The ongoing impacts on the sistergirl resulted in her committing suicide (Kerry, 2018).

Generally, sistergirls set themselves apart from being transgender or lesbians. They see themselves as girls who want to settle down with a partner (preferably a male husband) with whom they can openly express their love. Since invasion, pressures have been placed on Aboriginal marriage practices (e.g. promised marriages and polygyny) by missionaries, church doctrines, government policy and later the state. Marriage equality for gay men, lesbians, bisexual men and women and sistergirls and brotherboys may be extremely problematic to navigate in numerous Aboriginal and Torres Strait Islander communities. The work of Kerry (2018) found that sistergirls found it difficult because they still have their own cultures and the community may not accept them for who they are in their gender-defined identity as an Aboriginal and Torres Strait Islander male or female.

Aboriginal and Torres Strait Islander males have a role as custodians of reinforcing the values of customs, beliefs and spirituality and, most of all, affinity with the land. They are not accustomed to talking about the subject of sexual health, so it is frequently neglected in public health discussions. Relatively little attention has been paid to understanding the lived realities of males, including how they conceptualise health, the major factors that influence their health and how they respond to health problems (Adams, 2016).

In some instances, homosexual male nurses and Aboriginal health workers are employed as sexual health workers in Aboriginal and Torres Strait Islander community controlled health services and state-operated health clinics. Most are well grounded, having grown up with families, relatives and friends in these communities. However, some Indigenous elderly males in communities have grown up with a heteronormative male perspective and are not accustomed to, nor have they had much association with, homosexual males.

CASE STUDY

Practising cultural safety

Imagine you are a gay Aboriginal male nurse employed in a health clinic situated in a remote Aboriginal community where strict 'male business' is practised. An elderly male (relative) is referred to you with a complaint of STI symptoms. He is worried, frightened and confused about not knowing what he has, or what problems it will cause him. He is escorted into the treatment room where you are waiting, but once he sees you he seems to be immobilised. His body language tells you that he does not want to talk to you and refuses to let you examine him. He tells the Aboriginal health worker what he thinks is wrong and the story has changed from him having an STI concern to having flu symptoms. All he appears to want to do is get some medication and remove himself from being near you and the clinic.

QUESTIONS FOR REFLECTION

- This is a culturally safe environment yet the elderly male does not feel safe in this location, in particular with your presence. How would you feel?
- You have grown up and are conversant with Aboriginal ways of living, lore and culture. What would you do in this situation where there is a conflict between sexuality and culture?
- What would be some possible support mechanisms that you could identify to ensure males would feel culturally safe and comfortable to come and be attended by you?
- How would you approach this elderly male to hold future conversations?
- What do you know about how Aboriginal people use the terms 'male' and 'men'? You might need to find this out.

Conclusion

Aboriginal and Torres Strait Islander women and men are acknowledged to be the most socially and economically disadvantaged group in Australia. They have the poorest health outcomes. While gendered understandings of Aboriginal and Torres Strait Islander men and women are now acknowledged in many documents and reports, they do not appear to be broadly rolled out into practice.

The cultural traditions that separate women's business and men's business within Aboriginal and Torres Strait Islander communities must be acknowledged and understood. They have important implications for culturally safe healthcare practice, particularly in settings in which individuals receive support with the basic activities of daily life.

While is it important to adopt a gendered perspective of health and to understand the different health needs of men and women, this approach is not sufficient for addressing the health disparities experienced by Indigenous men and women. The health of Aboriginal and Torres Strait Islander men and women needs to be addressed from a gendered position that also examines the differences between their health and the health of the broader population. In that way, actions can be taken to address the health gaps that continue to exist. It is important to remember that Aboriginality underpins the health and wellbeing of Aboriginal people, and gendered realities are embedded within that Aboriginality.

Learning activities

1. Can you identify any gender-specific health services in your region?
   - Why are they needed? What role(s) do they fulfil?
   - How do they cater for Aboriginal and Torres Strait Islander men or women?
   - Do they meet the needs of people from varying cultural and sexual identities? If so, how? If not, why not?
2. Can you identify any Aboriginal and Torres Strait Islander-specific health services in your region?
   - Why are they needed? What role(s) do they fulfil?
   - Do they have gender-specific services within the health service? If so, what are they? If not, what might be missing?
   - Where do you think Aboriginal and Torres Strait Islander people who do not identify as having a male or female gender identity might receive their health services? Why?
3. What might be the reasons Indigenous men and women choose to attend gender-specific health services that are available for all people, in preference to an Indigenous-specific service?

FURTHER READING

Department of Health (2010). *National Women's Health Policy 2010*. Canberra: Department of Health.

Department of Health (2019). *National Men's Health Strategy*. Canberra: Department of Health.

Department of Health (2019). *National Women's Health Strategy*. Canberra: Department of Health.

Department of Health (2013). *National Aboriginal and Torres Strait Islander Health Plan 2013–2023*. Canberra: Department of Health.

Visit the companion website at www.cambridge.org/highereducation/isbn/9781108794695/resources to see further online resources.

REFERENCES

ABS (2007). *The Health and Wellbeing of Aboriginal and Torres Strait Islander Women: A Snapshot, 2004–05*. Canberra: ABS.

ABS & AIHW (2008). *The Health and Welfare of Australia's Aboriginal and Torres Strait Islander Peoples 2008*. Canberra: ABS & AIHW.

Adams, M. (2007). Sexual and reproductive health problems among Aboriginal and Torres Strait Islander males. Unpublished PhD thesis, Queensland University of Technology.

Adams, M. (2014). *Men's Business: A Study into Aboriginal and Torres Strait Islander Men's Sexual and Reproductive Health*. Canberra: Magpie Goose.

Adams, M. (2016). *My Journey Through the Academic Mist*. Canberra: Magpie Goose.

AIHW (2015). *The Health and Welfare of Australia's Aboriginal and Torres Strait Islander Peoples 2015*. Canberra: AIHW.

AIHW (2018). *Aboriginal and Torres Strait Islander Health Performance Framework (HPF) Report 2017*. Canberra: AIHW. Retrieved from www.aihw.gov.au/reports/indigenous-health-welfare/health-performance-framework-new/contents/tier-1-health-status-outcomes/measure-1–12

AIHW (2019a). *Acute Rheumatic Fever and Rheumatic Heart Disease in Australia*. Canberra: AIHW. Retrieved from www.aihw.gov.au/reports/indigenous-australians/acute-rheumatic-fever-rheumatic-heart-disease/contents/summary

AIHW (2019b). *Profile of Indigenous Australians*. Canberra: AIHW. Retrieved from www.aihw.gov.au/reports/australias-welfare/profile-of-indigenous-australians

Angus, S. & AWHN-TC (2009). *Submission on National Issues, Barriers and Recommendations Concerning the Health Status of Aboriginal Women for the Development of the 'National Aboriginal Women's Health Policy' as Identified by Aboriginal Women, Community Women, Partners and Service Providers*. Melbourne: AWHN.

AWHN (2009). *Submission to the Development of a New National Women's Health Policy*. Melbourne: AWHN.

Baker, A.G., Blanch, F.R., Harkin, N. & Tur S.U. (2016). *Bound and Unbound: Sovereign Acts II*. Adelaide: Yungorendi First Nations Centre, Flinders University. Retrieved from www.finders.edu.au/yunggorendi/unbound/unbound_home.cfm

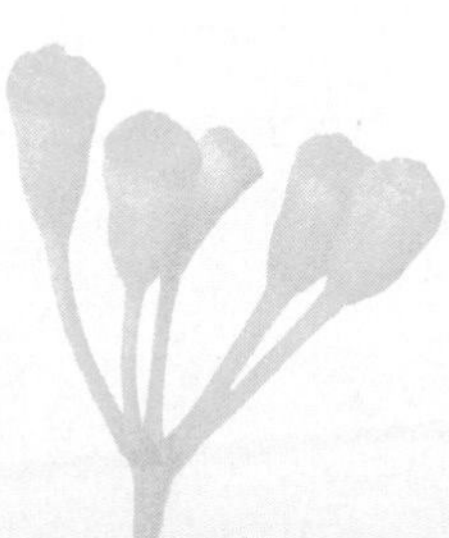

Bessarab, D. (2006). A study into the meanings of gender by Aboriginal people living in urban (Perth) and regional (Broome) settings. Unpublished PhD thesis, Curtin University.

Best, O. & Lucashenko, M. (1995). Women bashing: An urban Aboriginal perspective. *Social Alternatives*, 14(1), 19–22.

Clarke, A. (2015). Meet the transgender 'sistergirls' of the Tiwi Islands. *Buzzfeed*, 26 August. Retrieved from www.buzzfeed.com/allanclarke/sistergirls-of-the-tiwi-islands

Daylight, P. & Johnstone, M. (1986). *Women's Business: Report of the Aboriginal Women's Taskforce*. Canberra: Australian Government Publishing Service.

Department of Health (2013). *National Aboriginal and Torres Strait Islander Health Plan 2013–2023*. Canberra: Commonwealth of Australia.

DFAT (2013). *Sex and Gender Diverse Passport Applicants*. Canberra: Commonwealth of Australia. Retrieved from www.passports.gov.au/Web/SiteIndex.aspx

DHA (2009). *National Women's Health Policy: Consultation Discussion Paper*. Canberra: Australian Government Publishing Service. Retrieved from: www.health.gov.au/internet/main/publishing.nsf/Content/phd-women-consult-disc-paper

DHA (2010a). *National Male Health Policy: Building on the Strengths of Australian Males*. Canberra: Department of Health. Retrieved from www.health.gov.au/internet/main/publishing.nsf/Content/male-policy

DHA (2010b). *National Women's Health Policy 2010*. Canberra: Department of Health. Retrieved from www.health.gov.au/internet/publications/publishing.nsf/Content/womens-health-policy-toc

Fredericks, B. (2003). Talking about women's health: Aboriginal women's perceptions and experiences of health, well-being, identity, body and health services. Unpublished PhD thesis, Central Queensland University.

Fredericks, B. (2007). Australian Aboriginal women's health: Reflecting on the past and present. *Health and History: Journal of the Australian and New Zealand Society of the History of Medicine*, 9(2), 93–113.

Fredericks, B. (2008). Researching with Aboriginal women as an Aboriginal woman researcher. *Australian Feminist Studies*, 23(55), 113–29.

Fredericks, B. (2009). There is nothing that 'identifies me to that place': Aboriginal women's perceptions of health spaces and places. *Cultural Studies Review*, 15(2), 41–61.

Fredericks, B. (2010). Reempowering ourselves: Australian Aboriginal women. *Signs: Journal of Women in Culture and Society*, 35(3), 546–50.

Fredericks, B., Adams, K. & Angus, S. (2010). The National Aboriginal and Torres Strait Islander Women's Health Strategy. *Aboriginal and Islander Health Worker Journal*, 34(4), 32–4.

Fredericks, B., Adams, K., Angus, S. & AWHN-TC (2010). *National Aboriginal and Torres Strait Islander Women's Health Strategy*. Melbourne: AWHN.

Fredericks, B., Adams, K., Angus, S. & Walker, M. (2011). Setting a new agenda: Developing an Aboriginal and Torres Strait Islander Women's Health Strategy. *International Journal of Critical Indigenous Studies*, 4(2), 17–28.

Fredericks B., Daniels C., Judd, J. … Ball, R. (2017). *Gendered Indigenous Health and Wellbeing Within the Australian Health System: A Review of the Literature*. Rockhampton: CQUniversity.Retrieved from https://eprints.qut.edu.au/115966/1/

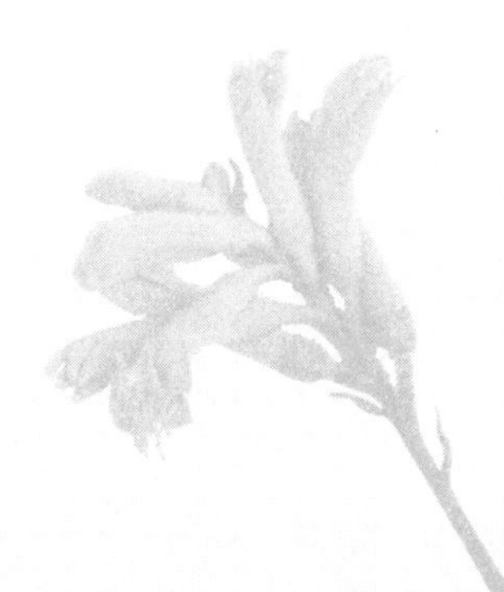

Gendered%20Indigenous%20Health%20and%20Wellbeing%20within%20the%20Australian%20Health%20System.%20A%20Review%20of%20the%20Literature.pdf%20%281%29.pdf

Fredericks, B., Longbottom, M., McPhail-Bell, K. & Worner, F. in collaboration with the Board of Waminda (2016). *Dead or Deadly Report: Waminda Aboriginal Women's Service*. Rockhampton: CQUniversity. Retrieved from http://acquire.cqu.edu.au:8080/vital/access/manager/Repository/cqu:13773

Harrison, J. (1991). *Tjitji Tjuta Atunymanama Kamiku Tjukurpawanangku: Looking After Children Grandmothers' Way*. Alice Springs: Nagaanyatjarra, Pitantjatjara Yankunytatjara Women's Council.

Huggins, J. (1994). A contemporary view of Aboriginal women's relationship to the white women's movement. In N. Grieve & A. Burns (eds), *Australian Women and Contemporary Feminist Thought*. Melbourne: Oxford University Press, pp. 70–9.

Kerry, S. (2018). Payback: The custom of assault and rape of sistergirls and brotherboys; Australia's trans and sex/gender diverse First Peoples. *Violence and Gender*, *5*(1), 37–41.

Kirby Institute (2017). *Bloodborne viral and sexually transmissible infections in Aboriginal and Torres Strait Islander people: Annual surveillance report 2017*. Sydney: Kirby Institute, University of NSW. Retrieved from https://kirby.unsw.edu.au/sites/default/files/kirby/report/KirbyInst_Indigenous_ASR2017-compressed.pdf

Lawrence, C., Prestage, G., Leishman, B., Ross, C., Muwadda, W., Costello, M., Rawstorne, P. & Grulich, A. (2004). *Queensland Survey of Aboriginal & Torres Strait Islander Men Who Have Sex with Men*. Sydney: National Centre in HIV Epidemiology and Clinical Research, Faculty of Medicine, University of New South Wales.

McPhail-Bell, K., Bond, C., Brough, M. & Fredericks, B. (2015). 'We don't tell people what to do': Ethical practice and Indigenous health promotion. *Health Promotion Journal of Australia*, 26(3), 195–9.

Moreton-Robinson, A. (2000). *Talkin' Up to the White Women: Indigenous Women and Feminism*. Brisbane: University of Queensland Press.

NAHSWP (1989). *A National Aboriginal Health Strategy*. Canberra: Australian Government Publishing Service.

NATSIHC (2001). *National Aboriginal and Torres Strait Islander Health Strategy, Consultation Draft*. Canberra: NATSIHC.

QAIHF (1999). *Corporate Plan*, Brisbane: QAIHF.

Ward, J., Bryant, J., Worth, H., Hull, P., Solar, S. & Bailey, S. (2013). Use of health services for sexually transmitted and blood-borne viral infections by young Aboriginal people in New South Wales. *Australian Journal of Primary Health*, 19, 81–6.

Wenitong, M., Adams, M. and Holden, C.A. (2014). Engaging Aboriginal and Torres Strait Islander men in primary care settings. *Medical Journal of Australia*, 200(11), 632–3.

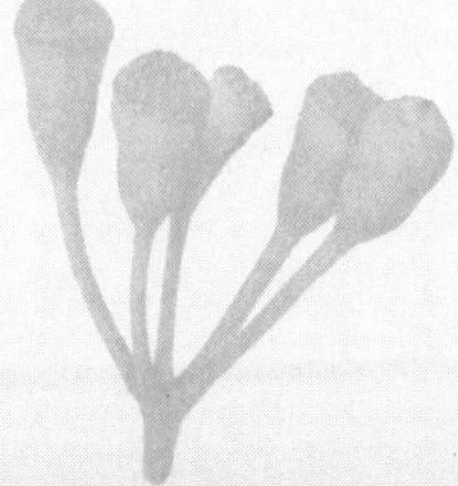

Community controlled health services: What they are and how they work

Bronwyn Fredericks, Odette Best and Raelene Ward

LEARNING OBJECTIVES

This chapter will help you to understand:

- The history and establishment of Aboriginal Community Controlled Health Services, through a case study of Brisbane's Aboriginal and Torres Strait Islander Health Service
- How Aboriginal community controlled health services work
- The role of nurses within Aboriginal community controlled health services
- The operation of community controlled services and how community controlled health services contribute to culturally safe healthcare
- The opportunities for community controlled health services in the future

KEY WORDS

community controlled health services
National Aboriginal Community Controlled Health Organisation (NACCHO)
Queensland Aboriginal and Islander Health Council (QAIHC)
self-determination

Introduction

community controlled health services Primary health services owned and managed by the communities in which they operate. Health service members are simultaneously owners and clients of the services.

This chapter explores Aboriginal and Torres Strait Islander **community controlled health services** and the important role they play in improving health outcomes for Aboriginal and Torres Strait Islander people. It is difficult to understand the Aboriginal community controlled health sector of today without considering how the sector developed. This chapter therefore outlines the conception and establishment of the services and the political realities facing Indigenous people at the time.

This chapter is organised around a case study of the Aboriginal and Torres Strait Islander Health Service in Brisbane, which celebrated its 40th anniversary in 2013. To complement the case study, the chapter includes an overview of the governance structures of the community controlled sector, as this is an area that can be difficult for health professionals to understand. The scenarios and questions focus on experiences that nurses might have working in an Aboriginal health service.

The need for community controlled, Indigenous-specific health services

The community controlled health movement grew against the harsh backdrop of racist and discriminatory policies such as protectionism and segregation (approximately from the 1890s to the 1950s, and longer in some jurisdictions). (These policies are discussed in Chapters 1 and 2.)

Aboriginal and Torres Strait Islander people who were living on reserves and missions often had access to small local hospitals. In these places, staffing was a key problem. White nurses and medical staff did not stay long, and qualified Indigenous staff were few and far between. These small local hospitals offered limited services, often in poor conditions. Many of the Indigenous people who lived on reserves and missions had been forcibly removed and placed in these places that were, in some cases, thousands of kilometres away from their homelands. They had little or no understanding of the traditional medicines available in these new lands. In addition, many missions were church affiliated, and traditional medicines were seen as the 'devil's work' (Huggins & Huggins, 1994; Rintoul, 1993).

Aboriginal and Torres Strait Islander people who lived in cities and regional settings experienced different problems. While healthcare was generally available in those communities, it was not always available to Indigenous people. In many cases, Aboriginal and Torres Strait Islander people were denied access to services. In some rural and regional settings, hospitals continued to operate segregated wards for Indigenous and non-Indigenous peoples (Rintoul, 1993). In Queensland, for example, segregated wards were still operating as late as the 1980s (Forsyth, 1990).

The poor health status of Aboriginal and Torres Strait Islander people became increasingly evident in the 1950s and 1960s. It began to attract both national and international attention. For example, a team of leading health experts from the World Health Organization (WHO) visited inner-city Brisbane in 1967 and prepared a report that condemned the appalling health conditions of Indigenous people (discussed by

Sam Watson in Best, 2004). Indigenous people in Melbourne, Sydney, Adelaide and other cities were experiencing similar health conditions and in the 1960s began to advocate for improved services (Fredericks & Legge, 2011). Knowledge of the health inequalities added strength to the activism of Aboriginal and Torres Strait Islander people as they fought for human rights, **self-determination**, sovereignty, land rights, equity and access to services.

self-determination The process of individuals determining how they manage their lives and what services they need. It is additionally utilised with regard to Indigenous-specific services, where the membership, governance mechanism and services are operated and managed by Indigenous Australians and are specifically for Indigenous Australians.

Increasing political activity and agitation occurred within Indigenous communities during the 1960s. Events such as the Freedom Ride in 1965 (National Museum Australia, 2007–08; Perkins, 1975) and the equal pay case of pastoral workers in the Northern Territory throughout the 1960s (Rintoul, 1993) were the breeding grounds for the establishment of a number of Indigenous community controlled services. In many communities, Indigenous activists became involved in the Federal Council for the Advancement of Aborigines and Torres Strait Islanders (FCAATSI).

> FCAATSI was formed in 1958 in Adelaide at a meeting of Aboriginal leaders, politicians, church and trade union representatives. FCAATSI became the first truly national lobby group that led the battle for equality and better living conditions for Aboriginals. The Council became an effective pressure group.
>
> (Watson, in Best, 2004, p. 58)

FCAATSI was the driving force behind the 1967 Referendum, which saw Aboriginal and Torres Strait Islander people recognised in the national census and gave the Commonwealth Government the power to make specific laws for Aboriginal and Torres Strait Islander people. FCAATSI was also a leading force in Indigenous politics. FCAATSI's members passed on national data to its state and territory members, who could then agitate for change at the local level. Many FCAATSI members were activists in their own communities, helping to establish Aboriginal organisations and services, such as health services.

Establishing the Aboriginal health service in Brisbane

In Brisbane, the early 1970s saw the emergence of activities that led to an independent health service for Aboriginal people. Sam Watson, a recognised community leader, activist and Elder who passed away in 2019, was a young community member at the time. He was highly active in establishing various Indigenous services in Brisbane and was also involved in establishing the Brisbane chapter of the Black Panther Party in 1972 (Black Panther Party, 1972). Watson spoke about the establishment of the Aboriginal and Torres Strait Islander Council in Brisbane:

> [T]he radicalisation of Indigenous people in Brisbane led to a small group of Aboriginal and Torres Strait Islander leaders holding a meeting in the upstairs room at a bank building in Stanley Street, Mater Hill in 1968. The purpose of that meeting was to talk about the situation of the black community in Brisbane and to formulate strategies to address the seemingly insurmountable problems faced by every Indigenous family and individual in the greater Brisbane area. In 1970, [Pastor] Don Brady, Denis Walker

> and their group set up the Aboriginal and Torres Strait Islander Council. They decided to have a governing committee of twenty people, all of whom had to be Aboriginal or Torres Strait Islander adults. The governing committee drew up the main areas of need and appointed a Tribal Councillor to be responsible for each portfolio. Jane Arnold was in charge of health.
>
> (Watson, in Best, 2004, p. 59)

The establishment of the Aboriginal and Torres Strait Islander Council added momentum to the push for an independent health service. The Brisbane community debated what could be done about the obvious lack of health services for the local Aboriginal and Torres Strait Islander population. They were concerned about what services were needed and how they could best be delivered. According to Watson:

> The late Jane Arnold and her small band of helpers enlisted sympathetic white doctors from the public hospital system and visited Aboriginal and Torres Strait Islander homes in the inner city suburbs and administered free medications and advice to the families they visited. This was the very first actual health program that was conceived, established and run by Aboriginal and Torres Strait Islander people to serve their own community.
>
> (Watson, in Best, 2004, p. 60)

The early 1970s was a time of protesting and rallying for the Brisbane Aboriginal and Torres Strait Islander community. Les Collins, now recognised for his commitment and long-term engagement in Indigenous health, was another young community member at the time (QAIHC, 2020b). Collins recalled:

> We started on the streets with a lot of protesting activities where Aboriginal people in Brisbane and throughout Queensland and Interstate would come together. What we were trying to do was redress some of the more obvious discriminatory practices for example the blatant denial of access to existing health care systems. This included talking to the Indigenous community, lobbying politicians and gaining political support from non-Aboriginal sympathisers, especially students and academics, and essentially we took it to the streets.
>
> (Collins, in Best, 2004, p. 55)

Civil rights marches began to occur on the streets of Brisbane from September 1971 and continued over several years. For example, on 23 November 1971, Indigenous men and women from the Tribal Council attempted to storm the Department of Aboriginal and Islander Affairs in George Street (Courier-Mail, 1971). The group was met by a wall of police who were there to stop the protestors from entering the building.

Members of the Australian Council of Churches, who were attending a conference on racism, joined the 1971 protest. The then Premier, Joh Bjelke-Petersen, blamed the Australian Council of Churches' representatives for getting involved and being part of the 'ugly scenes' (Aird, 2001; Courier-Mail, 1971). Former Catholic priest Richard Buchhorn recalled:

> It was traumatic experience for a lot of the people from the conference who saw the way the police behaved ... I remember a standoff in front of the Department

> of Aboriginal and Torres Strait Islander Affairs. Quite a number were arrested and taken off.
>
> (Buchhorn, in Aird, 2001, p. 113)

The 1971 protest resulted in a number of arrests. From this time, arrests became a regular occurrence and an expected aspect of Indigenous activism. For example, when reflecting on the preparations for a large rally held on 14 July 1972, Les Collins explained:

> Denis [Walker] said that the Government's getting really pissed off with us, doing these demonstrations. So you want to wear some protective gear. I know they are going to have the riot squads and everything there. He had the helmet, leather jacket and gloves. The riot squad moved in one part, near King George Square. They wanted to use their batons, so we had to defend ourselves somehow.
>
> (Collins, in Aird, 2001, p. 115)

The July 1972 rally attracted thousands of people and became known as the 'George Street Clash' (Collins, in Best, 2004, p. 56). The *Courier-Mail*'s photograph of Denis Walker in his protective gear, accompanied by Les Collins and others, is often used as an example of activism in that era.

Throughout the Aboriginal and Torres Strait Islander community in Australia, direct action was seen as an essential part of the struggle for the right to Indigenous services. Governments of the day considered the actions too political and militant in their execution, and the small amount of federal funding secured by the Tribal Council was withdrawn.

Even without funding, the Council continued to meet regularly. The Council believed that the scope and needs of the Indigenous population required 'specialist organisations to deal with areas of need in specific ways' (Watson, in Best, 2004, p. 62). The Council set up separate, purpose-built organisations to deal with three big problem areas: law, health and housing. In Queensland, this was the birth of community controlled Aboriginal and Torres Strait Islander services.

When the Brisbane community established this health service, it became the first community controlled health service in Brisbane (ATSICHS, 2020). It provided a new model for community healthcare in Queensland: Aboriginal and Torres Strait Islander people were now responsible for its establishment and held key roles in its structure. It was established by Aboriginal and Torres Strait Islander people specifically *for* Aboriginal and Torres Strait Islander people. Brisbane's service soon became known as the Aboriginal and Torres Strait Islander Community Health Service Brisbane Ltd (ATSICHS Brisbane).

From its base in Brisbane, the Aboriginal and Torres Strait Islander community supported other local communities in Queensland to establish their own health services, including the Bidgerdii Aboriginal and Torres Strait Islander Community Health Service Central Queensland Region. This pattern was replicated across the country, with the Victorian Aboriginal Health Services (VAHS) supporting the establishment of new services throughout Victoria and the Redfern Aboriginal Medical Service (AMS) helping other services to form in New South Wales. Australia's first community controlled health service was founded in July 1971 in Redfern.

Understanding the concept of community control

It is important to remember that the term 'community control' had not been articulated in Brisbane in the early days of Indigenous activism. A common Indigenous catch-cry throughout Australia in the 1970s was 'black affairs in black hands' (Collins, in Best 2004, p. 48) or 'by us, for us' (Fredericks & Legge, 2011). These ideas form the basis of what is now recognised as community control.

Within the health context, current understanding of community control refers to Aboriginal and Torres Strait Islander people 'being in control and participating in decision-making structures, administration procedures and service delivery' (Fredericks, Adams & Edwards, 2011, p. 86). This tends to involve Aboriginal and Torres Strait Islander people 'owning it, having a say about their own health and having the opportunity to provide feedback' (VACCHO & CRCAH, 2007, p. 1). Linked ideas include 'self-determination, reconciliation and providing culturally appropriate services' within the context of 'cultural history, cultural identity and having a "place" to identify with' (VACCHO & CRCAH, 2007, pp. 1–2). Through community controlled services, Aboriginal and Torres Strait Islander people are 'controlling their destinies and exercising responsibility for decision-making in health with their communities' (Fredericks, Adams & Edwards, 2011, p. 86).

Since the early days in the 1970s, Aboriginal and Torres Strait Islander community controlled health services have evolved in various ways to become incorporated Indigenous organisations initiated by local Indigenous communities, based within local Indigenous communities and governed by a group of Indigenous people who are elected by their communities. They deliver holistic and culturally safe health services to the communities that control them. Different communities have developed various versions of this broad framework. Some health services are referred to as Aboriginal Community Controlled Health Organisations (ACCHOs) and others are called Aboriginal Medical Services (AMSs). Within Queensland, often these services are called Aboriginal and Islander Health services, to represent Torres Strait Islander peoples establishing these services and usage of them. An example of this is the Brisbane Aboriginal and Islander Community Health Service.

Establishing a community controlled health service in Brisbane

In its early years, Aboriginal and Torres Strait Islander Health Service (ATSICHS) Brisbane relied heavily on fundraising and a group of volunteers. Watson recalled:

> There was only a very small group of us ... and we started to initiate funds through fundraising such as barbecues and the like. Basically we were able to with these funds hire an ex bookshop building up on Musgrave Road, Red Hill, Brisbane. We then had a few weekends transforming the shop into suitable space for the health service. Pastor Don Brady was a qualified cottages carpenter so he knew how to handle a saw and

> hammer. Then we constructed a list of voluntary doctors who could give 2 to 3 hours a week and in that way we were able to launch the clinic on 13th February back in 1973 as a voluntary run health service for the community.
>
> (Watson, in Best, 2004, p. 64)

Between February and May 1973, clinic staff saw 119 patients (DAA, 1973). Watson noted:

> In those first three months of 1973, whilst the Board waited for the funds to come through, they were able to set up a roster of voluntary doctors who came in for two to three hour sessions and provided general clinics. The word had to be passed around the community that doctors were available on certain days to see patients. People flocked to see the doctors and were content to wait for hours. The service was also provided with boxes of free drug samples, so they were able to operate a limited pharmacy.
>
> (Watson, in Best, 2004, p. 64)

While based at Red Hill, ATSICHS Brisbane delivered a broad range of services to the community, including general medical and dental, social work and field work support and advice, mobile clinics, a transport service, and outreach work to homeless people in South Brisbane and Fortitude Valley (ATSICHS, 2020). The breadth of services was remarkable, and at the time it was unheard of to have a health service provider offering services such as transportation and mobile clinics. ATSICHS was responding to a need articulated by the community, and helping to increase the community's access to health services (Best, 2004).

ATSICHS Brisbane has moved and grown from its original 1973 location in Red Hill. In 1976, it moved to South Brisbane, then to Woolloongabba in 1985. In 2006, ATSICHS moved to West End and then back to Woolloongabba in 2009. In 2009, ATSICHS Brisbane established clinics at Woodridge, Northgate and Acacia Ridge.

Today, ATSICHS Brisbane is one of the largest community controlled health services in the country and one of the largest Aboriginal and Torres Strait Islander community controlled organisations in Queensland. It provides a diverse range of health programs and services to the Aboriginal and Torres Strait Islander community of greater Brisbane. In 2013, its services included a general clinic, family and child health, antenatal and paediatric clinics, a youth clinic and services, women's health, men's health, dental care, optometry, hearing and podiatry clinics and a healing centre. ATSICHS Brisbane provides services to over 12,000 clients (ATSICHS, n.d.).

Working in a community controlled clinic

A community controlled clinic like ATSICHS Brisbane employs a large and diverse suite of professional staff – just like any other large health service. Aboriginal Registered Nurses were among the first health professionals employed by community controlled health services and remain the backbone of health service staff. One of these early Aboriginal Registered Nurses, Mary Martin, worked with ATSICHS Brisbane for several years from 1976 and has retained a connection with the community controlled health sector since.

In community controlled health services, Registered Nurses work as part of multidisciplinary teams that may also include enrolled nurses, midwives, Aboriginal health workers and other health professionals. Health service staff are often credentialled in additional areas, such as ear health, women's health, nutrition, sexual health and so on.

CASE STUDY

Marilyn improves care for young women at ATSICHS Brisbane

Marilyn [not her real name] is a Registered Nurse (RN) who worked at ATSICHS Brisbane. We have permission from her to share this story.

As a young Registered Nurse (RN), I was employed at the Aboriginal and Torres Strait Islander Community Health Service in Brisbane (ATSICHS Brisbane). I was attached to the Indigenous Youth Health Service, and worked in a team of five health staff: me as RN, a program coordinator, a part-time doctor, a drug and alcohol worker, and a youth worker. My role as RN was diverse and included venepuncture, dressings, health promotion, vaccinations and sexual healthcare.

One of my main jobs was to encourage young women to undertake sexual health checks. One morning, a young Indigenous woman told me that she would only have a pap smear if it could be done by one of the nurses. The part-time doctor in our team was male, and this was a problem for our young Indigenous women clients because of the Indigenous distinctions of women's health and men's health. Seeing the male doctor for a pap smear was not an option for our clients, and our clinic's female doctor (attached to the adult clinic) was completely booked out. None of the RNs in the service was authorised to conduct pap smears.

It was clear that the RNs and Aboriginal health workers needed to be trained in pap smear procedures. I spoke to the service coordinator, who wholeheartedly agreed that this was a gap in our services. The board agreed with the proposal, and we applied to Queensland Health for funding for the training. We received $7000 for the training, and the service soon became a reality for our clients.

The number of young, at-risk Indigenous women who accessed our services for sexual health checks immediately skyrocketed. I felt that I was helping to provide a very important service to my community. As a young RN, I was an active member of a health team that identified needs among our client group, gained support from the board, helped to secure funding, and were trained to provide better health outcomes for the community.

Marilyn's story is an example of a young RN advocating on behalf of her clients and collaborating with other health professionals to achieve positive outcomes for her client group. Staff in Aboriginal and Torres Strait Islander Health Services often need to take the initiative when they identify service gaps – by applying for funding and developing community-based solutions to problems. They frequently collaborate with other services and organisations to maximise services for Aboriginal and Torres Strait Islander people. At times, the programs offered by health services can be threatened by funding shortfalls or changes in government priorities. At other times, new opportunities may become available due to new government initiatives. Government funding cycles can make it difficult for health services to plan for long-term service delivery of some programs.

QUESTIONS FOR REFLECTION

- What steps did Marilyn take to address the problem she identified?
- What barriers did Marilyn face? What difficulties might she have needed to address?
- What was the nature of the partnership she established? How did it work?
- What was the outcome for Aboriginal and Torres Strait Islander women?

QUESTION FOR REFLECTION

- Identify some challenges you might face if you were working as a Registered Nurse within an Aboriginal community controlled health service.

The governance of community controlled health services

Aboriginal and Torres Strait Islander community controlled health services aim to provide high-quality, holistic healthcare in their local communities. The services are planned, managed and controlled by the communities they serve.

Most community controlled health services are managed by a board of directors or a management committee elected from the membership base. The members are usually Aboriginal and Torres Strait Islander people who live in the local area. Normally, elections for the board of directors are held at an annual general meeting (though some services may elect directors for longer periods). Some community controlled services invite other people to join the board – such as non-Indigenous people or Indigenous people from other regions who may have skills not available in the local community. An individual invited onto a board under these circumstances may be referred to as a 'skills-based director'.

The board of directors is accountable to the service's members and to the funding bodies. Most boards meet monthly and hold general meetings for all members at least once a year. The board may also organise special general meetings to discuss changes to the constitution or major planning issues. The board provides a full report to the members once a year and also provides reports to funding bodies.

The board operates under a constitution of the organisation's members. Working within the rules of the constitution, the board sets the overall direction of the health service and develops an annual plan of activities. The board is responsible for assessing the performance of the chief executive officer (CEO) or manager, reviewing the service's performance, assessing its risk management and ensuring that the service conforms to legislative and regulatory requirements. The board also reaches out to the wider community by advocating on behalf of the service, communicating with external stakeholders and monitoring the government and policy environments.

The day-to-day work of the service is coordinated by the CEO or manager. This person is responsible for liaising between the board and the staff: this person implements the board's plans and reports to the board about the work of the staff. Staff who work within the service are employed by the board and are answerable to the board through the CEO or manager.

Working within a community controlled health service means that the patients and clients of the service are likely to be general members and may even be members of the board. Even if they are not board members themselves, clients and patients probably know someone who is. In a sense, the clients in community controlled services are also the employers.

Most Aboriginal and Torres Strait Islander community controlled health services are members of a representative organisation, which provides advice and support to the services and advocates for them at the national level. They work to strengthen the community controlled sector, increase workforce development opportunities and provide leadership and advice within their jurisdictions. In Queensland, most Aboriginal and Torres Strait Islander health services are members of the **Queensland Aboriginal and Islander Health Council (QAIHC)** (an overview of its members is provided in the text box below); in New South Wales, they are members of the Aboriginal Health and Medical Research Council of New South Wales (AH&MRC NSW); in Victoria, they are members of the Victorian Aboriginal Community Controlled Health Organisation (VACCHO). Other states and territories have their own representative organisations (except for the Australian Capital Territory and Tasmania, each of which has only one community controlled health service). The different state organisations organise meetings for service board members and training for other staff. For example, Registered Nurses may be invited to attend state meetings regarding immunisation, women's health or other health-specific issues.

Queensland Aboriginal and Islander Health Council (QAIHC) A leadership and policy organisation established in 1990. It is the peak organisation representing 26 Aboriginal and Torres Strait Islander community controlled health services (CCHS) in Queensland at both a state and national level. The organisation is 'dedicated to achieving improved Aboriginal and Torres Strait Islander health outcomes in Queensland through the delivery of comprehensive and culturally appropriate primary health care'. (QAIHC, 2020a)

In Queensland, QAIHC represents 26 community controlled health services and has a number of associated members who 'share a passion and commitment to addressing the unique healthcare needs of their communities through specialised, comprehensive and culturally appropriate primary health care' (QAIHC, 2020b). QAIHC was originally established as the Queensland Aboriginal and Islander Health Forum (QAIHF). It was self-funded until 1996, when the Commonwealth Department of Health began to provide funding support. In 2004, it was reconstituted under the Australian Investment and Securities Commission and became known as QAIHC.

QAIHC membership

QAIHC membership is open to all Aboriginal and Islander community controlled health services (AICCHS) and Regional Aboriginal and Islander Community Controlled Health Organisation (RAICCHO) in Queensland. The members of Aboriginal and Torres Strait Islander Community Health Service Brisbane are:

- Aboriginal and Torres Strait Islander Community Health Service Mackay
- Apunipima Cape York Health Council
- Cherbourg Regional Aboriginal and Islander Community Controlled Health Services
- Bidgerdii Aboriginal and Islander Community Health Service Rockhampton
- Carbal Medical Services Toowoomba
- Charleville & Western Areas Aboriginal & Torres Strait Islander Community Health
- Cunnamulla Aboriginal Corporation for Health
- Galangoor Duwalami Primary Healthcare Fraser Coast
- Girudala Community Cooperative Society Bowen
- Goolburri Aboriginal Health Advancement Toowoomba
- Goondir Health Services Dalby
- Gurriny Yealamucka Health Service Yarrabah
- Injilinji Aboriginal and Torres Strait Islander Corporation for Children and Youth Services
- Kalwun Health Service Gold Coast
- Kambu Aboriginal and Torres Strait Islander Corporation for Health Ipswich
- Mamu Health Service Innisfail
- Gidgee Healing Mornington Island
- Mudth-Niyleta Aboriginal and Torres Strait Islander Corporation Sarina
- Nhulundu Health Service Gladstone
- North Coast Aboriginal Corporation for Community Health Sunshine Coast
- NPA Family and Community Services, Aboriginal and Islander Northern Peninsula Area
- Townsville Aboriginal and Islander Health Service
- Wuchopperen Health Service Cairns
- Yulu-Burri-Ba Aboriginal Corporation for Community Health Stradbroke Island.

REGIONAL MEMBERS

- Institute for Urban Indigenous Health Brisbane
- Northern Aboriginal & Torres Strait Islander Health Alliance Cairns

The state and territory organisations join together in a national organisation called the **National Aboriginal Community Controlled Health Organisation (NACCHO)** – Australia's national peak body for Aboriginal and Torres Strait Islander health. NACCHO describes its vision for Aboriginal peoples as follows:

> Sovereign Aboriginal peoples with a state of well-being, consistent with our holistic concept of health, at least equal to that which existed prior to invasion and colonisation, enjoying all the rights and responsibilities inherent in our unceded sovereignty.
> (NACCHO, 2012)

National Aboriginal Community Controlled Health Organisation (NACCHO) The national leadership body for Aboriginal and Torres Strait Islander health in Australia representing 143 Aboriginal Community Controlled Health Organisations (ACCHOs) that operate in over 300 clinics across Australia, delivering holistic, comprehensive and culturally competent primary healthcare services. (NACCHO, 2020)

NACCHO represents Aboriginal and Torres Strait Islander community controlled health services at the national level and presents a unified voice to government, institutions and organisations. It represents, advocates and campaigns for better health for Aboriginal and Torres Strait Islander peoples and communities, along with equitable funding for healthcare, high-quality care and comprehensive primary healthcare. NACCHO's long-term objectives and principles are broader and include the alleviation of poverty, the advancement of Aboriginal and Torres Strait Islander spirituality and recognition of human rights.

Cultural safety in Indigenous health

Aboriginal controlled health services working to close the health gap

The primary healthcare approach delivered by ACCHOs is more comprehensive and diverse than mainstream services. Multidisciplinary care teams are foundational, as is the fostering and development of long-term relationships. The culturally safe environment fostered by ACCHOs allows Aboriginal and Torres Strait Islander people to draw strength from their identity, culture and community. The Queensland Productivity Commission (QPC, 2017, p. xiv) notes that ACCHOs 'provide comprehensive healthcare within the cultural paradigm that makes services more accessible'. Moreover, they have 'reduced unintentional racism and barriers to health care access' and they demonstrate 'superior performance to mainstream general practice' (QPC, 2017, p. xiv).

Causes of death and chronic disease burden

Figure 6.1 shows the causes of mortality in Indigenous Australians from 2008 to 2012.

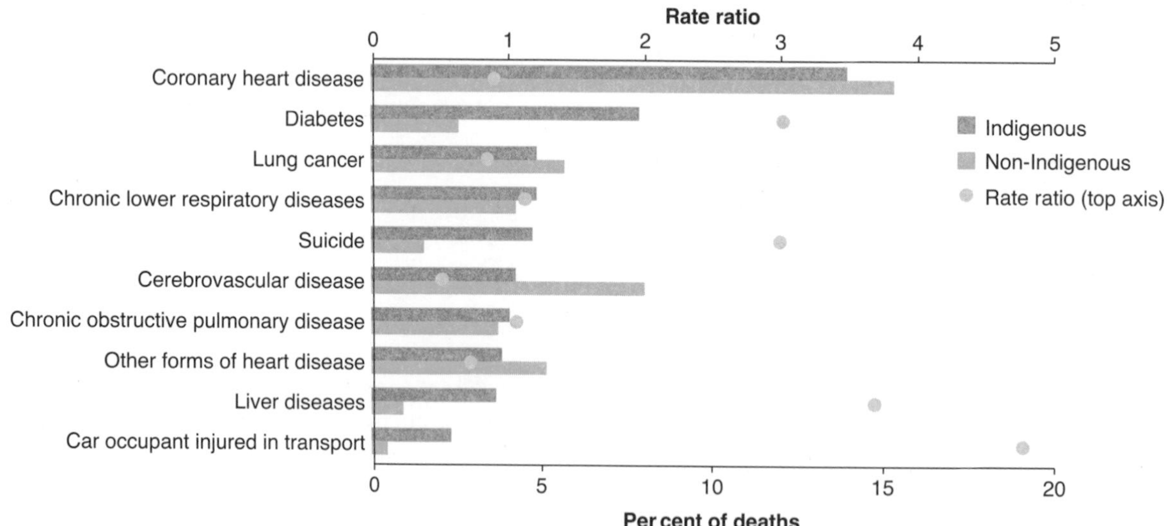

Figure 6.1 Causes of mortality in Indigenous Australians

Note: Data are for 2008–12 for New South Wales, Queensland, Western Australia, South Australia and the Northern Territory only.

Source: Reproduced from AIHW (2015, p. 115).

For the same period, NACCHO (2014) reports that chronic diseases were responsible for 70 per cent of the total health gap and for 64 per cent of the total disease burden among Indigenous Australians, with the five most significant disease groups being:

- mental and substance use disorders (19 per cent)
- injuries (including suicide) (15 per cent)
- cardiovascular diseases (12 per cent)
- cancer (9 per cent), and
- respiratory diseases (8 per cent).

Reducing exposure to modifiable risk factors may have prevented over one-third (37 per cent) of the burden of chronic disease. Such risk factors included tobacco and alcohol use, high body mass, physical inactivity, high blood pressure and dietary factors (NACCHO, 2014).

CASE STUDY

Aboriginal patients going back to their communities

This case study focuses on a 40-year-old Aboriginal patient who has a number of chronic diseases and has been receiving treatment in a large urban hospital. Recently, the patient sustained an infected foot that requires wound management and antibiotics. The patient is being prepared for discharge and it is your role to support their transition back into their community. You find out that your patient is originally from Cape York in North Queensland and will be discharged within a few days. As the primary nurse, you need to ensure that the patient is going to receive follow-up care when he returns to his community. The patient's medical history includes:

- hypertension and high cholesterol
- mild renal impairment
- myocardial infarction
- type 2 diabetes.

Additional health-related information:

- Has a family history of heart disease.
- Gave up cigarettes six months ago.
- Has a poor diet.
- Attends every six months for script renewals.
- Has stated that he does not have a full understanding of his chronic illnesses.
- In his community, he is surrounded by family and extended family. He is an active community member and is regarded as Uncle by many and is the current chair of the men's group.

Further actions are needed to develop an appropriate care plan for this patient. After talking with the patient, you discover that the main health service used by the patient

(cont.)

is called Apunipima Cape York Health Council. In your clinical decision-making, you need to find out how this service can support your patient upon his return.

QUESTIONS FOR REFLECTION

- What is Apunipima Cape York Health Council and what types of services does it provide?
- Identify the types of services that can support your patient's range of conditions.
- The patient has recently given up smoking and has expressed that he would like to lose some weight. Can you identify a number of issues for food security within this remote community that may impact his ability to reach his weight goal?
- Your patient has stated that he is yet to have his latest 715 (health check). Conduct an online search to find out what a 715 health check for Indigenous people is, along with the benefits and where to get one.

CASE STUDY

Planning for NAIDOC Week in a health service

Imagine you are a Registered Nurse working in a multidisciplinary clinic in an Aboriginal and Torres Strait Islander community controlled health service in a regional community. The health service has one large clinic and also offers two visiting clinics to smaller communities, two days a week. At the staff meeting this week, the CEO tells staff that the board of directors would like this year's NAIDOC Week celebrations to focus on the national NAIDOC theme and diabetes. The main clinic includes two Registered Nurses, two enrolled nurses and three Aboriginal health workers, and they have been asked to take the lead on this.

QUESTIONS FOR REFLECTION

- If you do not know what NAIDOC Week celebrations are, STOP working on this case study now and do some research about what NAIDOC Week is and what it means for Aboriginal and Torres Strait Islander communities across Australia.
- Identify why the board may have suggested diabetes as the health focus. *Hint:* undertake a search about the prevalence of diabetes among Indigenous Australians.
- Identify the clinical skills you and your team members will need before you may undertake diabetes checks.
- Identify some organisations that may be able to offer support or resources for a successful diabetes program in the community.
- What other health professionals may play a part in the diabetes program and why?
- What is a normal blood sugar level?

- Suggest a healthy food option to present to community members who have their blood sugar level measured. Why is it healthy?

NAIDOC Week can be an ideal time to focus on health issues with members of the Aboriginal and Torres Strait Islander community. There are other events held during the year that also offer valuable opportunities for health promotion. You might want to explore some of these to assist you in planning your work with Indigenous peoples and communities.

The future

The political reality of Aboriginal and Torres Strait Islander people's lives is changing. So too are the health services that seek to serve Aboriginal and Torres Strait Islander people. Community controlled services often rely on government funding, and they face increasing pressure from funders to achieve more with their money and to demonstrate improvements in health outcomes.

The health sector is also changing. New services and organisations have entered regional areas and are actively competing with Indigenous organisations for the right to provide services to Aboriginal and Torres Strait Islander populations. In some places, large general practice clinics are making active attempts to provide services to Indigenous people, and may even employ Aboriginal and Torres Strait Islander staff. This means that many regional communities now offer a wider range of health service options for the community, including the local Aboriginal and Torres Strait Islander population. Many Aboriginal and Torres Strait Islander people can now choose between Indigenous-specific health services and mainstream health services.

New services are also available through Medicare Locals, which operate as regional primary healthcare organisations that work to connect local health services. Medicare Locals are governed by local clinicians and community leaders, and their membership includes a range of organisations involved in providing health services. Some Medicare Locals have an Aboriginal or Torres Strait Islander person on the board or a subcommittee to address the needs of the region's Aboriginal and Torres Strait Islander people. Medicare Locals develop regional strategies that fit within the Closing the Gap campaign (see Chapter 2).

Aboriginal and Torres Strait Islander community controlled health services are beginning to organise themselves into regional groups and alliances built around common interests. One collaboration is the Institute for Urban Indigenous Health (IUIH), which was established in 2009 in response to the needs of Aboriginal and Torres Strait Islander people in Southeast Queensland. The IUIH includes four community controlled health services (ATSICHS Brisbane; Kalwun Health Service, Gold Coast; Yulu-Burri-Ba Aboriginal Corporation for Community Health, Stradbroke Island; and Kambu Medical Centre, Ipswich) and has a partnership with Queensland Health's Inala Aboriginal and Torres Strait Islander Health Service.

Conclusion

Aboriginal and Torres Strait Islander community controlled health services provide a strong model for delivering health services that meet their communities' needs and have demonstrated performance superior to general practice in delivering healthcare to Indigenous people (QPC, 2017). They are operated and managed by Aboriginal and Torres Strait Islander people, and provide services directly to the communities to which they belong. Community controlled health services play a vital role in improving health outcomes for Aboriginal and Torres Strait Islander people.

In tracing the development of ATSICHS Brisbane, this chapter shows how community controlled health services are grounded in the political reality faced by Aboriginal and Torres Strait Islander people. The community controlled health model provides flexibility and allows each service to develop responsive services that are specifically relevant to their communities. Each service operates differently and offers a different range of services. As the community's needs change, so does the health service.

For health professionals, community controlled health services provide an opportunity to deliver community based services that make a significant difference to the health outcomes of Aboriginal and Torres Strait Islander peoples. The work is diverse and rewarding. In many cases, working in a community controlled health service can provide opportunities for skills development that may not be available in other places. Nurses and midwives are encouraged to keep an open mind and think about working in the community controlled sector.

Learning activities

1. Define the role of self-determinism as the underlining principle in the development of Aboriginal and Torres Strait Islander community controlled health services.
2. Outline the significance of primary healthcare being embedded in Aboriginal community controlled health services.
3. Identify the structure of the board of an Aboriginal and Torres Strait Islander community controlled health service. Consider the board's relationship with the Indigenous community it represents.

FURTHER READING

Aboriginal Health & Medical Research Council (2015). *Aboriginal Communities Improving Aboriginal Health: An Evidence Review on the Contribution of Aboriginal Community Controlled Health Services to Improving Aboriginal Health*. Sydney: Aboriginal Health & Medical Research Council.

Adams, M. (2009). Close the Gap: Aboriginal community controlled health services. *Medical Journal of Australia*, 190(10), 593.

Mazel, O. (2016). Self-determination and the right to health: Australian Aboriginal community controlled health services. *Human Rights Law Review*, 16(2), 323–355.

Visit the companion website at www.cambridge.org/highereducation/isbn/9781108794695/resources to see further online resources.

REFERENCES

AIHW (2015). The health and welfare of Australia's Aboriginal and Torres Strait Islander peoples 2015. Cat. no. IHW 147. Canberra: AIHW. Retrieved from www.aihw.gov.au/getmedia/584073f7-041e-4818–9419-39f5a060b1aa/18175.pdf.aspx?inline=true

Aird, M. (2001). *Brisbane Blacks*. Brisbane: Keeaira Press.

ATSICHS Brisbane (2020). About Us. Retrieved from www.atsichsbrisbane.org.au/about-us/our-identity

Best, O. (2004). Community control theory and practice: A case study of the Brisbane Aboriginal and Islander Community Health Service. Unpublished Master's thesis, Griffith University.

Black Panther Party (1972). *Black Panther Party, Brisbane, Manifesto 1972*. Brisbane: Black Panther Party of Australia. Retrieved from www.qhatlas.com.au/photograph/black-panther-party-brisbane-manifesto-1972

Courier-Mail (1971). Aboriginals and police clash, *Courier-Mail*, 24 November.

Department of Aboriginal Affairs (1973). *Associations and Societies: Aboriginal and Islander Community Health Service Brisbane Ltd*. Brisbane: Department of Aboriginal Affairs.

Forsyth, S. (1990). Telling stories: Nurses, politics and Aboriginal Australians, circa 1900–1980s. *Contemporary Nurse: A Journal for the Australian Nursing Profession*, 24(1), 33–4.

Fredericks, B., Adams, K. & Edwards, R. (2011). Aboriginal community control and decolonizing health policy: A yarn from Australia. In H. Lofgren, E. de Leeuw & M. Leahy (eds), *Democratizing Health Consumer Groups in the Policy Process*. Cheltenham: Edward Elgar, pp. 81–96.

Fredericks, B. & Legge, D. (2011). *Revitalizing Health for All: International Indigenous Representative Group Learning from the Experience of Comprehensive Primary Health Care in Australia – A Commentary on Three Project Reports*. Melbourne: The Lowitja Institute.

Huggins, R. & Huggins, J. (1994). *Aunty Rita*. Canberra: Aboriginal Studies Press.

NACCHO (2012). Vision and Principles. Retrieved from www.naccho.org.au/about-us/vision-and-principle

NACCHO (2014). Indigenous health at a glance. Retrieved from www.naccho.org.au/wp-content/uploads/Key-facts-2-Indigenous-health-at-a-glance-FINAL.pdf

NACCHO (2020). *NACCHO*. Retrieved from www.naccho.org.au

National Museum Australia. (2007–08). *Freedom ride, 1965: Collaborating for Indigenous Rights*. Retrieved from www.indigenousrights.net.au/section.asp?sID=33

Perkins, C. (1975). *A Bastard Like Me: Autobiography of Australia's First Aboriginal University Graduate*. Sydney: Ure Smith.

QAIHC (2020a). About QAIHC. Retrieved from www.qaihc.com.au/about

QAIHC (2020b). Our role. Retrieved from www.qaihc.com.au.about/our-role

QPC (2017). *Final Report: Service Delivery in Remote and Discrete Aboriginal and Torres Strait Islander Communities*. Brisbane: Queensland Productivity Commission. Retrieved from https://qpc.blob.core.windows.net/wordpress/2018/06/Service-delivery-Final-Report.pdf

Rintoul, S. (1993). *The Wailing: A National Black Oral History*. Melbourne: Heinemann.

VACCHO & CRCAH (2007). *Communities Working for Health and Wellbeing: Success Stories from the Aboriginal Community Controlled Health Sector in Victoria*. Melbourne: VACCHO & CRCAH.

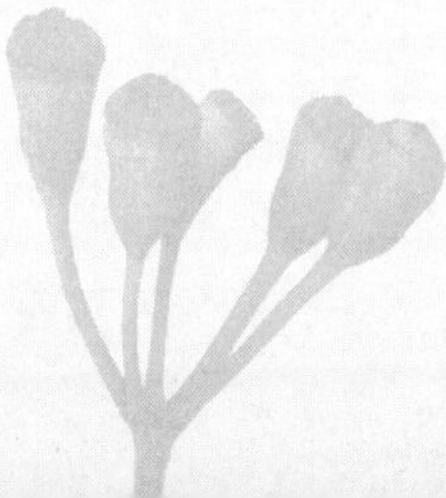

Midwifery practices and Aboriginal and Torres Strait Islander women: Urban and regional perspectives

Machellee Kosiak

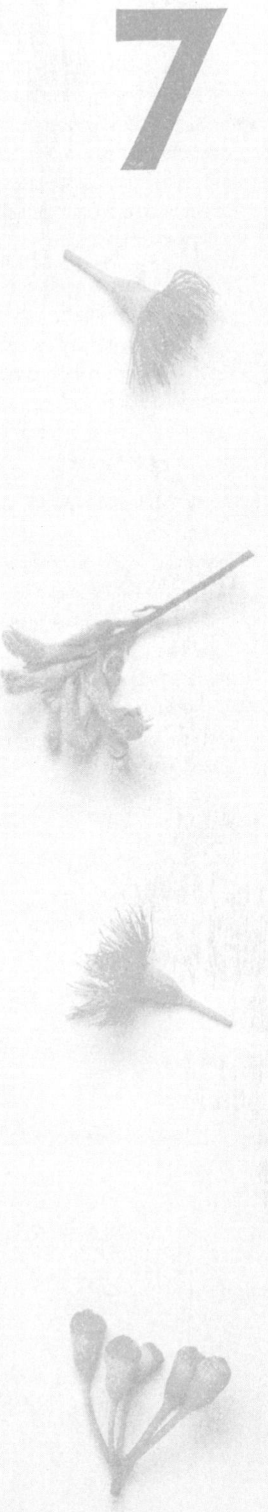

LEARNING OBJECTIVES

This chapter will help you to understand:

- Aboriginal and Torres Strait Islander birthing practices in urban and regional settings
- Traditional Aboriginal and Torres Strait Islander birthing practices
- Recent statistical trends in Aboriginal and Torres Strait Islander births
- Contemporary Aboriginal and Torres Strait Islander birthing practices
- The place of Indigenous-led maternity care services in Australian healthcare
- The role of Indigenous midwives in the workforce
- Maternity care options for Aboriginal and Torres Strait Islander families in urban environments
- Culturally safe maternity care for Aboriginal and Torres Strait Islander women and families

KEY WORDS

birthing on Country
cultural safety in midwifery care
sit down
urban and regional maternity settings
women's business

Introduction

urban and regional maternity settings Maternity services available in major towns and cities, including specialist services such as advanced neonatal, obstetrics and gynaecological services.

cultural safety in midwifery care An approach to nursing practice developed in New Zealand that recognises the importance of cultural understanding and seeks to practise in a way that provides a culturally safe service.

women's business An all-encompassing term used by Indigenous women to describe all things to do with women's social, spiritual, cultural and ceremonial beliefs across their lifespan. These include conception, puberty, menstruation, contraception, abortion, pregnancy, childbirth and menopause.

This chapter discusses the challenges that face Aboriginal and Torres Strait Islander women and their families in **urban and regional maternity settings**. It is written from the framework of **cultural safety in midwifery care** (discussed in Chapter 3).

Giving birth is a significant, intimate, personal and life-changing experience – for all women, across all cultures. It is also a topic of great debate among Indigenous and non-Indigenous health professionals, Elders, communities, women and their families. The debates centre on issues that are particularly relevant to Aboriginal and Torres Strait Islander women, such as accepted birthing and midwifery practices, where women choose to give birth (and whether they are able to choose the location) and whether they have the right to practise cultural and spiritual beliefs about **women's business**. To explore these issues, this chapter provides an historical perspective of birthing and midwifery practices among Aboriginal and Torres Strait Islander women. It then explores some contemporary issues and discusses some of the author's own midwifery experiences.

Giving birth in urban and regional settings: Specific issues for Aboriginal and Torres Strait Islander women

Urban and regional centres provide many specialist services that are important for pregnancy and childbirth, including advanced neonatal, obstetric and gynaecological services. The standard of care is usually high, but they are daunting places for many women, and can be particularly daunting for Aboriginal and Torres Strait Islander families

Although a wide range of services exist within urban and regional centres, they are not necessarily accessible to Aboriginal and Torres Strait Islander women and their families. Accessibility is about more than geographical location: it includes other aspects of physical accessibility, affordability, appropriateness and acceptability (that is, whether the service is culturally safe).

The Australian Institute of Health and Welfare (AIHW, 2019b) classifies rural, metropolitan, regional and remote locations according to population size (with a metropolitan centre having a population of over 100,000). Another interesting way to define towns and cities is to think about the population of Aboriginal and Torres Strait Islander people living there and the availability of culturally safe services – for example:

> major towns and cities, where the Aboriginal and Torres Strait Islander population is a minority within a larger total population, and where 'mainstream' (that is, not Indigenous-specific) health services exist either as the only available health services or as alternative to Indigenous-specific services such as Aboriginal Community Controlled Health Services.
>
> (Scrimgeour & Scrimgeour, 2008, p. 1)

Aboriginal and Torres Strait Islander women face many challenges when they encounter mainstream health services; these are linked to historical factors, colonisation, the healthcare system, family responsibilities and kinship. For example, Aboriginal and Torres Strait Islander women are linked to family, kin and the past in many different, spiritual ways. Family business always takes precedence over the individual's needs. Concepts of time and space are cultural, and are different from those that dominate in mainstream health services.

Aboriginal and Torres Strait Islander people prioritise relationships, so developing relationships between clients and services is vital. In addition, Aboriginal and Torres Strait Islander caregivers may use traditional knowledge that has guided and surrounded women's birthing practices for generations. These cultural differences mean that culturally safe midwifery practices require consideration and flexibility from mainstream health services.

Aboriginal and Torres Strait Islander women in all areas of Australia have a right to culturally safe and supportive birthing experiences. They are increasingly demanding that this cultural right be recognised by mainstream services. The historical lack of understanding was explained clearly by Hancock (2006, p. 4):

> There is inadequate comprehension of Aboriginal women's birthing and postpartum experiences. That is not to refute the significance of traditional knowledge and beliefs Aboriginal women hold, but to emphasise that Aboriginal women's preferences, feelings and encounters with the health system as it impacts on them and their family and community lives during pregnancy and after, are poorly understood and appreciated. Aboriginal women's voices are only infrequently heard, their choices are limited if any, and they are required to adhere to expectations about what is 'good' care for them during pregnancy, birth and after the baby is born. That they do not always 'comply', are often seen as 'difficult' and choose to 'abscond' from medical and hospital care must be recognized as inadequacy of the health system not Aboriginal women's negligence. There is an urgent need for rethinking of the axis of maternity care as it relates to Aboriginal women.

This is changing, however, and there is a slow move from Australian governments and healthcare services to deliver more appropriate maternity services for Aboriginal and Torres Strait Islander women.

In 2012, Australia's Birthing on Country workshop was held in Alice Springs – in part as a response to the National Maternity Services Plan. Women's business and birthing traditions are strong in Central Australia, so Alice Springs seemed a fitting place to hold this discussion about **birthing on Country**. The author was privileged to attend the workshop.

The workshop's keynote speaker was Djapirri Mununggirritij Yirrkala, a respected Elder from East Arnhem Land. She stated:

> Birthing is the most powerful thing that happens to a mother and child ... our generation needs to know the route and identity of where they came from; to ensure pride, passion, dignity and leadership to carry us through to the future; BoC [Birthing on Country] connects Indigenous Australians to the land.
>
> (cited in Kildea, Dennis & Stapleton, 2013, p. 6)

birthing on Country Birthing within the woman's home community and providing care that is culturally and spiritually safe for that woman and her family.

The workshop participants agreed that birthing on Country provides 'the best start in life' for Aboriginal and Torres Strait Islander families. 'Allowing Indigenous women to birth where they live or at their chosen cultural location' (Kildea et al., 2013, p. 12), irrespective of whether the location is urban, regional or remote, is seen as essential. Developing cultural models of care is a fundamental requirement for all birthing services (Kildea et al., 2013).

The National Maternity Services Plan (2010–2015) was completed in 2016. This led the Council of Australian Governments (COAG) Health Council to consult with the Australian Health Ministers Advisory Council (AHMAC), tasked with developing an enduring National Framework for Maternity Services (COAG Health Council, 2017). The National Maternity Services review commenced in 2017, with a review completed in 2019. This review led to the publication of two documents showing encouraging change in strategy development to support improved maternity services for First Nations women and families: *Woman-centred Care: Strategic Directions for Australian Maternity Services* (COAG Health Council, 2019) and *Growing Deadly Families: Aboriginal and Torres Strait Islander Maternity Services Strategy 2019–2025* (Queensland Health, 2019), prepared under the auspices of the COAG Health Council and Queensland Health. These reports particularly investigated and aimed to develop a strategy that would ensure sustainable improvements for Indigenous mothers and babies. It is expected that the review and subsequent reports will support the emergence of continuity of care models for women and more specifically for Aboriginal and Torres Strait Islander women in the rural, remote and urban settings. This will be discussed further into this chapter.

Historical midwifery practice

It seems likely that traditional birthing and midwifery practices varied across Australia according to the traditions of each clan and the resources they had available. Birthing practices were passed on from older women to younger women. These practices were part of women's business that was not shared with men.

Early records suggest that colonisers recognised and valued the birthing practices of Aboriginal and Torres Strait Islander people. In a speech celebrating International Nurses Day in 2009, historian Helen Gregory noted that the traditional knowledge of Indigenous women was highly valued among the colonisers:

> Dame Mary Gilmour reported that many women in many parts of Queensland preferred Aboriginal accouchement assistance to that of unhygienic white doctors and nurses. Puerperal fever resulting from unhygienic obstetric and midwifery practices whether conducted in hospitals or in patients' own homes were the scourge of childbirth in European societies. In contrast, Aboriginal people in north-east Queensland for example, knew nothing of this problem. In that area, women in labour were attended by experienced senior women who ensured that placentas were burnt or deeply buried rather than left to rot in buckets under beds as was often the case in English hospitals.
>
> (Gregory, 2009, p. 3).

This high regard for traditional Aboriginal and Torres Strait Islander practices continued in rural communities until relatively recently. For example, Mawn Young, an Aboriginal nurse, was trained in the 1950s. She recalled growing up on a rural property with her great-grandmother, who was a traditional midwife. She had childhood memories of non-Indigenous cattlemen riding to her lodgings to urgently seek the assistance of her great-grandmother in the birthing of non-Indigenous station owners' wives and their babies (Best, 2012). Mrs Young remembered this continuing until at least the 1940s.

Colonisers sought Indigenous midwives because their birthing practices were by women and were 'safe'. It seems likely that maternal and infant death rates were minimal among Aboriginal women at the time. During the colonial period, records of Indigenous births were not kept by white men. Consequently, birthing was interpreted through the lens of cultural difference and inadequacy. The records could not have provided a complete or accurate view of traditional birthing (Collins, 2004).

In 1791, Lieutenant David Collins recounted the traditional birthing practices of the Eora peoples. His work provided the first recorded account of the birth of an Indigenous baby:

> This is an important record of traditional birthing practices among the Eora people. Only women were present at the labour of War-re-weer. Though they did not manually assist with the delivery, the women provided crucial moral and ritual support, plus a measure of pain relief (cold water poured on the abdomen). After the birth, the Europeans cut the umbilical cord – this was probably a shock to the mother, who may have preferred to ease into a period of separation. After delivery [of] the child and placenta, the mother was 'smoked' with herbs to aid her recovery, and indeed she quickly returned to her usual duties, with her baby by her side.
>
> (Collins, 2004, n.p.)

Although traditional birthing practices were highly valued within local communities, they gradually disappeared during the colonial period. The forced relocation of Aboriginal and Torres Strait Islander people during the Acts of Administration saw the demise of many of the traditional ways of knowing and doing. Any traditional midwifery practices in use today are very different from those used before colonial times.

Not all descriptions of traditional birthing practices during the colonial era were appropriate or accurate. For example, Bates' (2014) recollections of writings from the 1930s and Roth's (1897) discussion of the 1890s demonstrated gross ignorance and highly derogatory language. In Roth's anthropologically derived writings, birthing among Aboriginal women was placed in the section on ethno-pornography.

QUESTIONS FOR REFLECTION

- If traditional birthing practices were valued by Australia's colonisers, why did they disappear over time?
- Why are there few remaining records of traditional birthing practices?

Aboriginal and Torres Strait Islander peoples: An overview of maternal and neonatal statistics today

Population and location

Today's Aboriginal and Torres Strait Islander populations are diverse. Indigenous people live in many different places and have varied lifestyles (Eckermann et al., 2010). Australia remains one of the world's most highly urbanised yet sparsely populated countries – two people per square kilometre (ABS, 2018), The majority of the population (86 per cent) live in urban areas with almost two-thirds residing in capital cities (ABS, 2018). Currently, 3.3 per cent of Australia's population identifies as Aboriginal and/or Torres Strait Islander. A large majority of Aboriginal and Torres Strait Islander people live in urban, metropolitan centres – not in rural and remote areas of Australia as commonly assumed (AIHW, 2016). Areas noted to be experiencing significant growth are not surprisingly all coastal areas, such as Perth in Western Australia, the Gold Coast, Sunshine Coast and Townsville in Queensland, and Newcastle in New South Wales (ABS, 2018). This urban concentration is strongly linked to the historical dislocation of families, which has been discussed in previous chapters.

Australia's Aboriginal and Torres Strait Islander population is relatively youthful. In 2016, the median age of Indigenous people was 23.0 years, compared with 37.8 years for non-Indigenous people (ABS, 2018).

Fertility

Aboriginal and Torres Strait Islander people have a higher fertility rate than other Australians. Data presented by the ABS show the total fertility rate for Aboriginal and Torres Strait Islander women was estimated to be 2.37 babies per woman, compared with 1.74 babies per woman for all women in Australia (ABS, 2019). According to data from the AIHW (2020c), the higher fertility rate is explained by the age spread of the Aboriginal and Torres Strait Islander population: the younger overall population indicates higher fertility rates. In addition, deaths among Indigenous Australians – both women and men – occur at younger ages than among non-Indigenous Australians.

The fertility rate for Aboriginal and Torres Strait Islander women has fallen in recent decades, from around 5.8 babies per woman in the 1960s to 2.4 babies per woman in 2007. In 2010, it had risen to 2.57 babies per woman, which is higher than the fertility rate for the total Australian female population (of 1.89 babies per woman in 2010). In 2010, 75 per cent of births to Aboriginal and Torres Strait Islander women were to women aged under 30 years, compared with 45 per cent of births to all Australian women (ABS, 2012).

In 2018, the mean age of Aboriginal and Torres Strait Islander mothers was 26.0 years, six times younger than mean age of all other mothers (31.4 years); however, the teenage (15–19) fertility rate for Aboriginal and Torres Strait Islanders women was five times the teenage fertility rate for all Australian women (Figure 7.1).

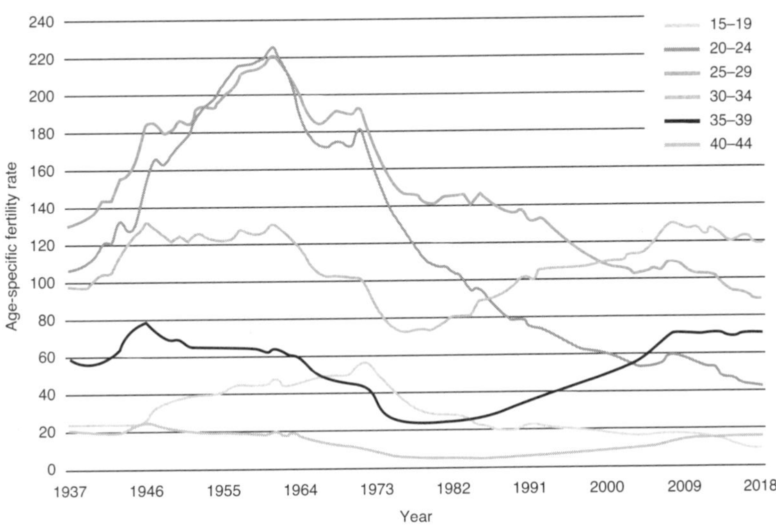

Figure 7.1 Age-specific fertility rates, 1937 to 2018; births per 1000 women

Source: ABS (2019).

Anecdotally, First Nations fertility rates appear to be declining due to a possible increase in teenage awareness and uptake of contraception (Figure 7.2). More accurate statistics will not be available until the next census, scheduled for 2021.

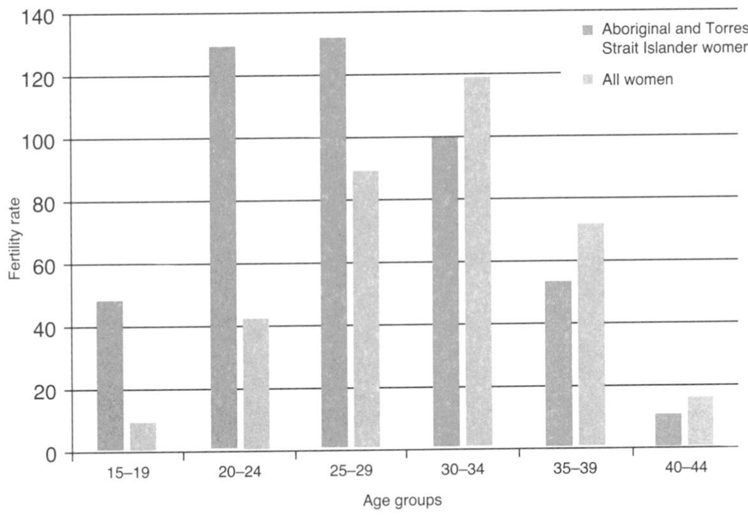

Figure 7.2 Age-specific fertility rates, Aboriginal and Torres Strait Islander women and all women – 2018; births per 1000 women

Source: ABS (2019).

Life expectancy and maternal health

The life-expectancy gap between Aboriginal and Torres Strait Islanders and other Australians is significant. Life expectancy is reported in three-year cycles. In 2015–17, Aboriginal and Torres Strait Islander life expectancy was estimated to be 75.6 years for females and 71.6 years for males, a lower life expectancy of 7.8 years for females and

8.6 years for males compared with other Australians. As discussed comprehensively in Chapter 2, between 2010–12 and 2015–17, there was a small, non-significant reduction in the difference of 1.9 years for females and 2.5 years for males (DPMC, 2020).

Life expectancy is partly influenced by the maternal risk factors encountered by Aboriginal and Torres Strait Islander women, such as smoking, harmful consumption of alcohol, illicit drug use, poor nutrition, diabetes and exposure to violence (AIHW, 2011). These risk factors can lead to pre-term births (prior to 37 weeks of gestation), which brings the risk of a range of adverse neonatal outcomes. In 2010, 13.5 per cent of babies born to Aboriginal and Torres Strait Islander women were pre-term, compared with 8 per cent of babies born to non-Indigenous women.

Birthweight

Pre-term birth (before 37-week gestation) is linked to greater risk of significant morbidity and mortality in newborn babies (AIHW, 2020b; Li et al., 2012). Many babies born to Aboriginal and Torres Strait Islander women have low birthweight (Figure 7.3), which brings significant and well-recognised health risks. Birthweight is a key indicator of immediate and future health for the newborn. Infants born with normal birthweight are less likely to develop chronic disease in later life. According to the latest national perinatal statistics (AIHW, 2014; Li et al., 2012), low birthweight occurs at twice the rate among Aboriginal and Torres Strait Islander women than it does among other Australian women. Approximately 12 per cent of live-born Aboriginal and Torres Strait Islander babies had low birthweight, compared with 6 per cent of those born to non-Indigenous women. However, in the recently updated report by the AIHW (2020b), *Australia's Mothers and Babies 2018*, these statistics were slightly lowered for babies of Indigenous mothers, with 14 per cent born pre-term compared with 8.5 per cent of babies of non-Indigenous mothers and 11.7 per cent being of low birthweight (AIHW, 2020b). See the Further Reading section at the end of the chapter for a link to the full report.

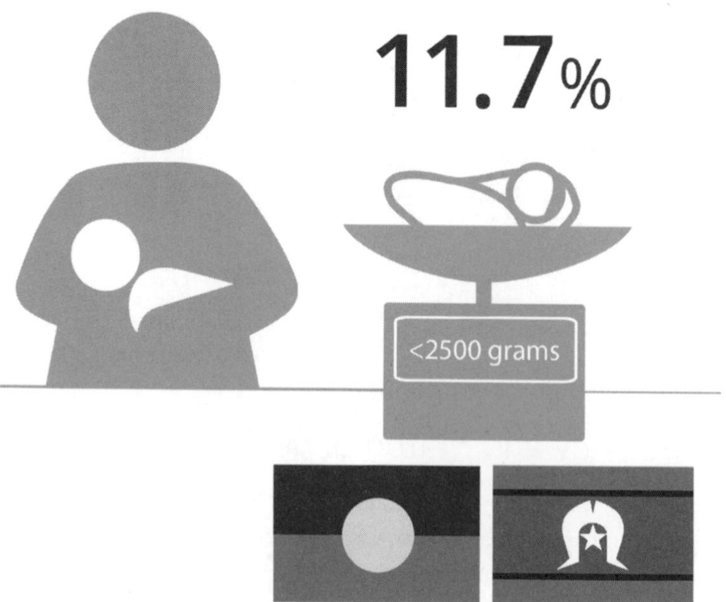

Figure 7.3 Proportion of low-birthweight babies of Indigenous mothers in 2018
Source: AIHW (2020b, p. 47).

Low birthweight (LBW) is shown to be increased with remoteness. This is directly related to the lack of maternity and Indigenous-related services (AIHW, 2020b; DPMC, 2020); however, it continuing to be relatively high, at 10.6 per cent, in urban areas (AIHW, 2020b) (Figure 7.4).

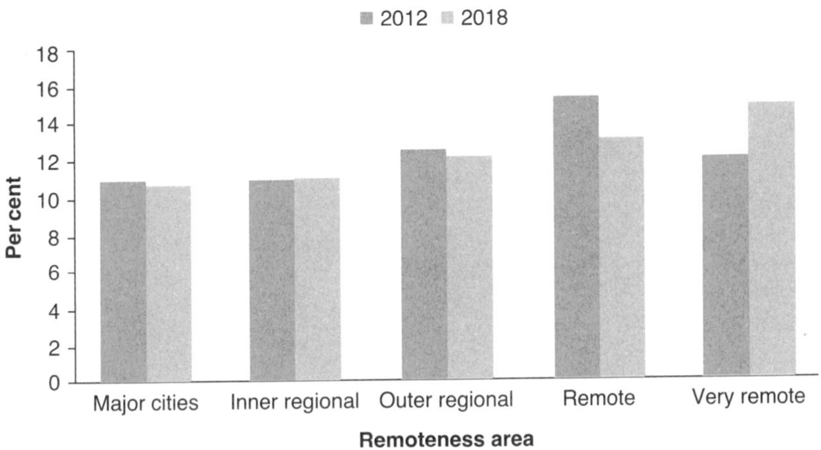

Figure 7.4 Low birthweight of liveborn babies of Indigenous mothers, by remoteness, 2012 and 2018

Source: AIHW (2020b, p. 48).

The AIHW (2020a) summarises the risks associated with low and high birthweight as follows:

- Low birthweight babies (less than 2500 grams) are more likely to die in infancy or to be at increased risk of illness in infancy. Low birthweight is closely associated with pre-term birth – almost three in four low birthweight babies were pre-term, and more than half of pre-term babies were of low birthweight in 2017 (AIHW, 2020a). Babies may also be low birthweight because they are small for gestational age, while some low-birthweight babies may be both pre-term and small for gestational age.
- High birthweight (4500 grams or more) is also of concern. Data from twelve high, middle and low-income countries indicate that higher birthweight was associated with increased odds of obesity among children aged nine to eleven years (AIHW, 2020a; Qiao et al., 2015).

The AIHW (2020d) reported that as of June 2019, 86 per cent of Indigenous babies in the previous year had a normal birthweight. Rates of normal birthweight were highest in Queensland and South Australia (both 89 per cent), and in major cities and inner regional areas (both 88 per cent), and lowest in Victoria/Tasmania (82 per cent combined) and remote areas (82 per cent) (AIHW, 2020d).

Interestingly, infant birthweights are increasing across Australia and so is women's Body Mass Index (BMI). For non-pregnant women, the healthy BMI (defined as the ratio of weight and height (kg/m2)) range is 18.5 to 24.9. While increases in BMI are expected during pregnancy, a BMI of 30 or more at the first antenatal visit is considered obesity during pregnancy (AIHW, 2020b) (Figure 7.5).

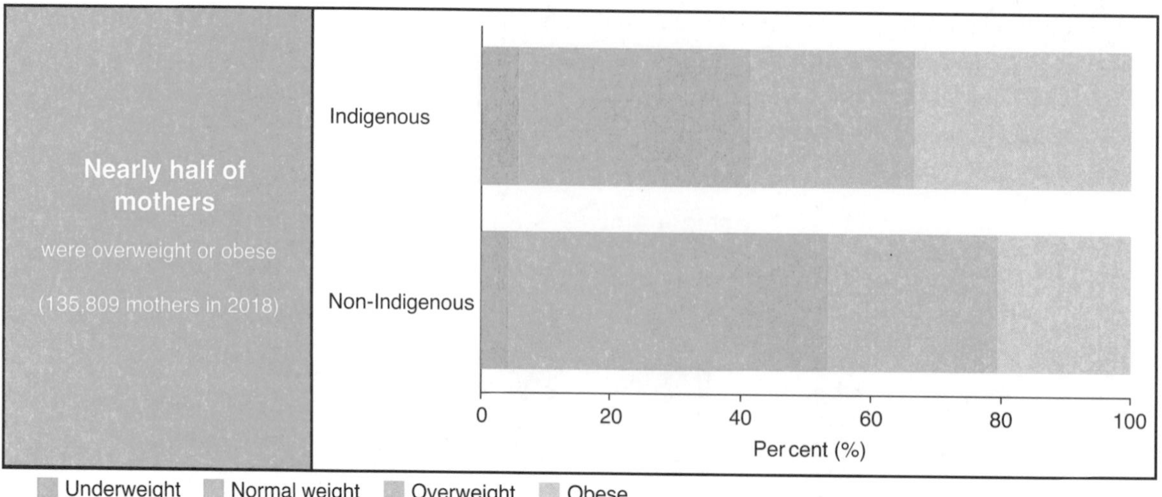

Figure 7.5 BMI by Indigenous status of mother, 2018

Notes

1 Age-standardised percentage calculated after excluding records with Not stated values. Care must be taken when interpreting percentages.
2 Percentages are directly age-standardised using the 30 June 2001 Australian female Estimated Resident Population (ERP) aged 15–44 as the standard population. Five-year age groups are used for age-standardisation. The lowest age group was 15–19 years and the highest was 40–44 years.

Source: AIHW (2020c).

QUESTIONS FOR REFLECTION

- What are the health implications for high or large for gestational age babies?
- Why would a baby be of a high birthweight? Consider the implications for both mother and baby.

Maternal health BMI risk factors: Gestational diabetes

Diabetes affecting pregnancy can be pre-existing (type 1 or 2), or it can develop during pregnancy (gestational diabetes) (AIHW, 2019a). Gestational diabetes mellitus (GDM) is a form of diabetes that occurs in pregnancy, which can lead to type 2 diabetes It can have significant complications and affect pregnancy outcomes (AIHW, 2019a).

Diabetes is a significant maternal risk factor for Aboriginal and Torres Strait Islander women (Figure 7.6). The disease can have an impact on both women and their babies – affecting neonatal birthweight and the lifelong health of mother and baby. Aboriginal and Torres Strait Islander mothers are more likely to develop type 2 diabetes and are of greater risk of GDM than non-Indigenous mothers (AIHW, 2020b). The AIHW (2019a) estimates that diabetes affects three to four times more Indigenous women than non-Indigenous women. Data show pregnant Indigenous women have an elevated risk of diabetes, metabolic problems and high blood pressure (ABS, 2012; AIHW, 2019a). Aboriginal and Torres Strait Islander women are more than ten times more likely to have type 2 diabetes during pregnancy and 1.5 times more likely to have GDM compared with other Australian women. More than 50 per cent of Indigenous women with GDM are under 30 years of age, compared with less than one-third of other Australian women with GDM (ABS, 2012; AIHW, 2019a).

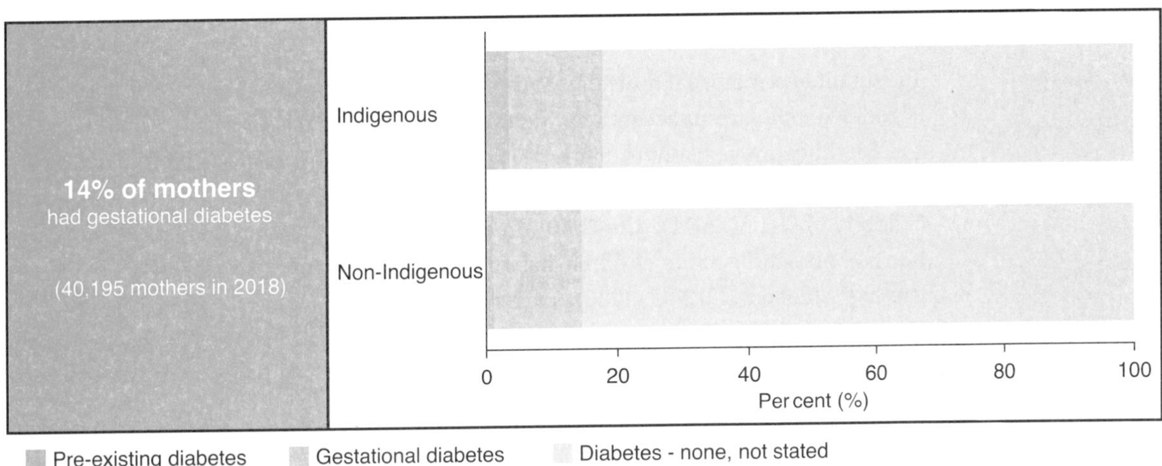

Figure 7.6 Diabetes status and Indigenous status of mother, 2018

Note: Percentages are directly age-standardised using the 30 June 2001 Australian female Estimated Resident Population (ERP) aged 15–44 as the standard population. Five-year age groups are used for age-standardisation. The lowest age group was 15–19 years and the highest was 40–44 years.

Source: AIHW (2020c).

Positive trends for Indigenous mothers

An increase in services providing culturally safe maternity care in urban, regional and remote areas has seen a rise in First Nations mothers accessing antenatal care at earlier gestations (AIHW, 2020b). It has been noted that early antenatal care and engagement have positive consequences and lead to improvements to maternal and infant health outcomes for Indigenous mothers and babies (Kildea et al., 2019).

Women-focused and culturally safe antenatal care includes targeting areas such as reduction or cessation of smoking, lifestyle concerns (e.g. weight), preventing and managing chronic conditions including diabetes mellitus and GDM, social and emotional factors, perinatal mental health, the link between domestic violence and gestational age at birth, birthweight, and work in stillbirth and neonatal deaths.

Recent years have also seen improvements in antenatal care attendance during the first trimester (from 49 per cent in 2012 to 65 per cent in 2018) and a reduction in smoking at any time during pregnancy (from 49 per cent in 2010 to 44 per cent in 2018). The proportion of babies who were small for gestational age born to Indigenous mothers also decreased from 14.4 per cent in 2013 to 13.8 per cent in 2018 (AIHW, 2020b).

QUESTIONS FOR REFLECTION

- Have you cared for a woman with GDM?
- Consider and list three implications of maternal and neonatal outcomes for an Aboriginal woman with GDM.
- What would be some identified risk factors? Consider BMI.
- As a health practitioner, if you saw an Aboriginal woman being stereotyped in the clinic at which you are working, what would you do?

Infant mortality and morbidity

The infant and maternal mortality and morbidity rates of Aboriginal and Torres Strait Islander people are unacceptably high. Aboriginal and Torres Strait Islander babies are 2.1 times more likely to die in their first year of life (AIHW, 2018) In addition, their mothers are twice as likely as other Australians to die during pregnancy and childbirth (AIHW, 2011). The 2020 *Closing the Gap Report* documents 'the mortality rate for non-Indigenous children has improved at a faster rate and as a result, the gap has widened' (DPMC, 2020), suggesting that this shows no significant change to infant mortality and morbidity rates. These data show that maternal health is a key driver of health outcomes for mothers and children; they include health and social determinants such as obesity, diabetes, smoking and alcohol use (DPMC, 2020).

It is significant that some Aboriginal and Torres Strait Islander women believe giving birth in hospital causes infant mortality. They believe babies get sick and die because of a 'weakened spirit' because they are not welcomed into the world with the appropriate ceremonies (such as smoking ceremonies), which may be custom within a woman's community (Aunty Pamela M. Connolly, personal communication, 2015).

For all these reasons, and with the support of Elders and community, increasing the number of trained local women to be midwives to enable more birth on country will make a difference to maternal and neonatal health outcomes. Indigenous midwives supporting Indigenous women will make a significant difference to our long-term life expectancy. Positive outcomes will occur when Aboriginal and Torres Strait Islander women have access to a known midwife, in a culturally safe continuity model.

Indigenous identification

The accuracy of data describing the health of Aboriginal and Torres Strait Islander people is questionable. One major contributing factor is that those who attend health services may not be asked whether they identify as being an Aboriginal or Torres Strait Islander person. When women give birth, they are often not asked whether they 'identify as Indigenous' and they are frequently not asked about their partner's Indigenous status. It is critically important that an initial clinical assessment includes socio-demographic and cultural assessment in addition to the more fundamental and observation-based clinical assessments. Without this basic information, we cannot hope to provide culturally safe healthcare. Identifying the newborn as Aboriginal and/or Torres Strait Islander is essential for acknowledging the child's Indigeneity and for accurate data collection.

QUESTIONS FOR REFLECTION

- Why is it important to know whether a woman and/or her partner identify as Indigenous?
- How might this knowledge influence your midwifery practice?
- If you were from another country, how would you feel when you saw a person from your country? Would you consider yourself to be safe?

Contemporary midwifery practice

Contemporary approaches recognise that birthing and midwifery practices are important aspects of connection to Country and identity for Aboriginal and Torres Strait Islander people. There is an increasing move to give women greater choice about where and how they give birth.

Aboriginal and Torres Strait Islander women typically give birth in mainstream health services. Those living in remote communities are transported to large regional centres. (See Chapter 8 for an extended discussion of the birthing and midwifery issues relevant to people who live in remote communities.)

For many Aboriginal and Torres Strait Islander women, attending hospital for their baby's birth is a frightening and alienating experience. Some Aboriginal and Torres Strait Islander women believe that their relationship with the land is established through the birthing experience and is vitally important to their culture. For these women, giving birth in hospitals where they do not feel culturally safe can present major difficulties, both culturally and spiritually.

In many situations, current healthcare practices for Aboriginal and Torres Strait Islander women do not take into account their community or cultural wishes for childbirth. Some women wish to give birth on their own terms, surrounded by their choice of family and support people in a culturally safe environment. Many women want to be as close as possible to their home communities. The 2008 initial Maternity Services Review (Department of Health, 2009) highlighted the importance of developing culturally safe care for Indigenous women.

In 2005, the Queensland government released a report titled *Re-Birthing, Report of the Review of Maternity Services in Queensland* (Hirst, 2005). While the report did not include recommendations for Aboriginal and Torres Strait Islander women in urban centres, it did highlight three priorities for change: improving the poor outcomes for Aboriginal and Torres Strait Islander people; care of women who live in rural and remote locations; and establishing postnatal care services. Unfortunately, these priorities for change were not implemented.

Four years later, the Improving Maternity Services in Australia Report (Maternity Services Review, 2009) included a discussion of the different needs of women who live and give birth in urban and regional areas (Kildea & Wardaguga, 2009). In this report, the Queensland government recommended principles for the development of local maternity care that *feels* local and *feels* as though it is owned by the women who use it. This approach reflects a theme commonly expressed by Aboriginal and Torres Strait women across Australia: that 'Elders, who are the cultural custodians of birthing skills, knowledge and practices are passing away without having the opportunity to hand down this knowledge' (Kildea & Wardaguga, 2009).

The Grandmothers, traditional custodians of women's Business, believe it is important to act quickly to ensure that Aboriginal and Torres Strait Islander women have the opportunity to provide care, on their Country, in their own way (Kildea & Wardaguga, 2009). Many Aboriginal and Torres Strait Islander Australians believe that removing women from their home communities to give birth contributes to poorer long-term social, emotional and physical health. Indigenous women leave their communities in early pregnancy, going to an urban setting to '**sit down**' while awaiting the birth of their baby (discussed below and in Chapter 8).

sit down A term that refers to the period of time women spend away from their home awaiting the birth of their baby. They usually stay in a hostel.

A similar circumstance was experienced by the Canadian Inuit peoples (Van Wagner et al., 2007). It has been particularly evident with a lack of, or reduction in, the maternity services that were previously available within Australian Indigenous communities.

Providing control at the community level brings opportunities for positive community outcomes to occur. Birthing on communities may be a way to positively engage the support of partners, family members and the wider community in order to bring about the social change that is needed in order to grow physically, spiritually and emotionally strong Indigenous communities.

Indigenous-led urban and regional models of care

This section introduces urban and regional models of care using the example of two specific Indigenous-specific clinics that have been set up at the Mater Misericordae Public and Caboolture Hospitals in Queensland.

The Murri Clinic at Mater Mothers' Misericordiae Public Hospital, Brisbane

It was a privilege for the author, as an Indigenous midwife, to help a friend, Denise Watego, a Noonuccal Elder from Stradbroke Island, to establish the first Indigenous-specific antenatal clinic for Aboriginal and Torres Strait Islander women in an inner-city tertiary hospital. Denise, an indefatigable champion of efforts to improve maternal and infant health, launched the service in the basement of the old Mater Mothers' Hospital in Brisbane. She provided continuing support in her role as Indigenous liaison officer, and thus the Murri Clinic at the Mater Mothers' Hospital was born.

Sadly, Denise has passed away, but she would be proud of the work we are doing to increase care for women and support the Indigenous midwifery workforce. A specific antenatal clinic for Murri women has been in operation since 2004 in response to an identified need to provide culturally safe care to Indigenous childbearing women and their families attending the Mater Mothers' Hospital. It is structured as a midwifery-led medical collaboration.

The clinic provides Indigenous women with an environment in which they feel comfortable and believe they will be treated with respect and dignity. Partners and other family members, including grandmothers and children, are encouraged to be present.

As concerns arise during a woman's care, they are resolved with the active involvement of the hospital's Indigenous liaison staff. One outcome of this practice has been a noticeable decrease in active one-on-one consultations between women and the social worker. Complex issues are discussed through *collaboration* between the Indigenous liaison staff, midwives, doctors, social workers and, if relevant, child protection liaison officers. Through a collaborative and collegial process, the staff work as a team and form an action plan to benefit both the mother and baby.

Following a successful evaluation of the Murri Clinic in October 2013, the Mater Mothers' Public hospital extended the clinic's services by launching an Indigenous midwifery group model of care. This program aims to close the gap in maternal and infant health outcomes in the Brisbane urban Aboriginal and Torres Strait Islander community. The Mater has partnered with the Institute of Urban Indigenous Health and the Aboriginal and Torres Strait Islander Community Health Service, Brisbane, to launch this initiative. The group includes four non-Indigenous midwives who work alongside Indigenous maternal and infant health workers and Indigenous liaison officers to offer continuity of care during the antenatal, birthing and postnatal periods.

Ngarrama Birthing Service at Caboolture Hospital, Queensland

Caboolture Hospital established an Aboriginal and Torres Strait Islander maternity service in response to the need for improved collaborative care for Aboriginal and Torres Strait Islander women, their families and the community.

The service was named 'Ngarrama' following community consultation with grandmothers and aunts in the area. *Ngarrama*, which means 'Guardian Birth Spirit', is from the Yuwaalayaay language. An Aunt gave permission from the traditional owners to use the name for the service to be provided at Kabul (the traditional Aboriginal name for Caboolture).

The maternity service is based on Queensland Health's goal to close the gap in health outcomes for Indigenous Queenslanders by 2033. Queensland Health highlighted the need for a midwifery-led, all-risk model of care. The Ngarrama maternity service is built on the premise that closing the gap in life expectancy is everyone's business – and this means changing practice.

Ngarrama maternity service is a specialty service offered to women of Aboriginal and Torres Strait Islander descent (or women whose partners are Indigenous). The service aims to better meet the needs of the growing numbers of Aboriginal and Torres Strait Islander women who live in the Caboolture area. The service is staffed by an Indigenous maternal and infant health worker, an Indigenous midwife and a non-Indigenous midwife. Care includes antenatal, birthing and postnatal follow-up, both in the hospital and in the community. The service also offers belly casting as an antenatal incentive. Belly casting is when a caste, usually made of plaster of Paris (gysum plaster), is made of the woman's pregnant belly; this birth art has proven to be a powerful healing tool for women and families.

This all-risk, midwifery-led model delivers comprehensive care to Aboriginal and Torres Strait Islander mothers and their babies. Women present with complex issues and histories that include obstetric, medical, social and family situations. Some women also present with chronic disease and psychosocial issues such as perinatal depression, domestic violence and child protection concerns. While the service is new, its successes in the local community are clear, with anecdotal evidence from the community and increasing attendance figures indicating increasing birth rates.

Both the Murri Clinic and Ngarrama birthing service offer choices for Aboriginal and Torres Strait Islander women in an urban environment. Not all Aboriginal and Torres Strait Islander women choose an Indigenous model for antenatal care, but for the first time the availability of these services allows them to make culturally safe choices. Staff members at these services have the benefit of appropriate education, which enhances the care provided and delivers a service that is welcoming, and both clinically and culturally safe.

Building an Indigenous midwifery workforce

The contemporary focus on training Aboriginal and Torres Strait Islander women to become midwives is helping to improve the extent of culturally safe care available for Indigenous women. This shift is happening both within Indigenous-specific services and in mainstream health services.

In addition to providing direct services for Aboriginal and Torres Strait Islander women, Aboriginal and Torres Strait Islander midwives are able to guide non-Indigenous, mainstream maternity service providers about their interactions with Indigenous women. Their work can help to ensure greater cultural safety, equity and increased access for Aboriginal and Torres Strait Islander women.

There remain many barriers for Aboriginal and Torres Strait Islander women entering tertiary education. Some of these include family commitments and community expectations, geographical remoteness, reduced access to transport, literacy issues, self-doubt, low self-esteem and lack of confidence. The government scholarships available to Aboriginal and Torres Strait Islander women usually do not sufficiently cover the incidental and ongoing expenses associated with studying an intensive three-year tertiary program. The combination of highly demanding academic study and extensive practice placements poses challenges for many students.

Despite the challenges, supporting Aboriginal and Torres Strait Islander communities to 'grow our own' midwives and healthcare professionals is essential to improving maternity healthcare and healthcare more generally. Supporting Indigenous students through midwifery training is a significant and necessary step towards improving perinatal outcomes for Aboriginal and Torres Strait Islander mothers and babies. Empowering Aboriginal and Torres Strait Islander women to participate in midwifery practice will encourage more widespread acceptance of culturally safe care and improve outcomes for Indigenous mothers and babies. In addition, empowering Aboriginal and Torres Strait Islander people through education will increase their skills, self-esteem and community status, and will contribute to an overall increase in the Indigenous workforce Australia wide.

The importance of recruiting and retaining Indigenous nurses and developing their ability to provide the most appropriate care for Indigenous people has been studied and described (e.g. Goold, 2006; West, Usher & Foster, 2010). However, there is little research discussing the Indigenous midwifery workforce. Health Workforce Australia identified only 60 Indigenous midwives across Australia in 2010 (AHMAC, 2011; AIWH, 2011). These limited midwifery workforce numbers suggest that both access to training and retention are important and significant issues (AHMAC, 2011). In 2017, the Indigenous midwifery workforce numbers increased to 293 midwives nationally. This is only 1 per cent of the total midwifery workforce (AIHW 2018). To make significant changes to maternal and infant mortality, a skilled Indigenous midwifery workforce is required. These numbers must be increased! it is hoped that significant improvement in workforce numbers will be seen after the 2021 census. Strategies by Australian universities to graduate midwives will be discussed later in the chapter.

A key recommendation for increasing the cultural safety of antenatal care is employing Indigenous midwives (Kildea et al., 2010). In remote Canada, the training of Indigenous midwives is thought to have contributed significantly to improved maternal and infant health outcomes (Couchie & Sanderson, 2007). There is good reason to believe that similar results could be achieved in Australia.

The Australian Catholic University recently commenced teaching a Bachelor of Midwifery (Indigenous) course, which had its first Indigenous midwifery graduates in 2013. Delivering programs that are specifically designed to address Indigenous midwifery issues and that provide the flexibility, creativity and resources needed by students from rural and remote locales are essential elements in increasing the numbers of Indigenous midwives working in Australia. Increasing the number of Aboriginal and Torres Strait Islander midwives practising throughout Australia – both in rural and remote communities, and in urban centres – will make a significant contribution towards providing better maternal outcomes for Indigenous women and their babies.

Cultural issues relevant to accessing maternity services

The importance of antenatal care

Availability of and access to quality antenatal care are universally recognised as predictors of perinatal and maternal outcomes. The gap between Indigenous and non-Indigenous health outcomes remains significant, and it is no coincidence that Indigenous women access antenatal care differently from other Australian women. The fear and mistrust that many Aboriginal and Torres Strait Islander people feel about health services can cause them to avoid mainstream care; this includes antenatal care until late in pregnancy, where the mother may either attend irregularly or not at all. Among Aboriginal and Torres Strait Islander women, late presentation for antenatal care is common. The first antenatal appointment is often at 24 weeks' gestation or later. Fewer antenatal visits follow. Poor birth outcomes are often associated with inadequate or compromised antenatal care.

Research confirms that providing culturally safe antenatal care that is well used by women and providing a healthy environment for the mother can improve the chances that her baby is a healthy birthweight (Herceg, 2005). Antenatal care may be especially important for Aboriginal and Torres Strait Islander women because of their higher risk of low-birthweight babies and greater exposure to other risk factors such as anaemia, poor nutritional status, hypertension, diabetes, smoking, and genital and urinary tract infections (de Costa & Child, 1996).

A variety of factors, in effect, prevent Indigenous women from presenting early for antenatal care. Geographical location is an obvious one, but historical barriers, such as the dislocation of families, removal of children and intervention by the Department of Child Safety are also significant. Many Aboriginal and Torres Strait Islander women are suspicious about antenatal care. In addition, socioeconomic and educational factors, transportation, the availability of local clinics and cultural safety are all factors that work against strong take-up of antenatal care.

Birthing on Country

For women living in rural and remote communities, travelling to urban centres for healthcare increases the burden for them and their families. Even today in most rural and remote communities, Indigenous women are taken from their community at 36 weeks of pregnancy to 'sit down'. Even those women who are considered 'low risk' are taken to be cared for in large urban centre. If women are considered 'at risk', they may be admitted to hospital (this applies equally to urban Aboriginal and Torres Strait Islander women, who may be admitted to a large hospital in their home city).

Many women are sent to health services located far away from their homes and communities and during this time do not have family support or a familiar person to guide them. They may never have been away from their community before, and this may be their first baby. They are likely to be alone and frightened. Quite possibly, English is not their first language.

These women may have to leave other children behind, be alone in a strange place and navigate an unfamiliar health system. All of the many little things that most Australian women find joyous about having a baby can be diminished, and the women may be burdened with psychological, emotional and financial stresses, and deep anxieties. When a woman is relocated to an unknown and unfamiliar place to give birth, her basic, culturally significant learning processes are fractured.

Women living in urban locations may also feel torn, as they may have been forced to move from their communities for work, study or a variety of family reasons. In addition, urban Indigenous families often face distinct challenges related to marginalisation and transgenerational trauma (Atkinson, 2002). They have been dislocated from their land, their culture, their community and often their own families. As a result of many levels of loss and trauma, the current generation is left with anxiety, rage, depression and a sense of helplessness in the face of conditions over which they feel they have no control.

In contrast, the traditional practice of birthing on one's own Country provides access to physical and spiritual support. Within their community, young women observe other women in the family. Birthing on Country helps young women to learn 'women's ways', see other women having babies, learn to cope with motherhood, be supported physically, spiritually and emotionally, and learn how to build a strong community.

QUESTIONS FOR REFLECTION

- How might an urban system that is alien to women from rural and remote communities provide safe cultural and spiritual care at such a significant time in their life?
- How might access to antenatal care be improved and promoted for Aboriginal and Torres Strait Islander women?
- How might women who are removed from their homes and families for the birth of their babies become strong women for their children? How might their cultural traditions about birthing be maintained?

Providing culturally safe midwifery care

Recent literature builds on the guidelines developed by the Australian College of Midwives (ACM, 2003) and details ways in which midwives might provide effective care for Aboriginal and Torres Strait women. Important considerations include:

- having a specific location for women and children that provides a safe, welcoming and flexible maternity service
- providing continuity of care and integration with other Indigenous and non-Indigenous services
- including home outreach (antenatal and postnatal) visits
- basing midwifery practice on communication, respect, relationships and trust
- ensuring that health service staff and caregivers show respect for family involvement
- having an appropriately trained workforce – with training in cultural safety
- providing, whenever possible, Aboriginal and Torres Strait Islander women with female caregivers and Aboriginal and Torres Strait Islander caregivers
- providing community based and/or community-controlled services
- providing transportation, childcare or playgroups (Herceg, 2005, pp. 3–4).

In order to achieve healthier outcomes for Indigenous women and their families, continuity of care is a basic necessity during and after pregnancy and childbirth. Continuity of care and caregivers, particularly the continuity of one central staff member, can ensure that midwifery:

- integrates with other services (such as an Aboriginal Medical Service or the hospital)
- has a focus on effective communication, relationship building and trust
- demonstrates respect for Aboriginal and Torres Strait Islander cultures
- provides for family involvement and care of other children
- provides an appropriately trained workforce
- prioritises Indigenous staff and female staff
- ensures that women give informed consent and have the right of refusal (AHMAC, 2011; Dudgeon, Wright & Coffin, 2010; Herceg, 2005; Reibel & Walker, 2010).

Contemporary midwifery practices can be linked to traditional skills and cultural traditions. By recognising the skills of traditional midwives and the wisdom of culture, midwives are able to support Aboriginal and Torres Strait Islander women throughout pregnancy and childbirth. Continuity of the caregiver is particularly important. Cultural practices, such as the smoking ceremony to welcome a baby to the community after the mother has travelled a long distance for the birth, are still performed and respected. These practices are believed to keep the baby healthy, heal the mother and reinforce their connection to the land. For women who live in urban and regional areas, these practices may be equally important and must be considered.

Culturally safe midwifery practice

Cultural safety in health services happens when people feel fully able to use a service provided by people from another culture without risk to their own (Ramsden, 2002).

This section builds on the discussion in Chapter 3 about culturally safe nursing practice, with a particular focus on the specialised field of midwifery. Through case study examples of Indigenous women and their birthing experiences, this section discusses cultural safety as it is relevant to midwifery in the Australian context.

Reflecting on your own practice

In order to provide culturally safe care in their practice, midwives must recognise and understand the importance of self-reflection. As Cox and Taua (2013), p. 329) note, 'reflective practice is a critical aspect of providing culturally safe care'.

Reflective practice can seem difficult, but it is a powerful tool for ensuring culturally safe practice for clients. Reflective practice is not just undertaken for Aboriginal and Torres Strait Islander people: it must be practised by all midwives who are looking after clients who are different from themselves. As noted in Chapter 3, self-reflection can help to expose the cultural issues relevant to midwifery clients and their families, midwifery practitioners' own personal cultural assumptions and practices, and the space between the two. A key benefit of regular self-reflection about midwifery care is the opportunity it provides to think about and initiate changes in practice. The goal of self-reflection is to improve professional practice and develop skills in a way that provides cultural safety for clients. As midwives, in our self-reflective practice we need to be asking ourselves the following questions: Are our general interactions culturally safe? What might be our cultural biases towards our clients? What do we do if our biases, assumptions and stereotypes are identified in the care we provide?

When working as a midwife, it is essential to be alert to one's own cultural biases and to question whether one's practices are appropriate for clients and their families. It is important for the midwife to ask constantly whether their actions are appropriate in ensuring that the care provided is culturally safe and sensitive to the needs of the families being cared for. In the author's work as an Indigenous midwife, self-reflection has been a valuable tool, even though it is often difficult. Self-reflection can help to ensure that self-bias is not evident in the care provided.

CASE STUDY

Providing culturally safe practice in an urban hospital

While I was working as a midwife in a large urban hospital, I was asked to assist a family whose four-week-old child had been flown in from a remote community. At times, midwifery care may involve times of extreme grief for women and their families. This was one of those times.

This family was told that that no further treatment was available for the child, and that palliative care would be offered. Despite all the medical and traditional healing provided by the grandmother, the child would soon pass away.

The family held rich family traditions and cultural beliefs. After some discussion, the family decided that they would like to perform a traditional ceremony for their child. There was some resistance and concern among the hospital staff, particularly regarding the child's safety. However, the family did not share these concerns. Both the Indigenous liaison officer supporting the family and I as the Indigenous midwife stressed that we should do what we could to enable their wishes. Helping the family to perform a traditional ceremony was not only culturally safe; it was the most appropriate care we could give!

The family was able to take the child outside under some magnificent trees. The intensive care nurse maintained the child's breathing with a ventilator, which was hidden under a cloth of Indigenous print. The family then had the opportunity to place their little one onto mother earth and perform a traditional ceremony. They were able to not only welcome their child to Country, but also to ensure that their child would be tied to this land, 'to his Dreaming', as he passed away.

Even today, this story brings tears to my eyes. Helping the family to perform the ceremony was a powerful achievement. Using my own self-reflective practice, I can see that the family was given time with their child – not in the sterile, cold intensive care unit, but in fresh air with sunshine on his little face. It was indeed the correct and culturally safe care for the family. Yes, it caused some staff to be anxious, but the family will always remember the willingness and sensitivity shown to them that day, not the many long, lonely hours sitting by an intensive care bed.

This family will always be in my thoughts. Even though we were in a large, imposing urban hospital, we were able to support their cultural needs. We should do this for all our mothers and their families. All we need to do is ask ourselves, 'What is culturally safe care for this family?'

QUESTIONS FOR REFLECTION

- How do you reflect upon and respond to this story?
- What might culturally safe practice mean for you as a midwife? How might cultural safety influence your work?

Minimise power differences

Midwives hold an astonishing amount of power in their relationships with women. The power is cross-cultural and part of the role that midwives perform at a time when their clients are vulnerable. But for many Aboriginal and Torres Strait Islander women, the notion of power is also tied up with 'whiteness' – in most cases, people in a position of power are non-Indigenous.

The power differential between a woman and her midwife may be significant. Women may have limited knowledge, may be experiencing pain and fear, may require assistance with personal care, or could be experiencing an unfamiliar loss of self-control or self-determination. Midwives should recognise the power imbalance and strive to work in partnership with women during pregnancy, childbearing and parenting. The midwife's task is to help others, including the woman and her infant(s), in order to promote a healthy experience and prevent or reduce potential for harm. Midwives can actively preserve the dignity of women and their infants by recognising the potential for vulnerability and powerlessness of the women in their care, and by consciously practising kindness.

Historically, midwives worked on a one-to-one basis with women, but the shift towards the biomedical model, with hospital births and a team of health professionals on hand, has tended to depersonalise midwifery practice. The biomedical model is diametrically opposed to traditional Aboriginal and Torres Strait Islander ways of healing and birthing. For Aboriginal and Torres Strait Islander women, pregnancy and childbirth are part of women's business. Traditionally, communities were able to provide continuity of care and ongoing partnerships between experienced, trusted midwives and women giving birth.

Power differences can be minimised when care is provided by a known caregiver who has an ongoing relationship with the woman and her family. Midwives who work to help meet a family's needs and expectations over a period of time can provide support that is life changing (Homer, Brodie & Leap, 2008). Power imbalances can shift and equalise when midwives work in collaboration with women and are able to offer women informed choices.

CASE STUDY

Combining tradition and modern practice

Mabel is a fair-skinned Aboriginal woman who is expecting her second baby. She plans to give birth at an urban hospital close to her new home.

Mabel's family moved to the city from remote Queensland many years ago, after a long search for her brothers and sisters. Mabel's brothers and sisters were taken from her parents when Mabel was a young child.

Mabel presents early for antenatal care and regularly attends visits. Her antenatal period is uneventful; she labours well and has a healthy baby.

After the birth, Mabel asks to keep her placenta. She is asked many questions. Her attempt to remain true to her culture is not supported, and she is unable to return her placenta to her Country. Her placenta was discarded.

QUESTIONS FOR REFLECTION

- What strategies would you consider appropriate in this case?
- How and why is this a significant part of an Aboriginal and Torres Strait Islander woman's birthing experience? What did Mabel want to do with the placenta?
- What could be done by the midwife to promote culturally safe maternity care for Mabel and other Aboriginal and Torres Strait Islander women in this situation?

Ensure you do not diminish, demean or disempower

As discussed by fellow Aboriginal and Torres Strait Islander health professionals throughout this book, health services that are culturally safe particularly in maternity settings are most likely to have significant maternal and neonatal outcomes. It is essential that we as nurses and midwives are aware of our own biases, including stereotyping of individuals who are different in physical features or beliefs from ourselves. Nurses, midwives and other health professionals should consider that women and their families have many experiences through history and within the health systems that have been not only undesirable but detrimental to their long-term health. Racism can be subtle or intentional; however, as uncomfortable as this topic is, it important to call it out. As a nurse, midwife or health professional, you are in a position that can enable change. It is important to remember that how you speak, move, gesture or discuss women and families will impact their lives.

CASE STUDY

Culturally safe midwifery practices: Being with women – or not?

Drawing on my experience as a midwife, one example of stereotyping a young woman clearly comes to mind.

One of the challenges faced by Indigenous mothers is the dislocation from family for many reasons, but predominantly at the time of birth. One such reason may be when traditional women move to birthing sites.

As pregnancy and birth are significant periods in a woman's life, it is only natural that she will crave the presence of her family. Yet for many Aboriginal and Torres Strait Islander women, this time may be marked by fear and anxiety. This fear often is related to history, colonisation and the Stolen Generations. This is discussed in Chapters 1 and 14.

Whilst working in an urban hospital, I met Tina. She was expecting her sixth baby and was now 36 weeks pregnant. Usually birth occurs between 37 and 41 weeks. Tina had caught the bus from a local Aboriginal community some 70 kilometres away from the hospital. She left in the early hours of the morning as there was only one service in the morning leaving for the larger town and one in the afternoon to return to community. She was accompanied by Destiny, her middle daughter. When Tina arrived, my colleague stated, 'She's one of yours. I can't deal with the tribe today, and you can look after her.' Without thought, I instantly replied, 'You mean … she is an Indigenous woman so I will look after her!'

Soon the doorbell to the birthing suite rang. When I meet Tina, as she moved slowly into the birthing suite and was contracting strongly, she had only a small bag with her. She was slim in stature, looked tired and was obviously in labour. Destiny, happy and excited, stated that Mummy was having 'big boy'. Tina was well aware of

(cont.)

the risks of having a premature baby – her last baby had been born at 34 weeks, which is why she had presented to the hospital.

As is the practice, I greeted Tina and asked her history. While monitoring her baby (listening for the heartbeat and checking the baby's position), we discussed where her mob was from, how far she'd travelled and where my family/mob were from.

It was easy for me to make a connection with her and the relief on her face was very obvious when she realised I understood about the issues she faced – including transport, leaving her young family and the issues that accompanied this.

It was a delight for me to see how Tina seemed to instantly relax when she realised that I, as a fair skinned Indigenous woman, was indeed Indigenous. 'I thought you were' was her comment as she smiled widely.

We discussed how she'd seen the midwife in the closest town to her community 'several times'. She stated that she wished her partner could be here for the birth. This would be almost impossible as he has no transport. 'The little ones would be okay with my sister but … ' I tucked Destiny up in a warm blanket on the recliner chair to sleep.

After leaving Tina and Destiny in the room, I was confronted with many questions from fellow staff regarding Tina's care and options. Among these was the question of her drug and alcohol use and abuse (Tina was a non-drinker and non-smoker). The most significant and unsettling comments or assumptions were: 'Does she have all her children? Was there a child alert?'

This stereotype not only angers but shames me as a nurse, a midwife and an Indigenous woman. I work within a profession that values women and prides itself as providing respectful women-centred care. To me, these comments and value judgements are as far as they could be from that belief of 'women-centred care' (Homer et al., 2012).

It is evident from many comments in the workplace that assumptions are made about women from many cultures. Whether racism is subtle or unintentional, stereotyping, discrimination and marginalisation of women and families are unacceptable. As midwives and nurses, we need to be aware of our own biases and treat all women with respect and dignity. After all, this is what our codes of practice align with. As midwives, we are mandatory reporters and there are instances when children's safety is at risk and measures should be put in place to protect them. However, the lack of culturally safe practices and/or the understanding of cultural sensitivity is evident in mainstream settings. There is a strong disparity in maternal health outcomes for Aboriginal and Torres Strait Islander women and children, and an undeniable need for culturally safe services to address these disparities.

QUESTIONS FOR REFLECTION

- Aboriginal and Torres Strait Islander women report that when they are supported by a non-Indigenous midwife or a midwife who is culturally safe, their satisfaction in their care experience is increased. Discuss this and outline the reasons why this is important?
- Research why comments such as 'She's one of yours. I can't deal with the tribe today' and 'You don't look Aboriginal' are stereotyping and not culturally safe. Is this racism?
- Reflect on and research racism in the workplace. How can you put practices in place so you are not that racist midwife or nurse?

Conclusion

Maternity care and midwifery services must be viewed through a lens of cultural safety. For Aboriginal and Torres Strait Islander women, this means that their care needs to consider their cultural choices and their geographic location. There are important differences in the care needs of Aboriginal and Torres Strait Islander women who live in urban environments and those from rural and remote communities who travel to tertiary hospitals to give birth.

By reflecting on the appropriate models of care, health professionals can:

- be culturally safe practitioners
- increase opportunities to engage Aboriginal and Torres Strait Islander mothers
- discuss risky health behaviors (such as smoking, alcohol consumption and poor nutrition) to encourage foetal wellbeing and provide long-term health benefits
- provide collaborative care that includes Aboriginal and Torres Strait Islander women, their families and their communities
- promote empowerment and self-determination.

Cultural safety means that women experience less fear. This will improve health outcomes for a range of issues, including mother and baby health, and concerns related to sexual health, contraception and breastfeeding.

In order to improve health outcomes for Aboriginal and Torres Strait Islander women, their babies and their families, it is essential that women have access to culturally safe health services. Improving the health of mothers and babies will positively benefit the overall health status of Aboriginal and Torres Strait Islander communities.

Learning activities

1. View the following YouTube clip: youtube/kymu_pW_Z7Y (Aboriginal Australians talking about birthing on country and how important it is for Aboriginal culture', from *The Face of Birth DVD,* produced by Good Eye Deer, 2013). Consider these questions:
   - How important is birthing on Country?
   - What is culturally safe care? Describe several culturally safe approaches.
   - How might you include culturally safe care into your practice?
   - Is it possible for continuity of care to be provided in the urban setting?
   - Suggest advantages and disadvantages of continuity of care for your practice.
2. View the following YouTube clip: www.youtube.com/watch?v=phz7DwQ80w8 ('Your Mob: Aboriginal nursing', produced by NSW Health, 2012). Consider these questions:
   - Write down ways in which you, as a health professional, might assist Indigenous people.
   - Comment on the cultural and clinical issues raised in the clip.
   - Reflect on the cultural safety shown in the clip.
   - What community supports may be available in this situation?

3. Explore ways in which Aboriginal and Torres Strait Islander women in urban and regional locations might gain access to appropriate care. What strategies would you use to assist these women? What strengths do you bring in caring for these women?
4. Imagine you were seeking to give birth in a large urban hospital (choose a specific hospital for your case study). You have recently moved to town from a remote area.
   - Where could you seek help? What help is available?
   - What community services and supports may be available? How might you find out about them?
   - Ask yourself: how will your pregnancy and your interactions with the hospital affect you and your family? How will the support services affect or support your social and cultural needs?

FURTHER READING

AIHW (2020). *Australia's Mothers and Babies 2018: In Brief.* Canberra: AIHW. Retrieved from www.aihw.gov.au/reports/mothers-babies/australias-mothers-and-babies-2018-in-brief/contents/table-of-contents

Aird, M. (1963). *Brisbane Blacks.* Brisbane: Keeaira Press.

Brown, A.E., Fereday, J.A., Middleton, P.F. & Pincombe J.I. (2016). Aboriginal and Torres Strait Islander women's experiences accessing standard hospital care for birth in South Australia: A phenomenological study. *Women Birth*, 29(4), 350–8.

CATSINaM, Australian College of Midwives & CRANAplus (2016). *Birthing on Country Position Statement.* Canberra: Congress of Aboriginal and Torres Strait Islander Nurses and Midwives. Retrieved from http://catsinam.org.au/static/uploads/files/birthing-on-country-position-statement-endorsed-march-2016-wfaxpyhvmxrw.pdf

DPMC (2020). *Closing the Gap Report 2020.* Retrieved from https://ctgreport.niaa.gov.au/sites/default/files/pdf/closing-the-gap-report-2020.pdf

Fredericks, B. (2008). 'We live in urban streets and suburbs too': The growing number of Aboriginal and Torres Strait Islander people living in urban areas. In L. Finch (ed.), *Seachange: New and Renewed Urban Landscapes, Proceedings of the 9th Australasian Urban History/ Planning History Conference, Maroochydore, 6–9 February.* Retrieved from http://eprints.qut.edu.au/13412.

Fredericks, B. (2013). 'We don't leave our identities at the city limits': Aboriginal and Torres Strait Islander people living in urban localities. *Australian Aboriginal Studies*, 1, 4–16.

Homer, C, Brodie, P. & Leap, N. (2008). *Midwifery Continuity of Care: A Practical Guide.* Sydney: Elsevier.

Kelly, J., West, R., Gamble, J., Sidebotham, M., Carson, V. & Duffy, E. (2014). 'She knows how we feel': Australian Aboriginal and Torres Strait Islander childbearing women's experience of continuity of care with an Australian Aboriginal and Torres Strait Islander midwifery student. *Women Birth*, 27(3), 157–62.

Kildea, S., Tracy, S., Sherwood, J., Magick-Dennis, F. & Barclay, L. (2016). Improving maternity services for indigenous women in Australia: Moving from policy to practice. *Medical Journal of Australia*, 205(8), 375–9.

Rumbold, A. & Cunningham, J. (2008). A review of the impact of antenatal care services for Australian Indigenous women and attempts to strengthen these services. *Maternal and Child Health Journal*, 12(1), 83–100.

Wilson, G. (2009). *What Do Aboriginal Women Think is Good Antenatal Care? Consultation Report.* Darwin: Cooperative Research Centre for Aboriginal Health.

Visit the companion website at www.cambridge.org/highereducation/isbn/9781108794695/resources to see further online resources.

REFERENCES

ABS (2012). *Births, Australia, 2011.* Canberra: ABS.

ABS (2018). *Estimates of Aboriginal and Torres Strait Islander Australians.* Canberra: ABS.

ABS (2019). *Births, Australia, 2018.* Canberra: ABS.

ACM (2003). *National Midwifery Guidelines for Consultation and Referral.* Canberra: ACM.

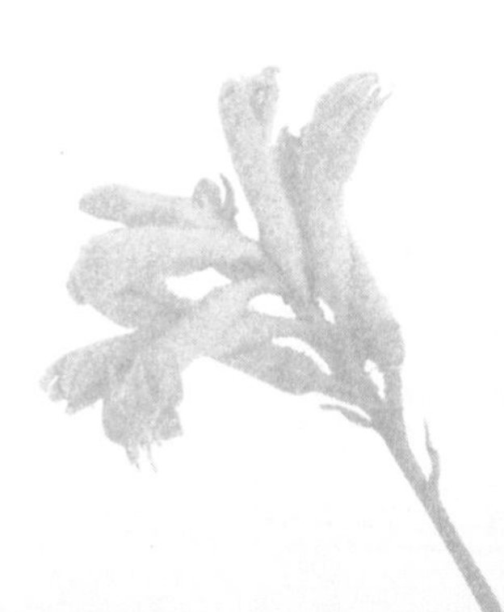

AHMAC (2011). *National Maternity Services Plan, 2011*. Canberra: AHMAC. Retrieved from www.health.gov.au/internet/publications/publishing.nsf/Content/pacd-maternityservicesplan-toc.

AIHW (2011). *The Health and Welfare of Australia's Aboriginal and Torres Strait Islander People: An Overview*. Canberra: AIHW. Retrieved from www.aihw.gov.au/publication-detail/?id=10737418989.

AIHW (2014). *Australia's Mothers and Babies: 2012*. Canberra: AIHW. Retrieved from www.aihw.gov.au/getmedia/674fe3d3-4432–4675-8a96-cab97e3c277f/18530.pdf.aspx?inline=true

AIHW (2016). *Indigenous Australians*. Canberra: AIHW. Retrieved from www.aihw.gov.au/reports-data/population-groups/indigenous-australians/overview.

AIHW (2019a). *Incidence of Gestational Diabetes in Australia*. Canberra: AIHW. Retrieved from www.aihw.gov.au/reports/diabetes/incidence-of-gestational-diabetes-in-australia

AIHW (2019b). *Rural & Remote Health*. Canberra: AIHW. Retrieved from www.aihw.gov.au/reports/rural-remote-australians/rural-remote-health

AIHW (2020a). *Australia's Children*. Canberra: AIHW. Retrieved from www.aihw.gov.au/getmedia/6af928d6-692e-4449-b915-cf2ca946982f/aihw-cws-69-print-report.pdf.aspx?inline=true

AIHW (2020b). *Australia's Mothers and Babies 2018: In Brief*. Canberra: AIHW. Retrieved from www.aihw.gov.au/reports/mothers-babies/australias-mothers-and-babies-2018-in-brief/contents/table-of-contents

AIHW (2020c). *Australia's Mothers and Babies Data Visualisations*. Retrieved from www.aihw.gov.au/reports/mothers-babies/australias-mothers-babies-data-visualisations

AIHW (2020d). *Indigenous Primary Health Care: Results from the OSR and nKPI collections*. Canberra: AIHW. Retrieved from www.aihw.gov.au/reports/indigenous-australians/indigenous-primary-health-care-results-osr-nkpi

Atkinson, J. (2002). *Trauma Trails, Recreating Song Lines: The Transgenerational Effects of Trauma in Indigenous Australia*. Melbourne: Spinifex Press.

Bates, D. (2014 [1938]). *The Passing of the Aborigines: A Lifetime Spent Among the Natives of Australia*. Adelaide: University of Adelaide.

Best, O. (2012). Yatdjuligin: The stories of Queensland Aboriginal Registered Nurses 1950–2005. Unpublished PhD thesis, University of Southern Queensland.

COAG Health Council (2017). *National Framework for Maternity Services*. Canberra: COAG Health Council. Retrieved from www.coaghealthcouncil.gov.au/Projects/National-Framework-for-Maternity-Services

COAG Health Council (2019). *Woman-centred Care: Strategic Directions for Australian Maternity Services*. Canberra: COAG Health Council. Retrieved from www.health.gov.au/sites/default/files/documents/2019/11/woman-centred-care-strategic-directions-for-australian-maternity-services.pdf

Collins, D. (2004 [1798]). *An Account of the English Colony in New South Wales with Remarks on the Dispositions, Customs, Manners, etc. of the Native Inhabitants of that Country*. London: T. Cadell & W. Davis.

Couchie, C. & Sanderson, S. (2007). A report on best practices for returning birth to rural and remote Aboriginal communities. *JOGC* (March), 250–4.

Cox, L. & Taua, C. (2013). Socio-cultural considerations and nursing practice. In J. Crisp, C. Taylor, C. Douglas & G. Rebeiro (eds), *Potter and Perry's Fundamentals of Nursing* (4th edn).Sydney: Elsevier, pp. 320–45.

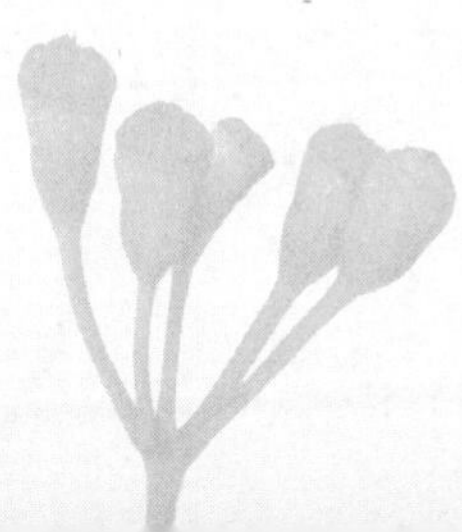

de Costa, C. & Child, A. (1996). Pregnancy outcomes in urban Aboriginal women. *The Medical Journal of Australia*, 164 (9), 523–6.

Department of Health (2009). *Improving Maternity Services in Australia: Report of the Maternity Services Review*. Canberra: Commonwealth of Australia. Retrieved from www.health.gov.au/internet/main/publishing.nsf/Content/maternityservicesreview-report.

DPMC (2020). *Closing the Gap Report 2020*. Retrieved from https://ctgreport.niaa.gov.au/sites/default/files/pdf/closing-the-gap-report-2020.pdf

Dudgeon, P., Wright, M. & Coffin, J. (2010). Talking it and walking it: Cultural competence. *Journal of Australian Indigenous Issues*, 13(3), 29–44.

Eckermann, A.K., Dowd, T., Chong, E., Nixon, L. & Gray, R. (2010). *Binan Goonj: Bridging Cultures in Aboriginal Health*: Sydney: Elsevier.

Goold, S. (2006). 'Gettin em n keepin em': Indigenous issues in nursing education. *Australian Aboriginal Studies*, 2, 57–61.

Gregory, H. (2009). Speech on International Nurses Day. Royal Brisbane and Women's Hospital, Brisbane.

Hancock, H. (2006). *Aboriginal Women's Perinatal Needs, Experiences and Maternity Services: A Literature Review to Enable Considerations to be made about Quality Indicators*. Alice Springs: Ngaanyatjarra Health Service.

Herceg, A. (2005). *Improving Health in Aboriginal and Torres Strait Islander Mothers, Babies and Young Children: A Literature Review*. Canberra: Australian Government Department of Health and Ageing.

Hirst, C. (2005). *Re-Birthing: Report of the Review of Maternity Services in Queensland*. Brisbane: Queensland Health.

Homer, C, Brodie, P. & Leap, N. (2008). *Midwifery Continuity of Care: A Practical Guide*. Sydney: Elsevier.

Homer, C.S., Foureur, M..J, Allende, T., Pekin, F., Caplice, S. & Catling-Paull, C. (2012). 'It's more than just having a baby': Women's experiences of a maternity service for Australian Aboriginal and Torres Strait Islander families. *Midwifery*, 28(4), E449–55.

Kildea, S. Dennis, F. & Stapleton, H. (2013). *Birthing on Country Workshop Report, Alice Springs, 4 July 2012*. Brisbane: Australian Catholic University and Mater Medical Research Unit on behalf of the Maternity Services Inter-Jurisdictional Committee for the Australian Health Minister's Advisory Council.

Kildea, S., Gao, Y., Hickey, S. ...Roe, Y. (2019). Reducing preterm birth amongst Aboriginal and Torres Strait Islander babies: A prospective cohort study, Brisbane, Australia. *eClinical Medicine*. 12: 43–51.

Kildea, S., Kruske, S., Barclay, L. & Tracy, S. (2010). 'Closing the Gap': How maternity services can contribute to reducing poor maternal infant health outcomes for Aboriginal and Torres Strait Islander women. *Rural and Remote Health*, 10, 1383.

Kildea, S. & Wardaguga, M. (2009). Childbirth in Australia: Aboriginal and Torres Strait Islander women. In H. Selin (ed.), *Childbirth Across Cultures*, Vol. 5. Dordrecht: Springer, pp. 275–86.

Li, Z., Zeki, R., Hilder, L. & Sullivan, E.A. (2012). *Australia's Mothers and Babies 2010*. Canberra: AIHW National Perinatal Epidemiology and Statistics Unit.

Maternity Services Review (2009). *Improving Maternity Services in Australia*. Canberra: Commonwealth of Australia.

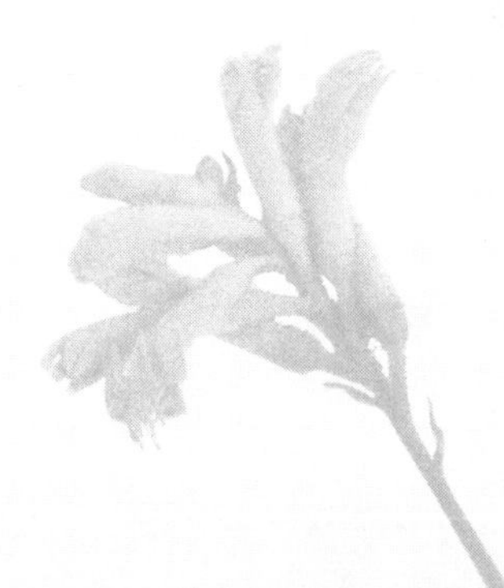

Qiao, Y., Ma, J., Wang, Y. … Hu, G. (2015). Birth weight and childhood obesity: A 12-country study. *International Journal of Obesity Supplements*, 5, S74–S79.

Queensland Health (2019). *Growing Deadly Families: Aboriginal and Torres Strait Islander Maternity Services Strategy 2019–2025*. Brisbane: Queensland Health. Retrieved from www.health.qld.gov.au/__data/assets/pdf_file/0030/932880/Growing-Deadly-Families-Strategy.pdf

Ramsden, I. (2002). Cultural safety and nursing education in Aotearoa and Te Waipounamu. Unpublished PhD thesis, Victoria University of Wellington.

Reibel, T. & Walker, R. (2010). Antenatal services for Aboriginal women: The relevance of cultural competence. *Quality in Primary Care*, 18(1), 65–74.

Roth, W.E. (1897). *Ethnological Studies Among the North-west-Central Queensland Aborigines*. London: E. Gregory.

Scrimgeour, M. & Scrimgeour, D. (2008). *Health Care Access for Aboriginal and Torres Strait Islander People Living in Urban Areas, and Related Research Issues: A Review of the Literature*. Darwin: Cooperative Research Centre for Aboriginal Health.

Van Wagner, V., Epoo, B., Nastapoka, J. & Harney, E. (2007). Reclaiming birth, health and community: Midwifery in the Inuit villages of Nunavik, Canada. *Journal of Midwifery & Women's Health*, 52(4), 384–91.

West, R., Usher, K. & Foster, K. (2010). Increased numbers of Australian Indigenous nurses would make a significant contribution to 'closing the gap' in Indigenous health: What is getting in the way? *Contemporary Nurse*, 36(1–2), 121–30.

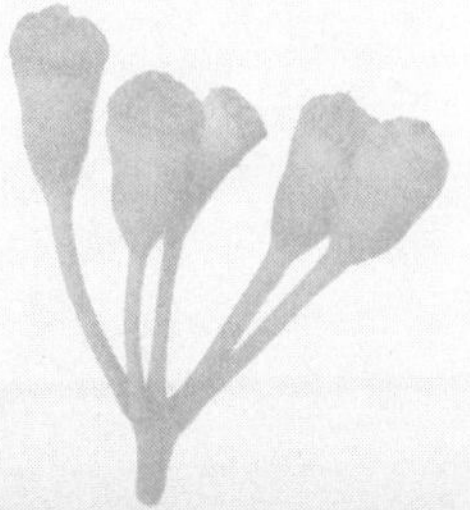

Indigenous birthing in remote locations: Grandmothers' Law and government medicine

Nicole Ramsamy

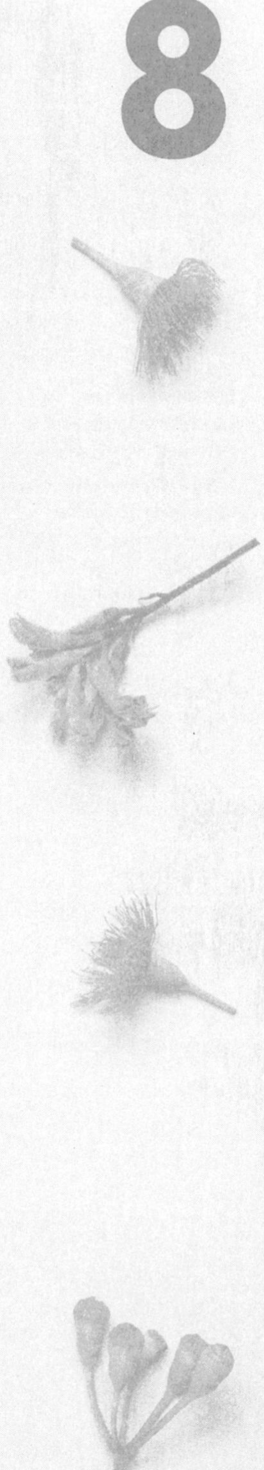

8

LEARNING OBJECTIVES

This chapter will help you to understand:

- Grandmothers' Law
- Historical issues relevant to midwifery practice in remote areas
- Current issues in remote area midwifery practice and hospital birthing practice, and their effects on remote Aboriginal and Torres Strait Islander women
- Cultural obligations during pregnancy and birthing

KEY WORDS

Grandmothers' Law
taboo

Introduction

The birthing experience is an event that can remain clear in a woman's mind for many years. It is a highly significant life event influenced by cultural traditions and family commitments.

Prior to colonisation, the traditional beliefs and birthing practices of Aboriginal and Torres Strait Islander people were carefully practised. Although birthing practices varied across the country, there were common themes of cultural obligation, ritual and **taboo**, and careful following of **Grandmothers' Law**.

taboo A custom that prohibits or restricts a particular thing or person. Traditionally, some foods were taboo during pregnancy.

Grandmothers' Law The traditional knowledge and experience of senior women in a community about attending to women during pregnancy, childbirth and postpartum.

This chapter explores the traditional midwifery and birthing practices relevant to Aboriginal and Torres Strait Islander peoples living in remote communities. It begins by exploring traditional approaches to birthing and explaining Grandmothers' Law. The chapter then draws on the author's experiences as a nurse practitioner/midwife in Pormpuraaw community in Cape York to explore some of the issues relevant to contemporary birthing practice for Aboriginal and Torres Strait Islander women and for the midwives who support them.

Traditional birthing practices on the homelands

For tens of thousands of years, Aboriginal women have kept Law and held ceremony in relation to the way in which they give birth (Apunipima Cape York Health Council, 1997). Many Aboriginal people around Australia believe that pregnant women visit a place where 'spirit' children live, and that one or more enter a woman's womb there.

Grandmothers' Law has been taught to traditional midwives by their grandmothers and Elders for generations and generations (CAAC, 1985; Gyia, 1986; Ward, 2018). Traditionally, these women were very well known and respected by their clan members, as they had much knowledge and experience in women's business and traditional medicine. While a lot of traditional birthing knowledge has been lost, some rituals continue to be practised today.

Traditionally, pregnant woman did not receive antenatal care or preparation for their births in the way that women do today, such as ultrasound examinations and other tests. Pregnancy was not announced until the woman felt the first movements of the baby inside her. Indigenous people consider pregnancy and birth to be a normal part of life, so little attention was given during pregnancy until labour was imminent.

Indigenous women in Cape York ate traditional foods, which were naturally rich in a variety of vitamins and minerals. Traditional Law about diet was strict for pregnant women. They were prohibited from eating 'big food' like kangaroo, emu, bird, barramundi, stingray and turtle. In some places, they were also prohibited from eating crab and some seasonal foods. In addition, they were not allowed to share their food with certain family members during their pregnancy. It was said that if they broke the Law by eating the wrong foods or sharing food with certain family members, it could result in complications during labour or birth, or the baby could be born with a deformity. The taboos were designed to ensure the health of mother and baby, and to avoid complications during birth.

Forbidden foods were taught according to the Grandmothers' Law, and varied between different clan groups and at different times of the year. For example, a pregnant woman could not eat carpet snake because it was thought that when she came to labour the birth would be impeded: the people believed that the snake would wrap itself around her abdomen, causing complications during birth. Similarly, pregnant women were forbidden from digging open the nesting mound of a scrub turkey, as it was likely to rip open her belly and the foetus might be harmed. Another taboo was for pregnant women to swim in lagoons to look for lily roots, because of the belief that a stillbirth could be caused by the rainbow serpent.

Traditionally, the surest way to avoid illness in pregnancy was to observe and practise the taboos associated with places, people and food, and to refrain from doing things that might lead someone to retaliate using sorcery.

Traditional midwives were highly knowledgeable about the bush medicines that were available locally and made use of them when necessary.

QUESTION FOR REFLECTION

- Reflect on your own cultural heritage and consider how it informs your beliefs about pregnancy and childbirth. Make a list of the activities, behaviours and health checks that are important during pregnancy. How have you learned about these things? How do your beliefs differ from the beliefs of your mother or grandmother?

Labour

During labour, only women who had given birth to a child were permitted at the birthing site. This was to preserve the secrets of Grandmothers' Law.

When labour commenced, the woman would seek assistance from her grandmothers and aunts, who would look after her over the next several weeks. In some clan groups, the labouring woman and traditional midwives would move to a camp some distance from the main camp for a time. They travelled by foot, with few resources.

The women's camp was prepared for the birth with wind barriers and fires for warmth, comfort and privacy. All the women would be naked and support was provided from behind the labouring woman in order not to disturb the natural flow of the birthing process.

Malpresentations would be corrected with massage and, in extreme cases, by manipulation. If there were complications, the grandmother might have sent a message to the father or a healer to perform certain rituals nearby. The labouring woman usually moved around freely during her labour, stopping during her contractions to lean against a tree or a rock.

Birth

Traditionally, Indigenous women of Cape York gave birth under trees, in bark huts or in caves, in a special place on their land away from the main camp. The woman's sisters and her mother would sometimes assist. It was believed that the presence of experienced traditional midwives to assist women in labour helped them to have easy births and healthy babies. Women from the husband's side of the family and the husband himself were not allowed near the birthing site unless invited by the grandmother.

Usually there would be two midwives at a birth. One would sit in front and the other at the back of the labouring woman, and they would rub her abdomen and back, and wipe her face and body. This all assisted in creating an easy birth.

When the labouring woman was ready to birth, she would be assisted to squat over a hollow depression on the earth. The baby would be delivered onto the ground. While this was happening, some traditional midwives would be singing in the background. Once delivered, the baby and the land became spiritually connected.

After the birth, the woman's grandmother and aunts would encourage the new mother to squat over smoking embers to assist with internal healing and prevent blood loss. After delivery, the newborn would be left on the ground untouched until they cried, and then would be lifted to the mother's breast. If the infant did not cry, showed no signs of life, was not looking strong or looked deformed in any way, they would be left untouched and buried at the place of birth. The baby would not be named. The newborn was not named until it was apparent that they would survive. The reason for this was that if the newborn died with a name, then saying that name within the Aboriginal culture would be disrespectful. It is also taboo for anyone to say the name or any name sounding like it.

There were a number of ceremonies surrounding the birth of a baby, particularly the cutting of the cord, the naming of the baby and burial of the placenta.

Afterbirth

Traditionally, midwives assisted in delivery of the afterbirth, which was then buried somewhere nearby. The placenta, membranes and blood products had a spiritual significance and were disposed of in traditional rituals. The placenta was buried where it was delivered (or nearby) and became a spiritual link with the land on which the newborn was delivered. Special care was taken to ensure it was tightly wrapped – for example, it might be wrapped in paper bark to protect it from animals.

The burial of the afterbirth connected the baby to its birth land and provided a special association with a family member. The person who buried the umbilical cord was allowed to apply native beeswax to the baby's umbilical stump for protection, and it would be her duty to protect the child. The grandmother traditionally separated the umbilical cord with her teeth or with crystal rock, a sharp shell or a stone knife. Warm sand was placed on the cord where the cut was made, to promote healing.

Smoking of the mother and the baby made sure the baby grew strong and the mother recovered quickly. Fire smoke and steam were used to assist the expulsion of the afterbirth and the healing of the tissues.

All the women remained at the birthing site for several weeks, during which time other ceremonies and rituals were carried out according to Grandmothers' Law, including the naming of the child. Men remained forbidden from the birthing site. However, the father was allowed to deliver food to the outskirts of the camp (certain foods remained forbidden).

The birthing place held special significance and provided a strong connection between the individual and their Country. The mother's and baby's blood were spilt on the ground during the birthing process, and this created the direct connection between the child and their Country.

In traditional practices and rituals, birthing involved more than the physical health of the mother and baby. Giving birth was a process of initiation and belonging to the culture that created spiritual links to that land and the ancestral Dreaming.

Breastfeeding and contraception

After the baby was born, a traditional midwife would search for a special tree from which to collect sap to help the mother's milk to flow. Some women would have to drink a liquid made from a black termite's nest. Women never questioned such customs, because they abided by Grandmothers' Law due to their position in the camp. If the midwife wished to have the newborn fed and let the mother rest for a time, she would find a close relative to breastfeed the baby.

During the first few months of life, a baby was considered to be especially vulnerable. Food taboos were followed while the mother was breastfeeding, and this could continue for up to three years. Some food taboos are related to a woman's nutritional wellbeing. For example, a woman may be prevented from eating a particular food associated with a deceased person's totem if she was a close kin of the deceased person, because the food would cause sickness.

Traditionally, there was no planned contraception, but the hunter-and-gatherer lifestyle, which included an extended period of breastfeeding, promoted lower fertility and assisted with contraception.

Meeting the father

When the mother had healed, the baby's father and his family were allowed to see the mother and the newborn. This was a very special time, when the family would smear the baby with their underarm moisture and smell.

Whether a father was able to see his baby depended on whether he was married to the mother. If the parents were not married, the father had to stay away from the child for several years, and the mother's family would make sure that he abided by this custom. If the parents were married, then the father would be able to see his baby after the mother had properly healed. This could be weeks after the birth, depending on the health of the mother.

The sex of the child also influenced the time at which the father and his family were allowed to see the child. If the newborn was a girl, the father had to wait several months to see her. If the newborn was a boy, the father would be allowed to see his son as soon as the mother was healed. The father was not allowed to wash or clean his daughter, but this was allowed for a son.

CASE STUDY

Grandmothers' Law and Nellie Benjamin

In Cape York Peninsula in Far North Queensland, Grandmothers' Law is all about women's business. It provides the laws related to pregnancy, birthing, afterbirth and breastfeeding ceremonies and rituals that occur on the local people's homelands. Grandmothers' Law is shared among Aboriginal women only – Torres Strait culture is different.

Knowledge shared with me by a Cape York Pormpuraaw Elder, Mrs Nellie Benjamin, was told to her by her Elders, mothers, aunts and grandmothers. Mrs Benjamin was born during the time of bush deliveries on her homeland. However, Mrs Benjamin's experiences of having her own children did not follow the traditional ways. Due to the effects of life under colonisation, she was unable to practise Grandmothers' Law and give birth on her homelands.

Mrs Benjamin was removed from Pormpuraaw seven months into her pregnancy. She was separated from her community, family, husband, children and cultural beliefs about Grandmothers' Law, and transferred to a remote hospital on Thursday Island to give birth. She was transferred to the metropolitan hospital in Cairns for the births of some of her other children.

Being transferred to hospital to give birth was extremely traumatic for Mrs Benjamin. She had no support person from her community. She had to give birth in the presence of men and women she did not know. Her babies were delivered by male obstetricians, even though it was a cultural taboo for her to have men close to her during birthing. She was required to stay in an unfamiliar environment, and was separated from her family for an extended time. She had to let other people care for her children during those times.

QUESTIONS FOR REFLECTION

- How do you feel about the conflicting issues that arise from women's desire to give birth on Country and the contemporary medical approach of ensuring clinical safety and best practice?
- Can you identify some of the cultural and health dilemmas in relation to pregnancy and childbirth faced by women who live in remote communities?

CASE STUDY

Kitty, Lizzie and baby

In 1887 or 1888, Violet Marshall's father accepted a position as resident surgeon at Port Douglas in North Queensland. Violet was thirteen years old. Her family had arrived from England in 1886. The hospital and residence were located on about 2 acres of ground, fenced all around and surrounded by high tropical growth. There was a dirt road winding away to the foot of a range.

One day, two Aboriginal women, Kitty and Lizzie, wandered into the kitchen saying that they were hungry. Violet gave them some flour. Tied to Kitty's back was Lizzie's tiny baby.

Violet was delighted to see a wee baby with tight little light brown curls and beautiful brown eyes. She wanted Lizzie and Kitty to let her bath and dress the baby. After some persuasion, Lizzie and Kitty agreed.

One evening, Violet heard the sounds of wailing and crying coming from the Aboriginal camp. The next day, Violet rode into the thick scrub to investigate. Suddenly she heard a piercing scream and saw a pack of mongrel dogs. Then four naked men appeared, with their spears pointed directly at Violet. Kitty screamed and tried to tell Violet to go home.

The local Aboriginal cultural belief was that babies should not be washed for some months after they were born, as they believed washing would lead to the baby's death. Violet had bathed the baby and the baby had since died. Violet had to pay for the death, and the Aboriginal men wanted to kill her.

If Kitty had not been present, Violet would have been killed. A massacre of the entire Aboriginal tribe would probably have followed.

Some weeks later, Lizzie arrived at the house with a small dilly bag around her neck. Violet wanted to know what was in the dilly bag. After much persuasion. Lizzie brought out a little dried hand. She was carrying her baby's hand and she carried it for good luck.

Story as told by Violet Marshall in the *Port Douglas Gazette*, 1997.

QUESTIONS FOR REFLECTION

- Write down your thoughts about why it was Violet's interpretation of the story that was published in the local newspaper?
- What message does this case study have for nurses and midwives today?

The impact of the missionaries

European settlement had a dramatic effect on Grandmothers' Law. Indigenous peoples' birthing practices were quickly disrupted and forcibly changed, most notably as a result of missionaries setting up dormitories on Aboriginal and Torres Strait Islander homelands.

Colonial policies had an immediate effect: Indigenous people were restricted and prohibited from practising their traditional culture. There was a rapid loss of cultural identity, with limited cultural knowledge passed on to future generations. This particularly applied to Grandmothers' Law.

The policy of segregation had a great effect on Indigenous people. It separated families and communities and denied parents of their right to be parents and to nurture their children. Government policies forced Indigenous people from their traditional lands and aimed to eradicate their culture by placing them in dormitories administered by many differing church denominations. The aims of the church were to civilise the 'natives', advocating for rejecting of culture and practices such as Grandmothers' Law. Traditional medicines used were often described as 'devil's work' by the colonisers, which demonstrated gross ignorance on their behalf. Many Indigenous community members were renamed and given British names and British clothes, and were forced to live on reserves with many different Indigenous clan groups and nations. They were prevented from practising and maintaining the traditional aspects of their cultures. Children were actively taught to reject their Indigenous heritage and to embrace the church and a white God. Punishment was fierce and swift if the newly introduced ways were not adhered to.

As discussed elsewhere in this text, colonial policies led to a rapid decline in the health of Aboriginal and Torres Strait Islander people. Mounting ill-health also led to a rapid decline in the Indigenous population. Many Elders died, and important rituals and traditions were lost along with them. As the health status of Aboriginal and Torres Strait Islander people declined and traditional health knowledge disappeared, pregnant women in communities began to adopt risky behaviours such as smoking tobacco and drinking alcohol. These factors led to an increase in low-birthweight babies, pregnancy complications and premature births.

Their diets were often less than optimal due to the history of being locked on missions and reserves and not being allowed to source traditional foods which were highly nutritious, unlike the highly processed introduced diets of white flour, sugar and tea. The diet was lacking in protein, calcium, vitamin A and vitamin C, and sometimes deficient in calories. It provided poor nourishment for pregnant women. Many women gave birth to low-birthweight babies. At birth, their babies had low body stores of nutrients, so their capacity to survive nutritional stress and infections was limited. After being weaned from breastfeeding, the children adopted the staple, nutritionally deficient diet of their settlement. By the 1970s, Indigenous women on Cape York Peninsula had no option but to go to Cairns to give birth. As a result, many Indigenous babies were not smoked and no longer had their placentas buried in the ground on their homelands. Connection to land was severed due to birthing on Country no longer being an option. Grandmothers' Law and local cultural traditions were irreparably disrupted.

During these missionary days, many women were reluctant to report their pregnancies or attend antenatal clinics. In the Indigenous worldview, pregnancy was not a health 'problem' that required medical and nursing attention, but a natural event of concern only to the woman's immediate family. Local belief systems provided a set of precautionary measures, mostly expressed as taboos that were designed to ensure the health of the unborn child.

Another reason Indigenous women from Cape York were unwilling to attend antenatal clinics was that they would have to leave their community to deliver their babies on Thursday Island or in Cairns. They usually left home at seven months of pregnancy. This process of birthing off Country was introduced to ensure that Western medical facilities were available to meet all kinds of birthing crises. Understandably, most pregnant women did not like the prospect of leaving their children, husbands and families for an extended time. Some tried to avoid the nursing sisters altogether and hid their pregnancies in the hope that their babies would be born at home in their community and on Country.

Birthing in the hospitals

In the 1920s, the Queensland government stated that there was to be no more birthing on the homelands. Indigenous women had no choice but to travel from their homes to give birth in hospitals hundreds of kilometres away. They usually travelled on their own, with little to no support from their mothers, grandmothers and aunts. This change in government policy and practice took place without consultation with the Indigenous women or their Elders. No cultural safety training was provided for hospital staff.

With birthing removed from the homelands, the traditional knowledge and experience of midwives was overwhelmingly lost. The traditional practices and cultural rituals of Grandmothers' Law could no longer take place. The transition to hospital was intended to ensure the safety of both mother and baby, and to provide the best medical care available. It also provided control for the government.

Indigenous women viewed hospital births with great fear and anxiety. Birthing became a traumatic experience. Indigenous women arrived at hospital with radically different beliefs about giving birth than the non-Indigenous staff, and they delivered their babies in a silent, fearful and unknown world. The mother's loneliness was exacerbated by the absence of familiar people, the use of English during labour, and the unknown and terrifying medical technology. Hospitals can be frightening places for Indigenous people who have lived all their lives in communities of no more than 1500 people, where everyone knows everyone else.

Between the 1930s and 1960s, women from the remote communities of Kowanyama, Pormpuraaw, Aurukun, Napranum, Weipa and Mapoon on Cape York Peninsula received their antenatal care from non-Indigenous midwives. They travelled by boat to Thursday Island in the Torres Strait to await the arrival of their baby and receive midwifery or obstetric care. During the 1970s, women were told that they could no longer give birth on Thursday Island, and were required to travel by air to Cairns to have their babies.

By the 1990s, the women of Cape York who had significant problems in their pregnancies were not being given anything like the standard of care expected anywhere else in the country. Most of the women had no idea how far along in their pregnancy they were, so it could be impossible to know whether they were going into labour spontaneously and prematurely, were in labour at the end of their pregnancy or there was a problem with their pregnancy. No one could balance the risks of delivering the baby because they did not know the maturity of the foetus. For obstetricians, it was difficult to make correct decisions in complex cases. Many of the women in remote communities had complex comorbidities, such as severe heart conditions related to rheumatic heart disease, diabetes and end-stage renal failure. These comorbidities meant that the women often required higher-level medical intervention rather than the usual standard care (Humphrey & Keating, 2004).

Today, some of the major health concerns for women in remote communities involve late antenatal presentation, sexually transmissible infection and pelvic inflammatory disease – all of which are linked to their lack of access to reasonable healthcare. Some women also experience infertility and chronic pain. Carcinoma of the cervix is thought to be five times more common among the Indigenous women of Cape York than it is in the Caucasian population of Australia. There are few professionally trained carers for pregnant women working in Cape York communities. There is only a handful of midwives in the entire area covered by Cape York Primary Health Care Centres (PHCC). There are few obstetrically trained doctors working in Cairns, which is the catchment area for all midwifery/obstetric care for the people of Cape York and Torres Strait Island Health Services.

Today, because most women give birth in hospitals, they are unable to carry out Grandmothers' Law. Tradition, culture and ceremonies provide meaning and significance to life events, and losing these threatens the health and wellbeing of Indigenous women and their babies.

CASE STUDY

Edna: Social and emotional wellbeing

Edna was 29 years old. She was expected to travel to Cairns from her community on Cape York Peninsula to have her seventh baby.

Edna had little antenatal care in the lead-up to the birth. She had anaemia and gestational diabetes, and was reported to child safety authorities because she had received little care despite many invitations to attend the clinic.

Edna did not want to leave the community to have her child because she had no one to look after her six children. She was concerned that her partner, John, would not be able to care for their children. She feared that he may not be able to get the children off to school and attend to all household chores because he also had to work. Edna was also worried that while she was away from the community, her partner may go looking for a girlfriend.

Edna felt that she could not rely on any other person in the community to help care for her children. She was anxious about her family and did not want to go to Cairns for long just to wait for the baby to arrive. She asked the doctor whether he could bring the baby on earlier, but he said that there was no medical reason to do so.

Edna waited out her time and was away from her community for six weeks in total, due to a complication during birth. When she returned to the community, everything seemed to be okay at first. But then she started hearing yarns about her partner seeing another woman. Edna was devastated, and soon found herself facing police charges for grievous bodily harm.

Now Edna is pregnant again and feels helpless. There is no one to help her to care for all her children. She has been reported to the child safety team as not being capable of looking after her children, who have skin infections and rarely attend school. The children are removed from her care and placed in government care outside of the community. Edna and her partner have limited visits with their children.

QUESTIONS FOR REFLECTION

- How did contemporary medical practices contribute to Edna's situation?
- What types of community support could help in a situation like Edna's?

Current midwifery practices in remote communities

When a woman presents to the primary healthcare clinic stating that she has missed her period and is feeling nauseated, it is strongly recommended that the health worker gets permission from her to collect a urine sample and perform a pregnancy test. At the same time, the woman should be offered opportunistic sexual health screening for trichomonas, chlamydia and gonorrhoea. If the pregnancy test is positive, it is important to request further tests such as the first pathology antenatal screening test. She should be referred to a midwife or doctor.

Midwives are in a unique position to promote optimal care for the women they see. They need a flexible approach to women's desires for alternative birthing practices while continuing to provide quality care. This is what underpins culturally safe service provision.

For midwives, showing consideration and flexibility in relation to birthing customs is simply an extension of their professional practice. Negotiation is a skill that can be incorporated into a discussion so the woman feels empowered even when discussing compromised, difficult and dangerous situations. Midwives can show cultural safety through some simple gestures, such as promoting the presence of support people such as mothers, grandmothers and aunts, or even allowing the woman to deliver her newborn into a box of soil brought in from her homeland and for the placenta to be transported back to her homeland for traditional burial. The key to providing culturally safe care is to foster the health of communities. The midwife needs to have undertaken deep reflective practice.

When providing one-on-one care to pregnant women, it is important to explore the most culturally safe approach to women's business and community-based care, during the antenatal and postnatal periods, and infancy and early parenting care, as well as through continuing support and health promotion. Midwives often liaise with the hospital, non-government organisations such as Apunipima Cape York Health Council, private health providers such as obstetricians and social healthcare providers. Their role is to ensure that there is collaborative continuity of care.

Midwives must aim to develop a meaningful partnership with the woman and her family. They must be careful not to compromise the relationship by judging the woman's behaviour and choices, which is culturally unsafe care. Midwives need to create a safe place for the woman to be honest about where she is at in her life and her decisions. Sometimes a consultation can take over an hour because the midwife needs to ensure that the woman feels she is in a safe place.

While childbirth is considered a normal and important event for Indigenous women, antenatal and postnatal care are not considered to be a high priority. Much of a remote-area midwife's work involves educating women about the importance of regular antenatal checks to reduce the incidence of complications.

Often, Indigenous women do not remember their medical, surgical or obstetric history, so the midwife may find it necessary to read through her medical charts, fill in any blanks and clarify details with the woman. The pregnancy health record, obstetric risk assessment, Safe Start and Edinburgh Depression Scale tools, plus the client's past history notes and the nurse's own midwifery knowledge and experience, are all useful in helping to carry out a comprehensive assessment of a woman at her first antenatal visit. Consultation and referral guidelines, the state maternity and neonatal guidelines, and any other resources available such as local support services are all useful to help alleviate any concerns. The midwife is responsible for planning the woman's care, in consultation with the woman. The midwife is also responsible for implementing that care, coordinating and collaborating with other care providers, scheduling appointments, organising pathology screening, conducting pap smears, administering and supplying medication, arranging nuchal translucency, organising morphology scans, and referring and liaising with other health service providers. The midwife can also help to arrange travel and accommodation.

The midwife's responsibility includes case management and communication with all the health teams involved in the woman's pregnancy care. The midwife liaises with the receiving hospital staff, including the antenatal clinic, obstetric services, liaison officers, radiology, pathology departments, medical records, diabetes centre, dieticians, diabetic educators, dentists, medical officers, mental health counsellors, alcohol and drug counsellors, patient travel officers and health workers. To maintain a professional relationship, the midwife needs to follow through on all communications in a timely manner.

Within the role, the midwife addresses the social and cultural determinants of health and talks to women about the safety of their environment, the adequacy of their income, meaningful roles in community, secure housing, and education and social support. The midwife also addresses public health issues such as promoting breastfeeding, stopping smoking, responding to situations of domestic violence, and drug and alcohol use. Providing referrals in remote areas has its challenges; support and allied health services are fewer than in regional and urban areas, and women often hesitate to access services in a small community where everyone knows everyone.

The midwife's clinical scope of practice includes performing basic obstetric sonography, performing an informal dating ultrasound, venipuncture for all blood tests in pregnancy, chronic disease and postnatal care, and treatment of sexually transmissible infections, urinary tract infections and anaemía. The primary clinical care manual and drug therapy protocols are useful guides for best practice. The midwife follows up the results from pathology collection and recalls the woman to let her know the results. If she is at risk, it may be necessary to discuss and counsel her about nuchal translucency tests if early in the gestation.

Many Indigenous women have longstanding health and social issues, so the midwife's work often focuses on healthy lifestyles to reduce perinatal and neonatal morbidity and mortality while addressing the social determinants of health at the same time. Having the support of an Indigenous health worker is crucial, as they tend to nurture the client's engagement with healthcare services far better than other health workers; this is because they are able to read the woman's body language from a cultural perspective (for more on Indigenous health workers, see Chapter 10).

Breastfeeding is the predominant infant-feeding choice for women in remote communities, so one challenge is to ensure that they have an adequate dietary intake. Women often need to support a current pregnancy while breastfeeding a toddler. If the woman wants to use infant formula, it is extremely important to make sure she can afford the ongoing costs and that she is educated about hygienic methods of preparing infant formula.

Women in remote communities often have low English literacy, so basic language and pictorial resources are useful in communicating with the women and their families. Better still is the development of resources in their languages, as many community members speak two to four Indigenous languages. Since maternal care is 'women's business', it is important to be careful to provide care in an appropriate setting in the clinic, away from men. Women's examinations, such as breast checks, need to be performed by female health practitioners so women are not embarrassed by having these tests completed by male doctors. Indigenous women from traditional and remote communities tend to make little eye contact and have minimal verbal communication; this is part of their cultural practice and needs to be respected, acknowledged and understood for it to be culturally safe care.

CASE STUDY

Transferring Jenny to Cairns

As the only midwife in Pormpuraaw community, it was up to me to recognise any urgent situation and respond appropriately. Jenny was a Gravida 9 Para 8 who attended the clinic having had no prior antenatal care. She was a diabetic and we were not sure when she had her last menstrual period.

Jenny's blood sugar level was high and the fundal height measurement was 37 centimetres. I knew that Jenny needed to be in Cairns, where she could be better assessed and cared for by specialist staff.

I arranged for Jenny to travel out of the community as soon as possible on the Royal Flying Doctor Service. It was difficult to encourage Jenny to travel so urgently. She had other children to consider and could not know how long she would be out of the community. This was quite concerning for her. She did not see that her immediate transfer was a priority and preferred to go after the weekend. However, as a health professional, I was aware of the health risks and complications that could arise.

QUESTIONS FOR REFLECTION

- How would you have responded to Jenny in this situation?
- Was immediate transfer to Cairns appropriate?

Building women's trust

A woman will not return to receive care if she does not get a good feeling for her midwife and if she hears negative things in the community about the midwife. She may not return even if the midwife is the only local healthcare provider. While the focus of practice should be to apply primary healthcare principles to educate women in making informed decisions for their own care, it is difficult to achieve this in an environment in which there is minimal community support to influence healthier lifestyles.

In order to influence women's health and wellbeing, gaining community involvement is paramount. The midwife's work involves promoting elimination or reduction in domestic violence, risky consumption of alcohol, smoking, drug use and sexually transmissible infection. This includes promoting healthy lifestyles with regular exercise and good nutrition. This work is difficult to achieve without adequate resources and a longstanding presence within the community.

The workload of a midwife in a remote community is hectic. In a community of 600 people, it is possible that ten pregnant women may need to be case managed at any given time. In addition to the role of midwife, a nurse in a remote community will need to do many chart reviews, follow up pathology and ultrasound tests, and liaise with the fly-in fly-out doctors, obstetricians and multidisciplinary team members. Working in a remote community makes it difficult to attend workshops and in-service professional development programs. Much of this needs to be done online to ensure that the midwife maintains her clinical knowledge.

The experiences of women in Pormpuraaw

Currently, all pregnant women living on Cape York Peninsula are transported to the nearest regional hospital, in Cairns, to deliver their babies. They are transferred at 36 weeks' gestation or earlier, depending on the perceived risks. The Patient Travel Subsidy Scheme (PTSS) pays for the women's transportation (by plane) and their accommodation in Cairns. However, if a woman chooses not to stay in the hostels, the PTSS will partially reimburse her for out-of-pocket expenses. Women who are under seventeen years of age or facing special circumstances are offered a support person.

Fortunately, in Cairns there is Mookai Rosie Bi-Bayan, an Indigenous family health and accommodation centre that offers support and education for pregnant women during their stay in Cairns. Mookai Rosie is staffed by Aboriginal and Torres Strait Islander people who are culturally supportive and safe.

There are times when women say that they cannot attend appointments due to family or community commitments, so it is important to work closely with them to ensure they have a negotiated outcome. This is culturally safe care.

When women are away from their homes for a minimum of four weeks to await the arrival of their baby, they can face enormous stress. They are surrounded by unfamiliar people, their baby is delivered in a strange environment, they worry for their other children and they are unable to undertake any of the traditional ceremonial activities during the birth of their baby. They may feel lonely and isolated from their family. They worry that their children will experience problems with other children in the community and that they cannot trust anyone in the community to look after their children (especially if they get sick). Many women feel that they should be able to take their children with them while they wait for the arrival of the new baby.

A return to birthing in communities

Many Aboriginal and Torres Strait Islander people feel that being born in hospitals takes away their birth rights and their land rights. There are plans to reopen the birthing centres of Cape York at Cooktown Hospital and Weipa Integrated Health

Service. Women from the surrounding communities will be able to give birth in these communities if they are deemed low risk. Women within the community are embracing this possibility and are starting to present early for antenatal care to ensure that they remain at low risk.

Birthing for Indigenous women in remote locations must be balanced with cultural safety that is inclusive of the social effects on families and communities. At current staffing levels, all communities struggle to develop and deliver culturally safe programs for antenatal education. If birthing closer to their homelands is going to be a choice for women, it must be introduced properly and resourced adequately, otherwise it could have a direct negative effect on the morbidity and mortality of women and their children. If anything goes wrong, families may blame the hospital or the midwife.

Birthing and maternity units need to promote cultural understanding by providing in-service education for midwives in relation to birthing customs. Women must be given back control over their birthing experience. If they wish to have a support person during labour, this should be encouraged and supported through the PTSS. Having support during labour can reduce fear and lower the rate of labour interventions, including caesarean section rates.

CASE STUDY

Minnie, Mary and Enid

In 1902, Minnie had a baby to a white man at Port Douglas. The baby was a beautiful, blue-eyed, blonde girl called Mary. Minnie was employed, but once she had a baby the Queensland government decided that she should be sent to Yarrabah mission, where she and her baby would be looked after by the church group under the *Aboriginals Protection and Restriction of the Sale of Opium Act 1897*. At Yarrabah, Minnie met her future husband and raised Mary and three other children.

When Mary was nineteen years old, she married Harry, who had been sent to Yarrabah from Mossman at the age of five. Mary and Harry were both children of the mission and they went on to have four children. Enid was their eldest child. At age ten, Enid was left at the mission. Enid remembered crying to go back home. She remained in the mission for nine years.

Throughout her time at the mission, the missionaries never spoke to Enid about where babies came from. As a child, Enid was told that fairies brought the babies to the hospital and gave them to new mothers. The meeting with the fairies was supposed to take place behind the dormitory, in a creek that had a waterfall. Enid and the other mission girls never had any education about women's business, such as sex, how babies were made, contraception and menstruation. The mission girls and boys were all very innocent. The boys' dormitory was close by the girls' dormitory, but both places had very high fences so girls and boys did not go into each other's areas willingly.

When Enid was in her teens, a priest called Father Brown asked Enid and her best friend Dulcie to become nurses. They both thought it was a good idea. Their training

(cont.)

as nurses got off to a good start, until one day they were asked to go and see a baby being born. Wow! They thought they were going to see the fairies bring a new baby from the waterfall.

Everything was going fine. The woman, Enid's cousin, had a good labour, and soon the baby's head appeared. Enid looked, screamed and ran out of the birthing room. That was the end of her nursing career. Dulcie went on to become a great midwife, delivering hundreds of babies over the years.

QUESTIONS FOR REFLECTION

- How would a traditional upbringing have prepared Enid for birthing?
- How does Enid's upbringing equip her to be a mother herself?

Conclusion

Aboriginal and Torres Strait Islander women are no longer able to give birth on their homelands or to practise their traditional birthing culture. Most women who live in remote communities are forced to leave their community for the birth of their babies in a city hospital that is many kilometres away from their children, husbands and families.

While much of the traditional knowledge has disappeared, some knowledge of Grandmothers' Law remains strong. Even though birthing now occurs off Country, strong Indigenous women have remembered some of their traditional practices and what they learned from their mothers, grandmothers and aunts. The traditional Indigenous laws that have survived despite Western practices need to be preserved and acknowledged in the biomedical model of care. Training in culturally safe midwifery practice is an important part of this. Many Aboriginal and Torres Strait Islander women give birth when they are young and have little education about mothering. They need support from their Elders, who often feel that the old ways of communicating and educating are breaking down and not being replaced. However, many women Elders say that times have changed and the young no longer listen to their Elders.

Learning activities

1. Compare birthing traditions in different cultures. You may like to choose two different cultures represented in your local community and compare their traditions and beliefs about pregnancy, birthing and the care of newborns.
2. Interview women who have given birth and ask about how their cultural traditions and beliefs influenced their pregnancy and childbirth experiences. If possible, interview women of different ages and from various cultural backgrounds.

3. Imagine that you are a Registered Midwife working at a health centre in a remote community. A woman in the early stages of pregnancy has approached you for advice about how to maintain her health and prepare for birth. What issues does your advice need to cover? How might your advice be different for a woman living in a remote community, compared with the advice you would give to a woman in an urban setting?

FURTHER READING

Dragon, N. (2019). Birthing on Country: Improving Aboriginal and Torres Strait Islander infant and maternal health. *Australian Nursing & Midwifery Journal,* 10 February. Retrieved from https://anmj.org.au/birthing-on-country-improving-indigenous-health

Gaskin, M. (1975). *Spiritual Midwifery*. Summertown, TN: Book Publishing Company.

Kildea, S., Gao, Y., Rolfe, M. ... Barclay, L.M. (2016). Remote links: Redesigning maternity care for Aboriginal women from remote communities in Northern Australia – a comparative cohort study. *Midwifery*, 34, 47–57. Retrieved from https://pubmed.ncbi.nlm.nih.gov/26971448

Visit the companion website at www.cambridge.org/highereducation/isbn/9781108794695/resources to see further online resources.

REFERENCES

Apunipima Cape York Health Council (1997). *Saving the Knowledge: Memories of Traditional Birthing in Cape York*. Bungalow, Qld: Apunipima Cape York Health Council.

CAAC (1985). *Borning Ampe mbwareke pmere alaltye: The Congress Alukura by the Grandmother's Law*. Report prepared by the Central Australian Aboriginal Congress, August 1985. Retrieved from: https://www.caac.org.au/uploads/pdfs/Borning-Ampe-mbwareke-pmere-alaltye-the-Congress-Alukura-by-the-grandmothers-law-report.pdf

Gyia, L. (1996). Congress Alukura by the Grandmothers' Law. *Aboriginal and Islander Health Worker Journal*, March, 14.

Humphrey, M. & Keating, S. (2004). Lack of antenatal care in Far North Queensland. *Australian and New Zealand Journal of Obstetrics and Gynaecology*, 44(1), 10–13.

Marshall, V. (1997). Aboriginal babies: A story of Port Douglas. *Port Douglas Gazette*, 24 December.

Ward, N.N. (2018). *Ninu Grandmothers' Law. The Autobiography of Nura Nungaka Ward*. Broome, WA: Magabala Books.

LEGISLATION CITED

Aboriginals Protection and Restriction of the Sale of Opium Act 1897

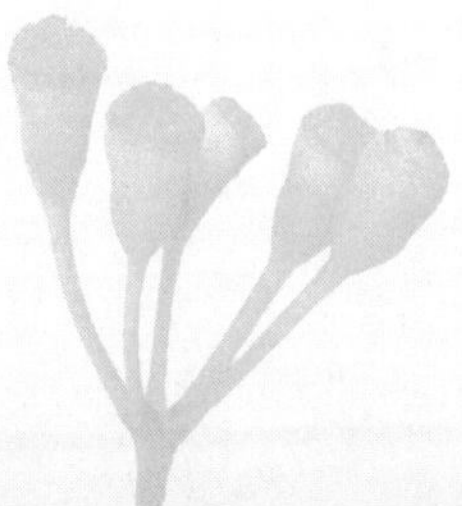

Remote area nursing practice

Nicole Ramsamy

9

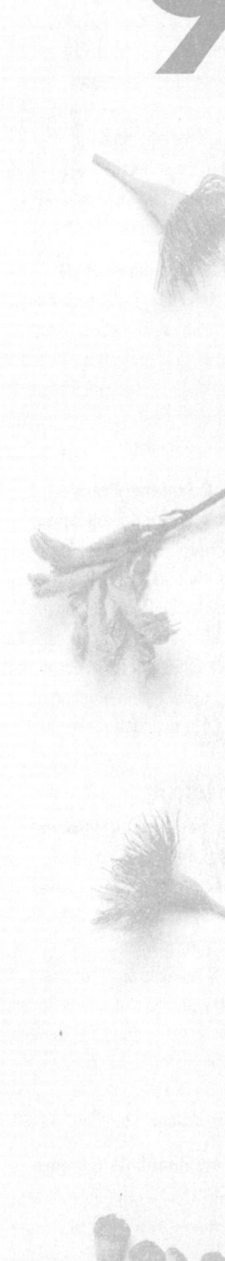

LEARNING OBJECTIVES

This chapter will help you to understand:

- The scope of remote area nursing practice
- The educational needs of remote area nurses (RANs)
- The cultural and socioeconomic issues relevant to remote area nursing
- Some factors that influence the ways in which healthcare services are organised and delivered in remote communities
- Some cultural obligations and practices relevant to remote area nursing

KEY WORDS

Deed of Grant in Trust (DOGIT)
Indigenous health worker (IHW)
Nurse Practitioner
Primary Health Care Centre (PHCC)
remote area nurse (RAN)
Remote Isolated Practice Endorsed Registered Nurse (RIPERN)

Introduction

Nurse Practitioner A Registered Nurse educated to Master's degree level who is authorised to work autonomously in an advanced and extended clinical role. Nurse Practitioners assess clients, manage their healthcare, refer them to other health professionals, prescribe medications and order diagnostic studies.

remote area nurse (RAN) RANs provide nursing services in remote Australian communities. Most RANs work in community-based health centres. They may have additional qualifications, in addition to being a Registered Nurse.

Remote Isolated Practice Endorsed Registered Nurse (RIPERN) RIPERNs are Registered Nurses with a Scheduled Medicines Endorsement by the Australian Health Practitioner Regulations Agency (AHPRA). They may provide a limited range of medicines in situations where there is limited access to a doctor or Nurse Practitioner.

Indigenous health workers (IHWs) IHWs provide a link between Aboriginal and Torres Strait Islander communities and healthcare services. They provide clinical services and promote primary care to individuals, families and community groups within their communities. They encourage Indigenous people to take an active role in managing their own health.

Primary Health Care Centre (PHCC) PHCCs offer a holistic approach to healthcare at the local level. The facilities available in a PHCC vary from community to community. The PHCC model emphasises equity, equality, affordability, appropriateness, accessibility and social justice. Each PHCC is uniquely designed to suit the culture of its host community.

In 2010, I became the first qualified Indigenous **Nurse Practitioner** in Queensland.

Becoming a Nurse Practitioner was a long and interesting journey. I completed a Bachelor of Nursing degree at the University of Newcastle in New South Wales in 1997, and the nursing graduate program at Mackay Base Hospital in Queensland in 1998. Venturing overseas, I worked in Newcastle upon Tyne (in England) for some time before returning to Queensland and working in remote communities at Cape York and Thursday Island. I returned to Cairns, where I was raised, to continue my studies, and completed the Master of Midwifery degree in 2003 at the University of Southern Queensland and Cairns Base Hospital.

While working in remote communities as a **remote area nurse (RAN)**, I became a **Remote Isolated Practice Endorsed Registered Nurse (RIPERN)**, and completed certificates in both immunisation and women's health. Together, these qualifications help to ensure that I am able to work in a remote healthcare centre and practise autonomously when there is no doctor available.

Remote area nursing is characterised by geographical, social and professional isolation. RANs must be specialist nurses in their remote communities. They coordinate and deliver a diverse range of healthcare services in an environment that is unique, challenging and demanding. Their clinical and operational duties are highly varied. RANs are able to work in a range of communities, including Aboriginal or Torres Strait Islander communities, or communities established around activities such as mining, agriculture, fishing, tourism and refugee detention.

The health profile of people living in remote Aboriginal and Torres Strait Islander communities is the poorest in Australia. There are great gaps in service provision. In addition, the relationships between the various health staff, such as RANs, **Indigenous health workers (IHWs)**, Registered Nurses (RNs), allied health staff and doctors can be strained due to unclear professional boundaries and other reasons. (See Chapter 10 for a discussion of the role of IHWs.) The scope and practice of each staff member need to be clarified.

This chapter reflects on my practice and experience of being a RAN. It explores the scope of RAN practice and discusses complexities such as cultural obligation, cultural safety, burden of disease and isolation when working in a remote Indigenous community. It reflects on my experience in different remote nursing roles: as a Clinical Nurse, Clinical Nurse Consultant and Acting Director of Nursing at the remote Aboriginal community Pormpuraaw, in its **Primary Health Care Centre (PHCC)**; as a Nurse Practitioner at the Napranum PHCC, an Aboriginal Community that services both Aboriginal and Torres Strait Islander people; and as a Nurse Practitioner in a mining town at the Weipa Integrated Health Care Service. All of these communities are located on Cape York Peninsula in Queensland.

Nurses are differentiated from other healthcare providers by their approach to patient care, training and scope of practice. Nurses practise in a number of areas, with different scopes of practice and levels of prescriber authority. They are permitted by most jurisdictions to practise independently in a variety of settings, depending on their training level and place of practice. Nursing education has undergone a process of change towards advanced and specialised credentials, and many of the traditional regulations and provider roles have been transformed. Rural and remote nursing is considered to be a specialist generalist role. Because rural and remote nurses lack medical support where they are located, they work in all aspects as primary caregiver, and at times beyond their scope of practice facilities (Mills, Birks & Hegney, 2010).

The Nurse Practitioner scope of practice in rural and remote communities includes the management of comprehensive primary healthcare, implementation of chronic disease care plans and attending to acute conditions. This service is the most convenient and financially sustainable option for enhancing health outcomes. The role of Nurse Practitioner has been introduced to respond to limited resources and meet the high demand of healthcare consumers and, most importantly, fill the gap in services.

The role of the Nurse Practitioner in remote and rural communities is explored throughout the rest of the chapter, using a series of case scenarios.

Collaborative multidisciplinary inter-agency team approach: Chronic disease

CASE STUDY

Lizzie

Lizzie (not her real name) is a 73-year-old woman of Torres Strait Island descent currently staying with her daughter. Lizzie has her own home but has decided to stay with her daughter due to a recent acute condition that has left her very anxious. When Lizzie is well, she travels between the communities to attend cultural festivities, sorry business and visit her extended family.

Lizzie is very mobile and has a medical condition consisting of type 2 diabetes mellitus, obstructive sleep disorder and a history of cellulitis due to a previous spider bite. Lizzie had just travelled out from her community for a family event and suddenly fell ill. She had symptoms of feeling very unwell: lethargy, chills, fever and not being able to walk. Taken to the general hospital, she was unable to provide a clear medical history of her chronic conditions or a list of medications to the treating doctor. The doctor admitted her to the hospital to treat the cellulitis on her left leg, uncertain of the cause.

The doctor reviewed her vital signs, which indicated tachycardia, tachypnea, nausea and confusion, and reviewed the pathology, which indicated an acute kidney injury secondary to dehydration with septicaemia. The doctor was very concerned about her prognosis and called for the family to be present (the Royal Flying Doctor Service was not an option at the time and Lizzie was too unwell to travel back to her community on a commercial flight). With the family at her bedside, the change in Lizzie was astonishing: her condition miraculously improved and she was able to return to her community by commercial aircraft.

(cont.)

Lizzie likes to visit a combination of services in her community that Queensland Health established many decades ago, and also Apunipima, an Aboriginal Community Controlled Organisation that started in 2010. When Lizzie returned to her community, she went to see the Queensland Health Nurse Practitioner, as she feels the service is comprehensive and culturally safe. Lizzie's recent hospitalisation required her to have follow-up for resolving cellulitis and acute kidney injury. The Nurse Practitioner reviewed Lizzie and discovered new symptoms: shortness of breath, hypertension, pitting oedema and a decline in her mobility. With further assessments of spirometry and an ECG and a referral to the Apunipima podiatrist, it was vital for Lizzie to be seen by physicians. With Lizzie's and her family's consent, she agreed to be transferred to the regional hospital to be reviewed by a multidisciplinary team of physicians – a cardiologist, respiratory specialist, endocrinologist, nephrologist, sleep study team and allied-health occupational therapist in view of medical aides. Due to the complexities of Lizzie's health issues, it was deemed best for her to be transferred and admitted to a regional hospital for the physicians to assess, implement and collaborate on the best care plan for her. Lizzie was discharged with an understanding of her current medical condition and told that the likely cause of her cellulitis was a spider bite she had had experienced seven years earlier. Lizzie is now more conscious of her medical history and medications, and continues to have regular health checks performed by her local Queensland Health PHCC.

QUESTION FOR REFLECTION

- What role did the Nurse Practitioner play in the care of Lizzie that would be beyond the scope of a general Registered Nurse?

Waiting for fly-in medical and allied health services from a number of partnership organisations, and then having to collaborate with everyone, can delay the delivery of care needed by people such as Lizzie, placing their health at risk and causing confusion and a lack of confidence in the service. When working across government and non-government agencies, nurses have a long history of being involved in care delivery, especially in areas that suffer social setbacks. They have a deep understanding of the cultures and values of the people living in remote areas, and this knowledge can be channelled appropriately and tailored to IT-based healthcare services.

Although Australia has one of the most stable and well-organised healthcare systems in the world, it is far from achieving the equality and equity that is desirable – despite deliberate efforts to address disparities in the health of Indigenous communities. The National Aboriginal and Torres Strait Island Health Plan 2013–2023 (DHA, 2013) provides long-term, evidence-based policy frameworks as part of the overarching Council of Australian Governments approach. The National Indigenous Reform Agreement 2008 (SCRGSP, 2009) established a framework and two of the targets involve closing the gap in child mortality by 2018 and in life expectancy by 2031. The way health services operate and are structured, the way care is delivered – including the patient's journey – and the clinical guidelines and pathways that are to be followed all determine the role of the Nurse Practitioner and their scope of practice in rural and remote communities. All these factors can contribute significantly to achieving these targets.

We must improve the integration between different service providers across primary healthcare, acute care, specialist care and particularly Indigenous care. Different trends in healthcare have made it possible for there to be a setting where patients and providers work together, and technology is constantly used for sharing communication and exchanging knowledge. Sharing of resources and ideas improves the way healthcare services are delivered and should eventually empower the healthcare providers to work more effectively.

Occasionally, I have found that the small work teams in remote communities can be challenging in many ways. For example, it can be trying for novice RANs, who may not have a broad scope of practice or set of clinical skills and knowledge. Their knowledge of the community and/or their clients' medical histories may be limited and their connections within community may not be strong. It is important for both experienced and novice RANs to do the best they can clinically and to adhere to their scope of practice. The novice RAN will learn over time what is required within their clinical context. It is essential that experienced RANs, while they undertake other operational and managerial roles, remain supportive of nurses presenting to these communities to work. We all have to start somewhere, and we all have to respect each other in order to work as a team.

Another challenge is that some nurses burn out or do not get along with others. Colleagues must remain supportive and respectful of each other as they work towards building their individual skills set – experience will follow. Remote area nursing may not be for everyone, and experienced RANs must be careful not to destroy a novice nurse's confidence or disempower them to the point where they leave the profession.

Mentoring was an important part of my learning to be a RAN. My early experience inspired me to be passionate and supportive in the nursing field when working with both clients and colleagues. As my career developed, I provided advocacy services for RANs at the regional, state and national levels and in the Indigenous communities where they worked.

QUESTION FOR REFLECTION

- This scenario identified mentoring as an integral part of learning to be a RAN. Reflect on the role of the RAN and consider why mentoring is so important.

Nursing in remote Australia

Living in a remote community: The example of Napranum

Napranum was officially gazetted as the place-name to replace Weipa South in September 1990 and the **Deed of Grant in Trust (DOGIT)** lands became known as the Napranum DOGIT in 1991. Napranum has become an increasingly prosperous community with modern facilities such as the Yepenyi-Awumpun art gallery, Mary Ann Coconut library and Indigenous Knowledge Centre, new Council offices, a health

Deed of Grant in Trust (DOGIT) A community land trust system established in Queensland to administer former reserves and missions. DOGITs were established in 1984 to allow community councils to own and administer former reserves and missions. The trusts are governed by local representatives who are elected every three years.

centre, a retirement home, a supermarket, a war memorial, workshops and many new houses being built over the past ten years (Napranum Aboriginal Shire Council, 2017).

Napranum, which means 'meeting place', has both Aboriginal and Torres Strait Islander people living in the community. It is located on the western side of Cape York Peninsula, approximately 800 kilometres north-west of Cairns. On a good travelling day, with decent road conditions, it is a nine-hour drive from Cairns. Most RNs take the 80-minute flight from Cairns. The airline's passengers are mostly non-Indigenous government employees working in mining and health fields. Other passengers include Indigenous people travelling for medical appointments, boarding school or family visits.

The Napranum community has a variety of facilities, such as:

- support services, including the PHCC, Home and Community Care (HACC), which offers limited services, child safety house and women's centre
- community facilities, including a library, arts and cultural centre, Uniting Church, child care centre, prep school, after-school care centre and ranger's office, grocery store and council office.

In terms of communication services, the community has public telephone boxes that sometimes work, free internet access in the library and a service for paid wireless internet and mobile telephones for use within the township.

The cost of food is consistently higher in remote communities than in urban areas, and food choices can be limited. Finding healthy food is often difficult because of the distances and freight costs. The recent Queensland Productivity Commission inquiry into service delivery in remote and discrete Aboriginal and Torres Strait Islander communities found that access to healthy food and food pricing was an issue for many remote communities (2017). These issues were further explored in a recent House of Representatives Standing Committee inquiry (2020) and were further exacerbated during the COVID-19 pandemic, as they are in natural disasters (see Fredericks & Best, 2020; Fredericks & Bradfield, 2021).

Much of the public housing in Napranum is of substandard quality and in need of extensive restoration in order to meet the needs of occupiers with disabilities. Housing is fundamental to people's health and wellbeing, and developing public policies and programs that provide sufficient, equitable, appropriate, secure housing is a continuing challenge. Housing has been raised as an ongoing issue in many remote communities (Queensland Productivity Commission, 2017).

Dogs are ever-present in Napranum. There are many broken fences, and dogs walk freely in and out of yards. They lie in the middle of the road in the streets and do not move for cars. People drive around them. Visitors have to be careful, because packs of dogs may see unfamiliar people as a threat and attack them. Some people regard their dogs as part of their family and, in some cases, as spirit dogs; this means that dogs are somewhat protected. There have been times when a dog has died after being hit by a car and the owner has asked for financial compensation. There is a fly-in vet service available on certain days in Weipa.

Napranum is remote, and the country around it is harsh. Anyone who ventures outside the township should advise someone about where they are going and how long they plan to be away. This country must be respected and explored with caution.

Remote areas make up 78 per cent of Australia's land mass (ABS, 2016). They are diverse, ranging from the huge central desert to the ski slopes of the south, the ochre mountains of the west and the crocodile-infested rivers of the north. Remote areas are often collectively described as 'the outback'. They are characterised by small and highly dispersed populations and limited access to all services. Roads are long, dusty and unsealed, with wandering stock and plenty of wildlife. In these conditions, a trip of 100 kilometres can take several hours (Smith, 2004).

RANs are Registered Nurses who live and work in remote communities and provide local healthcare services. Most have special qualifications for remote area work. There is a shortage of experienced and qualified RANs in Australia, as many have left this demanding practice due to retirement or personal health issues. Staff shortages of experienced RANs can limit the scope of services that RANs are able to offer and affect the health of people living in remote communities.

RANs come from a variety of career backgrounds, including rural hospitals, and emergency and community nursing roles. Usually their backgrounds have allowed them to gather diverse skills and experiences associated with a variety of clinical areas.

There is no such thing as a typical day for a RAN. Nurses working in rural and remote settings practise under enormous pressure to assume some of the functions that traditionally are in the realm of other disciplines. They must adapt to the community and to the needs of individuals, and act in ways that are often confronting, challenging, stimulating and rewarding. It is also imperative for RANs to have a well-grounded background in community and public health in order to better serve the rural and remote community, which has difficulty accessing and utilising care due to its geographical location and socioeconomic disparities. To provide safe and effective care to the patients, RANs must integrate knowledge, skills and attitudes in order to make sound judgements and appropriate decisions.

In remote communities, nurses and health workers provide critically needed services and community support. Successful nurses become active members of the community. For example, RANs and IHWs need to participate in the planning, organisation, operation and control of local healthcare services. They also develop activities to promote improvements in the available services and support the health of the community. They need to meet regularly with local stakeholders to advise them of community programs and learn about the community's health needs. For example, in some communities it may be relevant for nurses to develop specific programs that target petrol sniffing, skin conditions, influenza, homelessness, child safety or abuse, or domestic violence.

RANs need to be proactive in identifying and talking about community health issues. While they may be concerned about client confidentiality when they discuss the community's needs with stakeholders, it is often necessary to have these discussions without mentioning names. From the community's perspective, it is important to discuss emerging problems and promptly develop solutions so that issues can be resolved locally. A community cannot wait for organisations from outside to advise about what needs to be done. When problems cannot be resolved within the community, people are often removed and placed in an alien environment until something changes locally (and this may never happen). For example, Elders who are unable to care for themselves need various support services to work together in a way that will allow them to remain in their community with respect, dignity and safety. They may be sent out of their community until the appropriate environment is found. Often this does not happen, and the Elders are sent to residential care because family members are unable to provide the care they need.

Nursing in remote communities can be complicated by rapid staff turnover in many of the relevant support agencies. When staff are new to the community, have limited public health experience and have limited experience in working with Indigenous or remote communities, it can be almost impossible to build a service that is responsive to the needs of the local community. It is also very difficult to plan and sustain health-promotion activities or to seek support and commitment from government or non-government organisations for new initiatives. There is limited commitment at the policy level to providing support for remote health initiatives, developing culturally safe practice or exploring ways to create a sustainable workforce.

QUESTIONS FOR REFLECTION

- What aspects of nursing in remote areas are likely to be affected by rapid staff turnover?
- How can RANs support those who will take their place once their contract ends?

CASE STUDY

Mary and Aaron

Mary and Aaron live in the centre of Pormpuraaw, an Aboriginal community situated on the west coast of Cape York Peninsula. (This story is typical of many people in Pormpuraaw, but is not about actual individuals.)

Mary is 26 years old and Aaron is 28 years old. They have six children: Sarah (eleven), John (ten), Sian (eight), Jerry (five), Donald (three) and Jeremy (one). The family lives with Mary's mother, Dolly (aged 42), Mary's brother, Shaun (24), who is always in trouble with the law, and Mary's sister, Lily (20), plus Lily's three children, Jayden (four), Rhianna (three) and Brody (one). Their three-bedroom, low-set, brick house is home to five adults and nine children. The house has very little furniture and requires a lot of maintenance.

Mary's father passed away three months ago, at the age of 47. He had a heart attack and a history of diabetes mellitus type 2 (on insulin) and ischaemic heart disease. He rarely took his prescribed medication because he was frequently away, working on the roads for the community council.

Aaron's family lives within the community too, and sometimes family members come over to stay. That has happened less since Dolly came to live with them after the death of her husband and the closure of her house due to cultural obligations.

Mary and Aaron were both sent out of the community to attend high school. Neither finished Year 8; they were both suspended from high schools that were more than 2000 kilometres from their home community. Mary stays at home to care for the younger children, while Aaron works three days a week for the Community Development Employment Project (CDEP) in the parks and gardens work area.

Mary has hopes that her daughter, Sarah, will become a nurse at the local PHCC, but this would mean that she would have to leave the community to complete high school, attend university and work in the city before coming back home. Mary is concerned about the idea of Sarah being away from home so long that she might not want to come back to her community and family. In addition, Mary and Aaron do not have the money to support Sarah while she studies.

Mary and Aaron have very little furniture. They sleep on mattresses on the floor. There is nowhere in the community to buy furniture – except for plastic chairs and tables, which are expensive and do not last long. The house has built-in shelving. The screen doors and windows are all damaged, and their dogs come in and out of the house regularly. The yard is unfenced, overgrown with weeds and grass, and filled with broken toys and discarded things (like a rusty shower chair on the back veranda and a rusty old car in the front yard).

Mary says that she does not have time to look after her own health, and she struggles to make sure that all her children's health checks are up to date. Aaron does not think it is necessary for him and his family to have health checks; he avoids the PHCC because he believes that there is nothing wrong with him or his family.

Dolly is not permitted to leave her bedroom or have conversations with people for cultural reasons related to the passing of her husband. At some stage, the family will decide to undertake a 'house opening' of her house.

QUESTION FOR REFLECTION

- As the newly arrived non-Indigenous Nurse Practitioner in this community, where would you commence your provision of care in the above scenario?

This type of scenario is common in remote communities. People frequently live in overcrowded housing situations, with little furniture, poor sanitation, poor maintenance and dogs inside the house. Their basic needs are not met. They have limited access to cleaning products and equipment, and lack the self-determination needed to improve their basic health.

The work of remote area nurses

RANs deliver and coordinate health services in whatever manner they can, with whatever resources are available. When possible, they collaborate with a multidisciplinary team that visits the community for between one and five days at a time.

RANs are able to work alone, as the sole health practitioner in a community, or may be part of a small team based in a PHCC. The PHCC team may include a group of RANs, IHWs, child health nurses, midwives, mental health nurses, diabetic educators, aged care nurses, allied health staff and fly-in doctors. Some RANs hold multiple qualifications that enable them to be Registered Nurses, midwives, x-ray operators and public health workers. PHCC teams are not always co-located geographically. The staff members may all work independently, but collaborate across a region. Collaborative practice can be complicated and challenging because of transient clients, staff turnover, lack of resources and difficulties managing relationships.

RANs usually work on rostered shifts during business hours, and are on call for after-hours emergencies. RANs provide services 24 hours a day, seven days a week. The work involves a broad scope of health practice that provides emergency care and primary healthcare for individuals, families and the wider community. While RANs can experience personal and professional isolation, the scope of their practice and their broad skill set are unique in nursing and make being a RAN one of the most rewarding jobs in the nursing field.

A RAN who has additional notations on their AHPRA registration is highly regarded within remote communities and has excellent prospects for finding work. Examples of valuable additional qualifications include RIPERN, immunisation, emergency nursing, sexual health endorsements, midwifery, women's health pap smear provider, extended x-ray licence and training in public health. These additional skills allow the RAN to screen, detect and manage clients who present opportunistically at the service. Without these skills, RANs must constantly seek advice from distant doctors, such as the Royal Flying Doctor Service (RFDS), before commencing a treatment plan. Well-trained RANs can help to reduce the need for clients to travel out of the community and can also reduce the length of time clients need to wait for tests or treatment.

Additional qualifications are essential for RANs. Short courses or workshops such as advanced adult and paediatric life support, trauma care, plastering, remote emergency care, maternity care courses and cultural safety are all very helpful. Some RAN positions have extended responsibility in the practice of maternal and child health, mental health, women's health, men's health, community capacity-building, health promotion and chronic disease management. Any qualifications in these areas are helpful. Some health service districts have mandatory requirements for RANs to be certified in pre-hospital trauma life support (PHTLS), trauma nursing core course (TNCC), advanced life support (ALS) or paediatric life support (PALS). RANs also need annual training in fire and evacuation, manual handling, drug calculation, child safety and basic life support (CRANA, 2014).

The scope of a RAN's practice is regulated and affected by a range of workforce and legislative issues. Many of their qualifications need to be certified by the District Health Service and reviewed regularly. However, even with the extra training of RANs, there are still many gaps within the nursing system that affect their ability to provide holistic care. Nurse Practitioners are even more valuable to remote communities than RANs because their practice is autonomous and accountable. Nurse Practitioners provide a holistic view of health, with physical assessment skills, history-taking, illness-management skills and a primary healthcare perspective that provides a broad scope of practice.

The additional skills of a credentialled RAN

A trained and credentialled RAN is able to offer a level of healthcare that cannot be matched by RNs. (The following story is typical but is not about actual individuals.) For example, RN Sarah, who has no postgraduate qualifications and no remote area experience, attended to Maggie, a nineteen-year-old who presented with gradual onset of lower abdominal pain. Sarah took a history, made an initial assessment, contacted the RFDS for a management plan to help with Maggie's discomfort and supplied the medication prescribed by the doctor.

In another community, RAN Tina, with RIPERN, sexual health training, women's health training and five years of experience in remote area practice, attended to Rhonda, also a nineteen-year-old, who presented with gradual onset of lower abdominal pain. Tina took an in-depth history from Maggie and suggested that she had symptoms related to pelvic inflammatory disease. Tina was able to collect pathology and cytology to support her clinical assessment, and to supply medication and ensure that Rhonda was receiving the correct treatment with adequate follow-up within the community. Tina adopted a primary healthcare approach to best suit the needs of her client and her community. She was able to follow up with her client and provide a management plan for those involved (such as contact tracing if the pathology reports detected a sexual health condition).

The examples of Sarah and Tina illustrate the great advantage of qualifications and experience of RANs. The RAN with no endorsed qualifications must speak to a doctor for a treatment plan. In remote Indigenous communities, this can be an important distinction. Many Indigenous people have difficulty expressing their health history, and health practitioners can miss vital information. Having a broad health knowledge can help the RAN to take a thorough health assessment. Being known and trusted in the community also helps. Because Tina is the only available health professional in her community, and because her qualifications are sound, a RAN like Tina can assume some elements of a doctor's role.

The burden of disease and injury in remote communities

People who live in remote Aboriginal and Torres Strait Islander communities are exposed to an even higher burden of disease relative to non-remote populations, with a reduced life expectancy, increased rates of disability and reduced quality of life. This disparity is caused primarily by poor living conditions and limited access to health services. People in remote areas encounter many health challenges that are due to their living conditions, social isolation and socioeconomic disadvantage.

There are high rates of unemployment, low education levels and many overcrowded houses. Socioeconomic disadvantage places remote Indigenous people at high risk of chronic disease, communicable disease, infant mortality and morbidity, substance misuse, poor nutrition and emotional distress.

Cardiovascular disease (CVD), such as acute rheumatic fever and rheumatic heart disease, is the largest contributor to the health disparity and are the leading cause of death among Aboriginal and Torres Strait Islander people (AIHW, 2015; Penm, 2008). CVD risk factors include smoking, physical inactivity, poor nutrition, risky levels of alcohol consumption, hypertension, overweight and obesity, diabetes and chronic kidney disease. All of these risk factors are highly prevalent in remote Indigenous communities (AIHW, 2019; Penm, 2008).

Injuries and poisoning are responsible for 14 per cent of the health gap between Indigenous and other Australians, and are a major cause of hospitalisation of Aboriginal and Torres Strait Islander people (AHMAC, 2017). Injuries have three main causes: they may be inflicted by another person or persons; they may be the result of an accidental fall; or they may be due to self-harm. Social and economic disadvantage combined with feelings of despair can lead to self-harm, increasing the incidence of intentional injury. (For further discussion of social and emotional wellbeing and self-harm see Chapters 13 and 14.)

Complexities of the remote setting

As noted elsewhere in this book, Aboriginal and Torres Strait Islander people view their health differently from other Australians by adopting a holistic perspective. It is bound up in their communities' social, emotional, spiritual and cultural wellbeing. They place high emphasis on the land, dignity and community self-esteem (Smith, 2004). Nurses who work in remote communities need to understand this Indigenous concept of health. They must address the diverse needs of the entire community as they provide essential healthcare across the lifespan. Their work encompasses not only physical wellbeing, but also social, emotional, spiritual and cultural wellbeing.

Aboriginal and Torres Strait Islander people who live in remote communities have distinctive health concerns that relate directly to their living conditions, social isolation and distance from significant health services. In most cases, people who live in remote communities experience poorer health and wellbeing, and higher hospitalisation rates than those living in urban and metropolitan areas. They also have higher mortality and morbidity rates. The complexities of service provision within remote and discrete communities and accessing services, including health services, was identified in the recent Queensland Productivity Commission inquiry (2017) into service delivery in remote and discrete Aboriginal and Torres Strait Islander communities.

Aboriginal and Torres Strait Islander people in remote communities face several obstacles that reduce their access to adequate and appropriate healthcare. Part of the RAN's job is to help people to navigate the health system and get the care they need. When there are many obstacles facing a client, the person may delay seeking treatment until they feel the time is right. Sometimes clients simply refuse treatment and continue to put up with their health problems.

Many people who have grown up in remote communities have not completed school and have limited literacy and numeracy skills. They may not be able to read the instructions that explain how to prepare for a particular procedure.

In most cases, people who live in remote communities have to travel some distance for basic health assessments that are taken for granted in urban and metropolitan settings – including such basic services as radiology. Many people do not like travelling away from their communities. They may not be familiar with city life and feel that everything is too distant. They may worry about who will care for their children and family members in their absence.

RANs need to consider each client's circumstances and support clients by planning appointments in advance and providing support when it is needed. For example, the

RAN may need to plan appointments to minimise travel and to coincide with the client's payday (such as Centrelink payments) to make sure that the client is able to pay for transportation and meals. The client may need help to arrange care for children or other family members. The RAN may also need to make sure the client understands the reasons for the appointments, the tests to be conducted, any preparation required and the possible outcome. The client may need additional services, such as a support person or a liaison officer. They may need specific equipment when preparing for the procedure (such as a toilet close to the bedroom when preparing for a colonoscopy).

RANs can help to support clients who visit regional hospitals by putting them in touch with Indigenous Liaison Officers (ILOs) and any other support services available in the regional centre. ILOs can be a vital connection for community members who experience difficulties (particularly language difficulties) in hospital and other healthcare settings. ILOs can help the client to cope and adjust to the illness, explain hospital services and procedures, refer them to other support services, assist in problem-solving, provide practical assistance, assist with discharge planning, advocate for the client, provide education to other hospital staff, assist in accommodation, liaise with Centrelink if necessary and help to link clients to their families through letters and video-conferencing. Together, RANs and ILOs can make the health system workable and understandable for Indigenous people from remote communities.

QUESTIONS FOR REFLECTION

- Why is it important for RANs to understand Aboriginal and Torres Strait Islander views on health?
- Should RANs assume that once they have learned the views of one community, they fully understand the views of all Aboriginal and Torres Strait Islander people? Why or why not?

Cultural considerations

RANs who are living and working in remote Indigenous communities must be respectful of the cultural beliefs and obligations of the local people. RANs need to understand their place in the community, learn about what they can and cannot do, and come to understand the most effective ways to engage with their Indigenous clients.

One element of cultural respect is learning about the cultural significance of story places and recognising that particular parts of Country may be closed for a period due to cultural obligations. These are places of spiritual, historical or ceremonial significance that relate to a person's identity. Only people who are knowledgeable about the Country and the community's connections are able to identify these places. Often, they are off-limits to outsiders and other Indigenous families due to cultural restrictions, unless the family says that it is acceptable to travel to that Country.

Another element of cultural respect is learning the importance of storytelling. I discovered that storytelling is an effective method in health education. Listening to stories helps people to discover the truth for themselves and means that they are more likely to learn and remember. Stories make the message concrete and, because health messages are often abstract, it works well to give a health message in the context of concrete information about people and places. When stories are told properly, they use familiar surroundings and begin where people are before moving them on to where they need to be. Stories are most interesting when they are told in simple terms that leave the listener to fill in the details by asking questions and talking. I often tell a story about my own family:

> My mother and father have diabetes. I am likely to develop diabetes too, if I continue to eat and drink foods high in sugar and I don't exercise. Because I am careful about what I eat, how much I eat, and when I eat – including how much I exercise – my blood sugar levels remain normal ... My mother does what I do now and is very careful about the foods that she eats and tries to exercise regularly. Because of this, her blood sugar levels have returned to normal.

Anyone with basic health knowledge and some imagination can create stories. The essential ingredients are simple health teaching objectives and a scenario that evolves from the local culture.

Since Aboriginal traditions vary significantly from community to community, it is difficult to make generalisations about the cultural considerations that are important for RANs. It is a good idea for RANs who are new to a community to seek advice from an IHW, who will be able to give information about the community's practices. It is also important to identify a significant person within the community and to speak regularly to that person while being clearly respectful of cultural issues.

In some communities, it is important to observe each client's body language, and particularly to think about whether the client avoids or ignores the RAN. If this happens, it may be important to have another person present during the consultation to advocate on the client's behalf. It is usually important not to look clients in the eye or stare at them while talking, as this can be confrontational and offensive. Most RANs find that they are more successful if they do not look clients in the face when they ask questions. Questions can be overwhelming for Indigenous people. It is also important not to talk too loudly, as this can be shameful for the client – especially when there is limited space to talk within the health centre. Try not to confuse the client with too many words and remember that English is their second (or even their fifth) language.

IHWs can also help with other aspects of cultural difference. For example, in many communities it is disrespectful to say a deceased person's name or anything that sounds close to their name. At times, a local health worker may be unable to attend work or see clients because of their cultural obligations in relation to a deceased person.

Some people may not be allowed to speak to other people in the community due to their family connection. For example, it is possible that a woman may not be able to speak to her father-in-law and a man cannot speak to his mother-in-law. In some cases, a death in the community may 'poison' relationships within the community.

Cultural laws must be supported and respected. Cultural laws can change regularly, and must not be questioned by anyone. Questioning cultural laws will be seen as offensive.

In being respectful about cultural issues, if you are non-Indigenous you will need to:

- accept that you are in a different social and cultural world than you are used to
- respect the local cultural knowledge
- adopt a participatory rather than a controlling role
- allow time for people to think about suggestions and allow time for people to discuss things informally among themselves and in their own language
- analyse situations or problems carefully and in detail before providing an appropriate solution or outcome
- build enduring relationships with community people
- develop healthy working relationships with councils, communities, organisations and individuals
- promote goodwill and understanding between all parties
- encourage participation in discussions
- endeavour to be open, honest and sincere
- expect resistance to ideas and proposals that are incompatible with community values
- identify stakeholders in the community, including the chairperson, council members, Elders and respected younger people who possess higher education
- listen to people's views and take them seriously
- keep in mind that your perspectives and understandings may differ from those of others; give a little, listen a lot and learn a little to find out what the other party needs
- promise only what you can deliver or are capable of achieving
- respect people's customs, culture, values, religion, dignity and feelings
- talk in a way that is clear, understandable and free of jargon and acronyms; remember that English may be a fourth or fifth language for your clients; try to understand that Indigenous people tend to speak in a circular way
- understand cultural and community dynamics; avoid stereotyping, as each community is unique and will have different needs.

(DATSIPD, 2005)

In addition to these cultural considerations, you may also need to think about traditional healers. Traditional healers are not employed in PHCCs, recognised professionally or paid adequate remuneration in the same way that nurses are. A useful method is to let families approach traditional healers within their community by themselves. Be aware that inviting traditional healers into the PHCC at a family's request will not be eligible for government funding or support. Usually, it is up to families to pay for the healer's services, either with money or in other ways. Traditional healers are often an important part of remote communities, and RANs need to respect their work.

Cultural considerations are necessary if RANs are to gain the respect of their clients and their community. If clients feel culturally offended, it will be very difficult to regain their trust. They may never return to the health service for their own or their family's healthcare needs.

The final aspect of cultural consideration involves recognising your own culture. Health professionals need to reflect on their own cultural identities and recognise the effects of their culture upon others. A health practitioner's cultural values and beliefs can influence how they provide healthcare. (For more information on this topic, refer to Chapter 3.)

QUESTIONS FOR REFLECTION

- When entering a community for the first time, what steps can an RAN take to ensure they respect cultural traditions in their practice?
- Why is it important to avoid making assumptions?

Reflections of a Nurse Practitioner

Be prepared to help on the roadside

I was driving out of Pormpuraaw with my family to get to the airport in Cairns. I was planning to attend my Nurse Practitioner graduation ceremony in Ipswich. It was the early wet season, but we had managed to drive 140 kilometres in three hours, with slippery road conditions and in and out of flooded creeks. We encountered a vehicle that had turned onto its side. It was on the side of the road near some bushes. People were sitting on the side of the road and others were sitting over near the vehicle in the bushes. I could see tyre marks on the road that stopped at the point where the vehicle had rolled several times before landing on its side. There were things scattered around the vehicle and up the road.

I saw four people in total, two sitting in the shade by the vehicle and two on the side of the road beside a puddle. One person by the side of the road was lying down, and I could see that she was badly injured. My family and I stopped, and I used my satellite phone to call for emergency help. We stayed with the people for five hours until help arrived. Eventually, we were on our way again, with another twelve hours of driving in poor road conditions.

Cultural obligations

Concerned family members visited me at the PHCC, asking for a nurse to conduct a home visit as one of their family members was unwell at home. When I arrived at their home, the man refused to see me. He said he was using bush medicine to sort out his symptoms.

Two days later, the family returned to the PHCC, again asking for the nurse to come and see this man as he was no better. Again I visited, and again he refused to see me. I also offered other services, such as another health professional who he might prefer to see. Still he declined. I asked whether it was okay for the doctor to visit when he arrived the following day; again, the client declined any of the health services. I asked whether he wanted to be flown out of the community to seek medical treatment with an escort. He refused.

Three days after the fourth visit, the family awoke to find their loved one deceased. They came to the PHCC very distressed, saying that nobody did anything for him.

With the family's consent, the man's body was taken to the clinic and prepared to be flown out of the community for an autopsy the following day. When I was arranging the body for transfer that night, I found the deceased man's de facto wife hiding in the staff area. She was hiding from the man's family and was highly distressed. I approached her and asked what was wrong. She said that the family was after her and she was looking for somewhere safe to hide. She was also grieving the loss of her partner and wanted to see him. With knowledge of the community, I approached a family member and asked who would be the spokesperson within the family at this time. The family identified an Elder, who I approached to ask whether the deceased man's partner could please have some time with the deceased prior to transferring his body to the morgue. The Elder discussed this with a few of the family members and gave consent. I then safeguarded this process for both the family and the de facto wife within the clinic environment until his body was taken to the morgue. Next, I arranged a safe place at the women's centre for the woman to stay until she felt safe within the community. My job was to provide a culturally safe place for her to express her needs and also to respect the family's wishes.

Conclusion

RANs are typically hard-working, flexible, adaptable, resourceful and passionate health professionals. Their practice encompasses all the challenges and rewards that a remote setting can offer. Remote communities need qualified RANs, IHWs and doctors who can provide culturally safe health services within the local community.

Nurses are encouraged to think seriously about the rewards of working as a RAN. RANs and IHWs are also encouraged to:

- increase their professional skills and knowledge
- understand their own cultural boundaries and realities
- understand and be actively involved in health politics so changes can occur.

Working as a RAN is challenging. There is a risk that RANs might disassociate from metropolitan society and experience both personal and professional isolation. They tend to work very long hours in their communities. They face complex issues, including little on-the-ground support, poor infrastructure and operational issues.

Working as a RAN is also highly rewarding. RANs have an opportunity to develop a broad set of skills and work with great autonomy. They face responsibilities, challenges and rewards that will never be experienced in metropolitan settings. They also have opportunities to make a real, long-term difference to the health and wellbeing of people who live in remote communities.

Health belongs to everybody. Let's take care of it.

Learning activities

1. Imagine that you have accepted a six-month contract as a Registered Nurse in a remote community. How would you prepare for your role? What special training would you seek? How would you learn about the community?
2. Choose a remote community in your state or territory, and learn about its services and opportunities (a community's website will usually provide sufficient information). Compare this community with the community where you currently live. You could compare the overall population, employment opportunities,

socioeconomic data, availability of services, number of shops and number of health workers per person in the population. What does this comparison tell you about the experience of living in a remote community and managing your health needs?

3. Imagine that you are working in a remote Indigenous community and that your role includes health promotion. You decide to develop a promotional campaign about healthy eating, particularly targeting the community's young men. How would you begin to plan your campaign? What activities might you undertake? What can you realistically achieve with the resources available to you?
4. Imagine that you work in a remote Aboriginal community. You have just referred a 29-year-old woman, Angie, for a colonoscopy. She will need to travel to the nearest hospital, 350 kilometres away, for the test. How can you help Angie to prepare? What things about Angie's personal circumstances might you need to understand to ensure that Angie attends the test, is well prepared for the experience and does not find the trip traumatic?

FURTHER READING

Hegney, D., McCarthy, A., Rogers-Clark, C. & Gorman, D. (2002). Retaining rural and remote area nurses: The Queensland Australia experience. *Journal of Nursing Administration*, 3, 128–35.

Kruske, S., Lenthell, S., Kildea, S., Knight, S., Mackay, D. & Hegney, D. (2014). Rural and remote area nursing. In D. Brown, H. Edwards & T. Buckley (eds), *Lewis's Medical-surgical Nursing: Assessment and Management of Clinical Problems* (4th edn). Sydney: Elsevier, pp. 125–42.

Lethell, S., Wakerman, J., Opie, T., … Watson, C. (2009). What stresses remote area nurses? Current knowledge and future action. *Australian Journal of Rural Health*, 17, 208–13.

Yuginovich, T. (2000). A potted history of 19th century remote area nursing in Australia and in particular Queensland. *Australian Journal of Rural Health*, 8, 63–7.

Visit the companion website at www.cambridge.org/highereducation/isbn/9781108794695/resources to see further online resources.

REFERENCES

ABS (2016). *Remoteness Structure*. Canberra: ABS. Retrieved from www.abs.gov.au/websitedbs/D3310114.nsf/home/remoteness+structure

AHMAC (2017). *Aboriginal and Torres Strait Islander Health Performance Framework 2017 Report*. Canberra: AHMAC.

AIHW (2014). Remoteness and the health of Indigenous Australians. *Australia's health 2014*. Australia's health series no. 14. Cat. no. AUS 178. Canberra, ACT: Australian Institute of Health and Welfare, chapter 7. Retrieved from www.aihw.gov.au/getmedia/3fae0eb7-b2be-4ffc-9903-a414388af557/7_7-indigenous health-remoteness.pdf.aspx

AIHW (2015). The Health and Welfare of Australia's Aboriginal and Torres Strait Islander peoples: 2015. Canberra: AIHW.

AIHW (2019). *Rural and Remote Health*. Canberra: AIHW. Retrieved from www.aihw.gov.au/reports/rural-remote-australians/rural-remote-health/contents/summary

CRANA (2014). CRANAplus: Improving remote health website. Retrieved from www.crana.org.au

DATSIPD (2005). *Protocols for Consultation and Negotiation with Aboriginal People*. Brisbane: DATSIPD. Retrieved from www.rqi.org.au/wp-content/uploads/2012/01/protocols-for-consultation.pdf

DHA (2013). *National Aboriginal and Torres Strait Islander Health Plan 2013–2023*. Canberra: DHA.

Fredericks, B. & Best, O. (2020). On the long road to reform for food security for remote communities. *Croakey*, 3 May. Retrieved from https://croakey.org/on-the-long-road-to-reform-for-food-security-for-remote-communities/

Fredericks, B. & Bradfield, A. (2021). Food insecurity in uncertain times: Ways forward post-pandemic. *Griffith Review*, 71. Retrieved from www.griffithreview.com/articles/food-insecurity-in-uncertain-times/

House of Representatives Standing Committee on Indigenous Affairs (2020). *Report on Food Pricing and Food Security in Remote Indigenous Communities.* Canberra: Parliament of the Commonwealth of Australia. Retrieved from: www.aph.gov.au/Parliamentary_Business/Committees/House/Indigenous_Affairs/Foodpricing/Report.

Mills, J., Birks, M. & Hegney, D. (2010). The status of rural nursing in Australia: 12 years on. *Collegian*, 17(1), 30–37.

Napranum Aboriginal Shire Council (2017). Napranum Shire profile. Retrieved from www.napranum.qld.gov.au/community-information/shire-profile

Penm, E. (2008). *Cardiovascular Disease and Its Associated Risk Factors in Aboriginal and Torres Strait Islander Peoples 2004–05.* Canberra: AIHW.

Queensland Productivity Commission (2017). *Final Report: Service delivery in remote and discrete Aboriginal and Torres Strait Islander communities.* Brisbane. Retrieved from https://qpc.blob.core.windows.net/wordpress/2018/06/Service-delivery-Final-Report.pdf

SCRGSP (2009). *National Agreement Performance Information 2008–09: National Indigenous Reform Agreement.* Canberra: Productivity Commission.

Smith, J. (2004). *Australia's Rural and Remote Health: A Social Justice Perspective.* Melbourne: Tertiary Press.

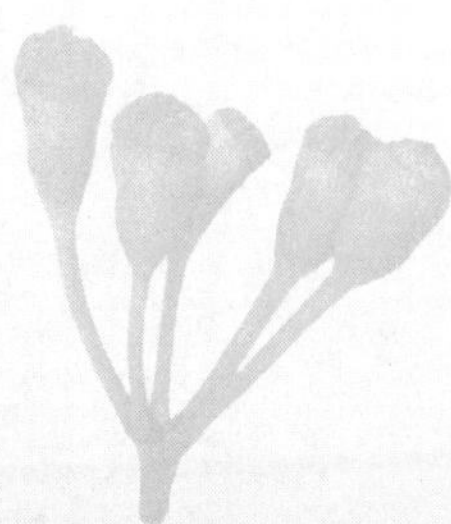

Working with Aboriginal and Torres Strait Islander health workers and health practitioners

10

Ali Drummond

LEARNING OBJECTIVES

This chapter will help you to understand:

- The development of the Aboriginal and Torres Strait Islander health worker role and the needs it was designed to meet
- The role of Aboriginal and Torres Strait Islander health workers in contemporary health service provision
- The emerging role of the Aboriginal and Torres Strait Islander health practitioner
- The relevant professional nursing and midwifery standards that guide collaboration with other healthcare workers
- The challenges and opportunities of interprofessional practice with Aboriginal and Torres Strait Islander health workers

KEY WORDS

Aboriginal and Torres Strait Islander health practitioner
Aboriginal and Torres Strait Islander health worker
accountability
competence
controlled medications
delegating
interprofessional practice
National Aboriginal and Torres Strait Islander Health Worker Association (NATSIHWA)
racialisation
racism
restricted medications
scope of practice
sociocultural
task-shifting
unregulated healthcare workers

Introduction

Aboriginal and Torres Strait Islander health worker An Aboriginal and/or Torres Strait Islander person who holds a minimum qualification in primary healthcare or clinical practice. This role supports numerous health practitioners, typically in cultural support roles; however, it is increasingly a clinical support role.

Aboriginal and Torres Strait Islander health practitioner A person who holds a minimum qualification of Certificate IV in Aboriginal and Torres Strait Islander Primary Health Care (Practice) and is registered by the Aboriginal and Torres Strait Islander Practice Board.

This chapter examines the role of the **Aboriginal and Torres Strait Islander health worker** (IHW) and the **Aboriginal and Torres Strait Islander health practitioner** (IHP), and discusses their relationships with nurses and midwives.

Nurses and midwives make a significant contribution to the health and wellbeing of Aboriginal and Torres Strait Islander people; they provide care across the healthcare continuum and throughout the human lifespan. However, barriers to access exist and are founded upon a history of strategic political disempowerment and contrasting ways of knowing, being and doing regarding health and wellbeing that continue to impede the quality and safety of nursing care experienced by Aboriginal and Torres Strait Islander people.

Providing training for Aboriginal and Torres Strait Islander people to participate in health service delivery has long been accepted as the most appropriate way to address these barriers. As shared in the epilogue, IHWs are part of the solution in terms of bridging the gap between Australian health services and Aboriginal and Torres Strait Islander people. There has been recent government investment to increase the participation of Aboriginal and Torres Strait Islander people in health professional roles such as nursing and midwifery, and the IHW role remains important to this.

IHWs contribute to the delivery of client-centred, holistic care for Aboriginal and Torres Strait Islander people, and provide guidance and leadership about cultural differences (Eckermann et al., 2010). The National Aboriginal Health Strategy asserts that the Indigenous heath worker

> bridges the "cultural chasm" separating traditional and western world views ... [relating] western beliefs to an Aboriginal conceptual framework, making it possible for Aboriginal patients to understand what is being said.
>
> (NAHSWP, 1989, p. 85)

sociocultural Refers to a broad range of factors that are both social and cultural. The two are interconnected as 'culture' refers to age, gender, ethnicity, class and so on, the meanings of which are dynamic and socially constructed. These factors include social norms within cultural groups and external social forces such as the social determinants of health.

Often, IHWs are members of the local Aboriginal or Torres Strait Islander community in which they work, so they draw on their inherent knowledge of the social, cultural and historical health determinants experienced by their community to advocate on behalf of their clients. Their **sociocultural** knowledge complements the usual information sought by medical and other practitioners, and results in healthcare that is more holistically responsive to the Aboriginal and Torres Strait Islander perspective of health and wellbeing. With their perspective of Aboriginal and Torres Strait Islander health and wellbeing that extends beyond the Western biomedically dominated understanding of health, IHWs frequently venture beyond the usual boundaries of health services to support the complex sociocultural needs of their clients (for example, they may look broadly at the social determinants of health, such as housing and legal issues) (Genat, 2006).

The IHW role is forging new territory in participating in healthcare in the acute hospital setting. IHWs have demonstrated that they are valuable for optimising communication between health professionals and patients, reducing Indigenous patients discharging against medical advice, improving the completion and continuity of health and increasing the recording of the Indigenous status of patients (Mackean et al., 2020).

Nurses and midwives have worked with IHWs since the health worker role was created. However, despite this long relationship, nurses and midwives continue to report some uncertainty about the role and capacity of IHWs. The introduction of the IHP role in July 2012 has increased the potential to further confuse nurses and midwives, and other health professionals. Uncertainty about roles has implications for interprofessional practice between nurses, midwives, IHWs and IHPs. It also has consequences for the quality of care provided and for patient outcomes (Eckermann et al., 2010). It is important for nurses and midwives to have a clear understanding of the roles of IHWs and IHPs so they may develop and maintain effective interprofessional relationships that nurture holistic and effective health services for Aboriginal and Torres Strait Islander people.

This chapter will introduce the IHW and IHP roles, as an understanding of them is important for nurses and midwives in order to optimise interprofessional practice with these practitioners. Furthermore, this chapter will discuss the application of nursing and midwifery professional standards to the interprofessional relationships between nurses, midwives, IHWs and IHPs.

The history of Aboriginal and Torres Strait Islander health workers

Community health workers have a long association with colonial administrations, internationally in the continents of Asia and Africa, as well as in Australia (Genat, 2006). In Australia, formal training of Aboriginal people began in the 1950s, with some missions and government reserves providing training for Aboriginal people to participate as healthcare assistants in local services (HRSCAA, 1979). Aboriginal people also supported the provision of healthcare in remote Australia, often providing transportation and assisting medical officers. They were often referred to as 'barefoot doctors', acknowledging their role in enabling Western medical care through their work assisting medical officers (Lockwood, 1966).

In the 1960s, the Western Australian government invested in the training and employment of a number of IHWs in the Kimberley region, to provide primary healthcare services to their local communities. A shift in national policy a decade later, which saw the emergence of Aboriginal and Torres Strait Islander self-determination and self-management policy eras, coincided with increased federal government investment in the growth of the IHW workforce (Genat, 2006). This was based on the belief that increased participation by Aboriginal and Torres Strait Islander people in healthcare delivery would increase the community's control over its local health services and help to break down barriers to access (NAHSWP, 1989).

The initial government intention was for IHWs to be supervised and trained by the nurses in their communities, with a goal that IHWs would eventually replace nurses (HRSCAA, 1979). However, this goal has not been realised. While training is recognised as an essential factor, inconsistencies emerged because training was a state and territory responsibility (Torzillo & Kerr, 1991). There were benefits to tailoring training so that it reflected the individual needs of each community; however, this brought about challenges such as practice inconsistency between IHWs from different communities, which limited their intra-state and interstate movement for work. This remains a challenge for IHWs today (Topp, Edelman & Taylor, 2018).

Shifts in national policy towards self-determination and self-management also resulted in the expansion of Aboriginal Medical Services (AMSs) throughout Australia (see Chapter 6). The philosophy underpinning the IHW role correlated with that of AMSs, and it is no surprise that AMSs became the major employer of IHWs (Genat, 2006). During this time, there were no Aboriginal or Torres Strait Islander doctors, and few nurses and nurses' aides (midwives were not counted separately). Few education and training providers made specific efforts to support Aboriginal and Torres Strait Islander people's participation in the health workforce (HRSCAA, 1979). By the end of the 1980s, however, there were fourteen doctors, 437 registered nurses, 392 enrolled nurses and 55 dental nurses who identified as being Aboriginal and/or Torres Strait Islander people (NAHSWP, 1989). However, these figures need to be scrutinised due to inadequate data on Aboriginal and Torres Strait Islander peoples, remembering that Aboriginal and Torres Strait Islander people were only included in the census from 1967, and that Indigeneity remained a valid reason for someone to exercise racial discrimination towards you. Despite these trained health practitioners, IHWs remained key staff in primary healthcare services, especially in remote areas of Australia.

Since the health professional workforce in remote Australia is limited, the capacity of health professionals working in these practice contexts has undergone strategic and opportunistic extensions in an effort to meet the needs of their clients and contexts. IHWs have not been immune to this, and IHWs in remote locations have greater clinical capability than their counterparts employed in regional and metropolitan health services. Publications such as the Northern Territory's Central Australian Rural Practitioner Association (CARPA) manual and Queensland's Primary Clinical Care Manual (PCCM) support extended practice by nurses and midwives, and IHWs (Murray & Wronski, 2006).

Murray and Wronski (2006) state that, due to the long history of strategic and opportunistic extensions of practice, clinical task delegation and interprofessional practice between health professionals have been developed, accepted and practised for many years in remote Australia. Internationally, it is a common practice in developing countries to optimise the limited capacity of the health professional workforce by delegating or shifting less complex tasks to less-qualified personnel (WHO, 2008).

Task-shifting

task-shifting Delegating less-complicated, low-risk tasks to local and often unregulated healthcare workers.

unregulated healthcare workers Healthcare workers whose roles are not regulated through required minimum training and competency assessments and whose work is not monitored by a professional board.

A common experience internationally for healthcare delivery in remote locations is poor access to a skilled workforce and inadequate resources. To address this, health service managers implement **task-shifting** to optimise the limited number of health professionals available and to delegate less-complicated, low-risk tasks to local, often **unregulated healthcare workers** (UHCW).

Internationally, UHCWs are usually provided with some education and training, but these are of a lower standard than the training received by the health professionals with whom they work. UHCWs often come from the community in which they are employed. They support the delivery of culturally safe care and become a pivotal conduit between the health service and the local community (WHO, 2008). Cultural safety is explored in Chapter 3.

Task-shifting of healthcare to UHCWs brings both advantages and disadvantages to the healthcare system and the professionals who work in it. From a nursing and midwifery perspective, being supported by UHCWs can lead to increased responsibility and more complex work. These advantages and disadvantages are summarised in Table 10.1.

Table 10.1 Task-shifting to UHCWs: Advantages, disadvantages and effects on the nursing and midwifery profession

Advantages	Disadvantages	Effects on the nursing/ midwifery professions
• UHCWs constitute a cheaper health workforce. • More health workers can be employed to provide care: this may lead to improvements in health outcomes. • Optimisation of the available healthcare workers is possible: nurses and midwives are able to care for those with the highest care needs.	• UHCWs often treat the most vulnerable. • It is common for conflicts to develop between UHCWs and regulated health professional groups. • The best distribution of UHCWs, their performance and associated costs are not easily determined or monitored. • The lack of clear policy, planning, monitoring and evaluation of task-shifting can limit effective, efficient and equitable coordination of care.	• There is an increase in nurses' and midwives' responsibility as trainers and supervisors. • More skilled health professionals are needed because the UHCW can generate an increase in patients (because healthcare becomes more accessible). • The complexity of health problems being treated by nurses and midwives increases, which may require further developed analytical, diagnostic and treatment skills.

Sources: ICN (2008); WHO (2008).

The international discussion about task-shifting to UHCWs clearly has parallels with the Australian experience for IHWs. The initial role of IHWs in Australia closely reflected international practice and emphasised their role as 'cultural brokers' who optimised the capacity of the health professionals. The specific focus on employing IHWs in remote locations where there is limited access to other health professionals also parallels the international experience (Genat, 2006).

Task-shifting is often seen by health professionals and managers as a convenient and low-cost way to 'shift' tasks that are considered simple. However, for IHWs, task shifting can leave them feeling like a 'jack of all trades'. It can create uncertainty about education and career pathways, can lead to workplace conflict if the capacity of their role is not understood and clarified, which may result in under-utilisation of IHWs' skills and can lead health workers to feel under-valued (Eckermann et al., 2010; Genat, 2006; Javanparast et al., 2018). Roles such as the UHCW, IHW and IHP are evidently quite disempowered compared with other health professionals.

Another comparable feature to the UHCW role is that IHW and IHP roles are recognised as 'the only Indigenous ethnic-based health workforce in Australia'

racism A social phenomenon that asserts the existence of different human races that are determined by physical and behaviour traits. This belief promotes a hierarchy of the supposed different human races, which historically have positioned white people at the top and black people at the bottom. Types of racism include interpersonal, institutional/systemic and scientific.

racialisation The act of applying the logic of racism to an individual or group of people.

National Aboriginal and Torres Strait Islander Health Worker Association (NATSIHWA) The peak national body supporting Aboriginal and Torres Strait Islander health workers.

(NATSIHWA, 2019, p. 2). The normal distribution of power among the health workforce thus highlights a significant problem, specifically because of the normalised disempowerment of IHWs and IHPs. This is an example of institutional **racism**, where Indigenous peoples have been racialised, and historically designated to the position within the broader health workforce with the least power.

Bond et al. (2019) found that publications about the IHW often highlighted the deficits of the role. Whether by design or not, these popular perspectives fail to see the deficits within the health systems that the IHW role was designed to improve for the benefit of Aboriginal and Torres Strait Islander people. The health system has failed to address the limitations embedded within the practice of task-shifting, including the **racialisation** of Indigenous peoples and marginalising them to roles of least power and influence.

In Australia, several developments have helped to refine the capacity of IHWs and created more certainty about their positions, including representation of IHWs by the **National Aboriginal and Torres Strait Islander Health Worker Association (NATSIHWA)**, regulation of IHWs in the Northern Territory and the creation of the IHP role. However, their disempowerment within the broader health workforce remains an ongoing issue.

QUESTIONS FOR REFLECTION

- History reveals a segregation of the health workforce, with Aboriginal and Torres Strait Islanders restricted to the lower-level jobs. Reflect on how you think this history of the health workforce might influence the relationship between a nurse and/or midwife and an IHW today.
- Task-shifting has been beneficial in remote locations of developing countries. In a developed country such as Australia, where education and training are accessible and there is an abundance of qualified health professionals, why do you think we still have roles such as the IHW?

The contemporary Indigenous health worker

IHWs are significant members of the primary and community healthcare workforce in Australia. In 2018, there were approximately 1600 IHWs employed in Australia (Industry Reference Committee, 2019). Most health workers are female (86 per cent of national IHW workforce) and aged between 35 and 54 years (66.8 per cent), with 42 years being the average age (Industry Reference Committee, 2019). Almost half of all IHWs are employed in remote and very remote locations of Australia (HWA, 2013).

A key part of the IHW role is to be a cultural broker who guides and protects the non-Indigenous health workforce (who are often short-term visitors to communities) (Eckermann et al., 2010). The IHW role has also expanded to include health program participation and management, and increased clinical capability that is driven by the needs of the client (HWA, 2011).

IHWs provide care across the human lifespan and work in numerous health programs. Their job titles vary enormously to reflect the focus of their roles. The Job Titles box summarises some of the job titles of IHWs.

Job titles held by IHWs

- Health worker (generalist)
- Aboriginal and Torres Strait Islander health practitioner
- Outreach worker
- Mental health worker
- Family health worker
- Sexual health worker
- Education officer
- Hospital liaison officer
- Oral/dental health worker
- Chronic disease worker
- Drug and alcohol worker
- Environmental health worker
- Community worker
- Healthy living worker
- Vascular health worker
- Pharmacy health worker
- Maternal and perinatal health worker
- Otitis media health worker
- Nutrition health worker

(NATSIHWA, 2012)

The scope of practice of IHWs and IHPs

Having a better understanding of the **scope of practice** of IHWs and IHPs may enable better interprofessional practice. The scope of practice of IHW and IHP professions spans the 'full spectrum of roles, functions, responsibilities, activities and decision-making capacities in which individuals who make up the profession are educated, competent and authorised' (NATSIHWA, 2019, p. 5). The scope of practice of individual IHWs and IHPs correlates with their level of education, authority and competency to perform (NATSIHWA, 2019, p. 5). This section will further explore the spectrum of the scope of practice of these professions. First it will explore the health needs of those in the client group, who are predominantly Aboriginal and Torres Strait Islander people, then the common practice context of these roles, then the level of **competence**, education and training, and finally, the relevant service providers policy.

scope of practice The accountabilities and responsibilities of regulated health professionals, whose registration is based on education and demonstrated competence. While not regulated, this also applies to the IHW role.

competence The combination of skills, knowledge, attitudes, values and abilities that underpins effective performance in a profession or occupation (NMBA, 2020d).

Health needs of the client group

IHWs are employed to work directly with Aboriginal and Torres Strait Islander people. It is well documented that there is a large gap in health outcomes and life expectancy between this client group and other Australians. This health gap is explored in other chapters in this text, particularly Chapters 1 and 2.

According to data from 2015–17, the life expectancy gap between Indigenous and non-Indigenous Australians is 8.6 years for men, and 7.8 years for women (DPMC, 2020). The five leading causes of death are circulatory disease; neoplasms; external causes (e.g. suicide and transport accidents); endocrine, metabolic and nutritional disorders; and respiratory disease (AHMAC, 2017, p. 88).

A significant percentage of the mortality experienced by Aboriginal and Torres Strait Islander people is considered avoidable – that is, from conditions that could have been avoided 'given timely and effective healthcare' (AHMAC, 2017, p. 91). This is particularly relevant for IHWs, as they are positioned within preventive healthcare work in primary and community healthcare settings.

Data from 2011–15 show that Aboriginal and Torres Strait Islander people experience more than three times greater avoidable mortality than non-Indigenous Australians (AHMAC, 2017, p. 91). The leading causes of avoidable mortality among Aboriginal and Torres Strait Islander people include ischaemic heart disease, diabetes, suicide, chronic obstructive pulmonary disease and cancer (AHMAC, 2017 p. 92). (For discussion of health disparities in relation to maternal and infant health, see Chapter 7.) Significant government investment in health education and prevention programs has attempted to address avoidable mortality. IHWs are involved in this work, and many have received relevant training to participate in these programs. Examples include smoking cessation (200 trained IHWs in 2011–12), reducing risky alcohol consumption, increasing opportunities for physical activity (with funding for sports and recreational activities), healthy eating programs, breastfeeding and healthy behaviour during pregnancy programs (AHMAC, 2012). Aboriginal and Torres Strait Islander people experience a high burden of chronic disease, and many IHWs are employed to care for patients with chronic diseases in the community setting.

The health needs of Aboriginal and Torres Strait Islander people are partly determined by the Aboriginal and Torres Strait Islander perspective of health and wellbeing. IHWs participate in providing care within the broad definition of health by coordinating the engagement of their clients across other social services (such as housing, employment, income and transportation). This is a good example of how IHWs achieve a holistic approach to healthcare (Genat, 2006). However, it can be difficult for IHWs to balance their engagement in sociocultural matters with their clinical support roles. While their health worker training provides education about health problems and treatments, health workers often find themselves attending to sociocultural matters rather than providing clinical care (Genat, 2006).

Practice context

Most IHWs are based in the primary and community health sector, particularly in AMS. They provide comprehensive primary healthcare for clients. This is described by the WHO's Alma-Ata Declaration as healthcare that

> is practical, scientifically sound and socially acceptable; uses technology to enable universal access for individuals, families and communities; is economically practical for the community and the country, emphasising self-reliance and self-determination;

> is an integral part of the country's health system and the overall social and economic development of the country; and, is the first level of contact with individuals, families and communities to where they live and work.
>
> (WHO, 1978)

In the context of Australia's Aboriginal and Torres Strait Islander health, the comprehensive primary healthcare approach may include clinical care, population health programs, facilitating access to secondary and tertiary care, and client and community assistance and advocacy. Given the high burden of chronic disease among Aboriginal and Torres Strait Islander people, primary and secondary prevention needs to be given appropriate attention (Dwyer et al., 2007).

In mainstream health services, IHWs are usually allocated to a specific health team, which confines their scope of practice. For example, in a Brisbane-based birthing on Country midwifery group practice, IHWs are important team members who provide support to Aboriginal and Torres Strait Islander women, including 'social and emotional well-being, smoking cessation, breastfeeding, and cultural support and advocacy' (Kildea et al., 2018, p. 233). In contrast, IHWs employed by an Aboriginal Community Controlled Health Service (ACCHS) report broader clinical scopes of practice – that is, IHWs employed in an ACCHS are often able to engage in more clinical practice (beyond education and patient support), which is enabled by expanded education and supportive health service policy (Topp et al., 2018). The practice context has a major effect on the education and training needs of IHWs. (For further discussion about ACCHSs, see Chapter 6.)

QUESTION FOR REFLECTION

- IHWs typically adopt a holistic and comprehensive perspective of primary healthcare that reflects the Aboriginal definition of health. From your experience, what value do you think the Western biomedical model places on investing in optimising primary and preventative healthcare?

Level of competence, education and training

The education pathway for IHWs is set out by NATSIHWA and is provided by various registered training organisations (Figure 10.1). The qualifications held by IHWs range from the Certificate II in Aboriginal and Torres Strait Islander Primary Health Care to the Advanced Diploma of Aboriginal and Torres Strait Islander Primary Health Care (Practice or Community Care) (NATSIHWA, 2012). Qualifications at Certificate IV level and above are available in two streams: Community Care, which focuses on community engagement and health promotion, and Practice, which focuses on clinical competency. Each qualification scaffolds from the previous one.

IHWs are also encouraged to participate in training throughout their careers; relevant courses are delivered by many organisations, such as the Council of Remote Area Nurses of Australia (CRANA) and Cancer Council Australia.

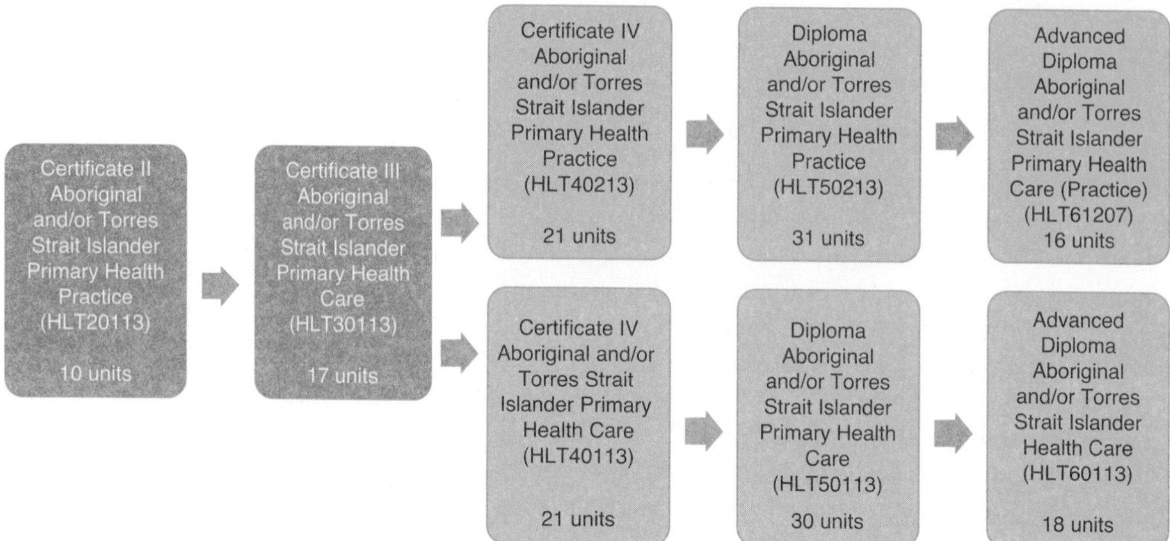

Figure 10.1 IHW education pathway. Each box includes the qualification name, code and number of units

Source: Adapted from training.gov.au.

NATSIHWA has developed a Professional Practice Framework for IHWs to help them, along with health professionals, health managers and communities, to better understand the scope of practice of IHWs according to the education and competencies they have accomplished. The framework identifies five *domains* of practice (Figure 10.2), each divided into *principles* that reflect the competencies associated

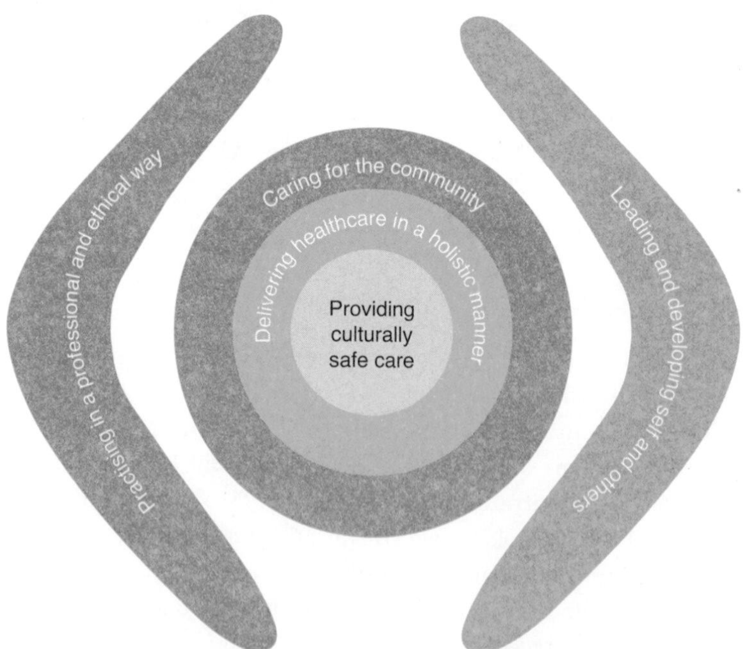

Figure 10.2 Domains of the Aboriginal and Torres Strait Islander Health Worker Professional Practice Framework

Source: NATSIHWA (2012, p. 7).

with the IHW's qualifications. These principles are further divided into *elements* of practice (Figure 10.3), which vary according to the IHW's experience (NATSIHWA, 2012). Note the final column, which highlights the competency standard code that reflects a unit of study in the IHW education pathway.

DOMAIN 1: PROVIDING CULTURALLY SAFE HEALTH CARE

PRINCIPLES	ELEMENTS		
	NEW	EXPERIENCED / ADVANCED As per 'NEW' with the following additional elements	COMPETENCY STANDARD CODE*
1. **Knowing and respecting our history, context, culture and customs**	a. Understand the context of local, regional, state, national as well as traditional and contemporary Aboriginal and Torres Strait Islander history b. Identify, consider and respect the local community values, beliefs, gender roles when providing health care to the Aboriginal and Torres Strait Islander people c. Understand the context of government policies, legislation on Aboriginal and Torres Strait Islander communities, families and individuals	a. Understand the context and identify the impact of government policies, legislation on Aboriginal and Torres Strait Islander communities, families and individuals	HLTAHW201B HLTAHW301B

Figure 10.3 Extract from NATSIHWA Professional Practice Framework. Domain 1: Providing culturally safe healthcare; Principle 1: Knowing and respecting our history, context, culture and customs

Source: NATSIHWA (2012, p. 9).

NATSIHWA's Professional Practice Framework is an essential tool for nurses and midwives to use when working with IHWs. It will assist in understanding the scope of practice of IHWs, particularly when considering delegation of activities. This will be explored later in the chapter.

In a unique circumstance, IHWs employed in some parts of Queensland deemed to be isolated practice areas (the Torres Strait and Cape York Peninsula) can undertake further education to become authorised to administer and supply **restricted medications** and **controlled medications** (Queensland Health, 2016). They must attain an isolated practice and/or sexual health authorisation by completing relevant training These extensions of practice through education and competency allow the IHW to administer medications in accordance with the 'Health (Drugs and Poisons) Regulation 1996, Drug Therapy Protocol – Indigenous Health Worker Isolated Practice Area'. Please refer to this for a detailed list of the approved medications and explanation of approved administration routes and relevant restrictions and conditions.

restricted medications Include Schedule 4 medications (prescription only), which include antibiotics and some analgesics.

controlled medications Schedule 8 medications, which have restrictions on manufacture, supply, distribution, possession and use due to the risk of abuse, misuse and dependence. Examples include morphine and fentanyl.

While there are opportunities for IHWs to increase their competency through education and training, practical barriers often prevent this from happening. The following are some typical barriers:

- Few teaching staff are available in rural and remote locations, so it is common for training to be delivered in urban areas, which may mean health workers need to relocate for training; they may experience a range of financial, accommodation and social problems through being separated from their families and community supports.
- Family commitments, such as attending funerals and caring for family members who are ill, consume time and are prioritised ahead of training.
- There are often difficulties finding backfill (replacement) staff when health workers travel to attend teaching blocks (often two weeks at a time).
- Poor role definition determines the types of courses undertaken by individuals.

- While proficiency in multiple languages may be common, poor English literacy is a barrier. This may reflect the poor early education opportunities often experienced in remote Australia.

(Davidson et al., 2008; Mitchell & Hussey, 2006).

There is a current need for more IHWs, particularly from the younger age group, to address the ageing population of the current workforce, and more men to meet the gendered health needs of the Aboriginal and Torres Strait Islander community (Wright, Briscoe & Lovett, 2019). Furthermore, there is a need for more opportunities for IHWs to engage in interprofessional education with other health professionals. Such an approach would nurture shared understanding of the different health professional roles and an increase individual confidence with contributing to interprofessional practice (Dettwiller et al., 2015).

Service provider's policy

Historically, the work of IHWs has generally been unregulated; however, NATSIHWA has increased its role in developing guidelines and frameworks to support local clinical governance of IHW roles. The lack of clarity about scopes of practice still persists, and creates greater flexibility in their work. However, for IHWs this flexibility can lead to uncertainty about how to contribute to healthcare, and can result in fragmented education and training pathways, and unrealistic workloads (Mackean et al., 2020). In some cases, a feeling of being unable to participate in healthcare activities can arise from a perception that IHWs are not able to contribute (the perception may come from themselves or from other health team members). The lack of guidelines at the local level may lead to this outcome (Si et al., 2006).

Tertiary hospitals are less familiar with the IHW role, so new programs such as birthing on Country midwifery group practice (Kildea et al. 2018) have experienced challenges with the integration of the role of the IHW in the tertiary setting. Mackean et al. (2020) found that IHWs in other tertiary health settings experienced similar challenges, including racism.

IHW roles within ACCHSs are often broader than those in mainstream health services. There is greater flexibility in the scope of practice of IHWs in ACCHS, which is a reflection of the range of health programs that aim to meet the holistic needs of their clients (Mitchell & Hussey, 2006).

NATSIHWA's (2012) Professional Practice Framework provides guidance for health service providers to support the ways in which they utilise their IHW workforce; however, its application varies. The history of arbitrary expansion of the roles and expectations of IHWs reflects this inconsistency in education, scope of practice and roles. NATSIHWA has recently published a template to support local planning of IHW's scope of practice for health promotion workers, alcohol and other drugs workers and child and maternal health workers, to name a few (NATSIHWA, 2020).

Regulation of IHPs

The regulation of various health professions aims to ensure the safety and quality of health services provided to the public. Regulation provides assurance to the public that each health professional who enacts authority through decision-making has the professional knowledge, experience and competency to do so (NMBA, 2020a).

Health professions are regulated through the *Health Practitioner Regulation National Law Act 2009* (Qld). It is enacted through various pieces of state and territory legislation and provides the basis for the National Registration and Accreditation Scheme (NRAS) and the establishment of various national health professional boards. The Nursing and Midwifery Board of Australia (NMBA), established in 2009, is an example of a health profession board.

Partially registered health professionals were assessed in 2010 to determine whether they were appropriate for inclusion under the NRAS. IHWs were included in this assessment because the scope of practice exercised by IHWs is registered in the Northern Territory. In that territory, IHWs were registered under the *Practitioners and Allied Professionals Registration Act 1986* (NT), and required to complete a Basic Skills Certificate in order to qualify for registration (Torzillo & Kerr, 1991).

Analysis of the role of IHWs for the NRAS aimed to determine whether their activities posed a significant risk of harm to the public. The assessment confirmed that eight high-risk activities are associated with the role of health worker. Based on this analysis, the IHW role as implemented in the Northern Territory was included under the NRAS. The title 'Aboriginal and Torres Strait Islander health practitioner' (ATSIHP) was established to distinguish individuals who were registered, and to recognise that the title of IHW is used nationally to describe varying roles.

The Aboriginal and Torres Strait Islander Health Practice Board was established in 2011 for this newly registered group of health professionals. The Board has a mandate to instil statutory regulations and develop professional self-regulation mechanisms for Indigenous health professionals to ensure public safety and quality. This includes the development and implementation of:

- registration and accreditation arrangements
- complaints-handling procedures
- conduct arrangements
- health and performance arrangements
- privacy and information sharing arrangements under the *Health Practitioner Regulation National Law Act 2009* (Qld).

In order to be registered by the Aboriginal and Torres Strait Islander Health Practice Board, individuals are required to obtain their qualifications through prescribed and accredited education providers and hold a licence to practise (Queensland Consolidated Acts, 2009). The Board has established a minimum education requirement for Aboriginal and Torres Strait Islander health practitioners as a Certificate IV in Aboriginal and Torres Strait Islander Primary Health Care (Practice).

There has been interest for IHWs and health service providers to increase the number of IHPs. Important aspects of successful upskilling of IHWs include the need to normalise the valued contribution of both the IHW and the IHP to patient care, and better coordination between education and health service providers in identifying ideal candidates for upskilling and ensuring their success (Hill et al., 2017).

In 2020, there were 812 IHPs registered within the Aboriginal and Torres Strait Islander Health Practice Board of Australia (ATSIHPBA) with the majority of them working in the Northern Territory (27 per cent), New South Wales (22 per cent), Western Australia (19.7 per cent) and Queensland (18 per cent) (ATSIHPBA, 2020, p. 4). Most IHPs are female (77.6 per cent), and a small majority are between 50 and 54 years of age (n = 102); however, the age distribution of registered IHPs is steady between 25 and 59 years of age (ATSIHPBA, 2020, pp. 5–6).

Cultural safety practitioners

The holistic practice of IHWs is considered to be inherently culturally safe (Eckermann et al., 2010) and aligned with the Aboriginal definition of health. However, caution is needed here in thinking that Indigenous identity is synonymous with being culturally safe. This section expands on the discussion of cultural safety in Chapter 3 of this text, to explore issues of cultural safety that are relevant to the work of IHWs. In particular, it focuses on the three steps 'towards achieving cultural safety': cultural awareness, cultural sensitivity and cultural safety (Ramsden, 2002, p. 117).

The first two steps do not emphasise the need to be aware of or sensitive to other cultures. On the contrary, they are about an understanding what culture is, and developing awareness of one's own culture, which Ramsden (2002, p. 117) believes includes 'the emotional, social, economic and political context in which people exist'.

Maintaining culturally safe practice is challenging for all health professionals. When working with Aboriginal and Torres Strait Islander clients, it may be beneficial to include an IHW in all aspects of healthcare delivery, including assessment, planning, implementation and evaluation of nursing and midwifery care. While the dominant biomedical model inevitably determines the structure and process of healthcare delivery in Australia, a culturally safe practitioner uses their knowledge to navigate the system and apply flexible processes to ensure that they meet the needs of Aboriginal and Torres Strait Islander patients. Culturally safe health practitioners are aware of cultural issues within the context of local health service protocol and policies.

There are many assumptions about the needs of Aboriginal and Torres Strait Islander clients. However, culturally safe practice requires flexibility and an interest in changing practice in order to meet the needs of individual clients and their communities. In some instances, clients will prioritise the skills of a health professional ahead of their cultural background. Some clients like to see IHWs who are members of their community, while other clients prefer a health professional who is not part of their community fabric. Trust and established relationships are strengths of the IHW; however, their membership as part of the community fabric may not always be a strength (Topp et al., 2018).

As a culturally safe practitioner, one must not rely just on the IHW to constantly solve the problems of all Indigenous patients and family members. This is a common frustration for IHWs (Topp et al., 2018). In exercising interprofessional collaboration, all health professionals must develop their knowledge and skills about culturally safe practice; this includes investing time in developing trusting relationships.

Cultural brokers

IHWs have long been valued for their roles as cultural brokers. They often accompany patients on their healthcare journey, within both Aboriginal and Torres Strait Islander-specific and mainstream health services (Dwyer et al., 2007). While the cultural broker role is generally recognised as a positive one, there has been some criticism that IHWs may nurture dependence in clients (Genat, 2006).

When nurses and midwives work alongside IHWs, it is possible that they will achieve better rapport with clients and provide more culturally safe care. Some Aboriginal and Torres Strait Islander patients have difficulty establishing rapport with nurses and midwives, perhaps because some patients are aware that nurses and midwives were instrumental in the forced removal of children from their parents during the Stolen Generations (HREOC, 1997).

IHWs are often established members of their communities and may have an innate understanding of the community – including relevant historical, social and cultural factors (Ridoutt & Pilbeam, 2010). This expert knowledge comes from lived experience that cannot be taught in the same way that biomedical competencies are taught (Bond et al., 2019). Their local knowledge means that they have established relationships in the community. Relationships are critical to providing care for Aboriginal and Torres Strait Islander clients, but may not be considered as important by non-Indigenous health professionals (Eckermann et al., 2010). The shared experience and understanding of culture, history and values of giving back to the community can establish a values connection that non-Indigenous health professionals may never be able to develop (Etowa et al., 2011).

Female IHWs are highly valued as members of maternity teams, and their cultural understanding gives a maternity team a great advantage. Aboriginal and Torres Strait Islander clients identify the availability of IHWs as an indication that a maternity team is appropriate and reliable (DHWA, 2012). When the relationship between the midwife and the health worker demonstrates mutual respect and intercultural partnership, clients experience both clinical and cultural benefits, and are more likely to make use of the services (Hartz et al., 2019; Stamp et al., 2008).

Experiences of racial discrimination

The Australian Human Rights Commission (AHRC, 2012) identified that racism against Aboriginal and Torres Strait Islander people continues to be reported regularly. A Victorian study recently found that 97 per cent of Aboriginal and Torres Strait Islander participants had experienced at least one form of racism in the previous twelve months; almost 30 per cent of participants identified health settings as the source of the racist experience (Ferdinand, Paradies & Kelaher, 2013).

Experiences of discrimination are relevant for both clients and IHWs. Ridoutt and Pilbeam (2010) found that IHWs frequently observed racism in the workplace and/or experienced it themselves. They suggested that the discrimination was often due to the lack of value placed on cultural understanding, identifying nurses as the main perpetrators of discrimination (Ridoutt & Pilbeam, 2010).

Genat's (2006) research identified divisions between nurses and IHWs. In this research, nurses expressed their 'disgust' at assertions that IHWs might one day take over the role of the nurse within health services. One of Genat's interviewees uncovered a perception that Indigenous nurses underwent a process of assimilation through their training, and became 'less Aboriginal' when they became nurses.

The historic racialisation and marginalisation of Indigenous peoples into the lowest-level role in the multidisciplinary health team, and the general perpetuation of this structure, remains a significant issue for addressing racism experienced by IHWs. A better understanding of their role, and optimising their contribution to interprofessional practice, can benefit all health professionals and particularly the patient.

QUESTIONS FOR REFLECTION

- Cultural safety is described as healthcare delivery that is culturally safe from the perspective of the recipients of healthcare. There is an assumption that Aboriginal and Torres Strait Islander workers always provide culturally safe care. Describe the flaws in this assumption.
- Similarly, there is a common belief that culturally safe care for Aboriginal and Torres Strait Islander peoples is the responsibility of Indigenous health professionals, such as the IHW. Describe the flaws in this assumption.

Working with Indigenous health workers

interprofessional practice Occurs when two or more autonomous and accountable professional groups work together with care recipients to achieve a common goal. In this approach, health professionals promote each other's contribution to ensure optimisation of healthcare.

For nurses and midwives, working with an IHW can bring great opportunities for **interprofessional practice** and improved community healthcare. When they work together, nurses and health workers can improve the quality of healthcare provided, the resources used and the outcomes for patients (Gwynne & Lincoln, 2017; Zwarenstein, Goldman & Reeves, 2009).

Interprofessional practice requires each health professional to clarify who is doing what, for what purpose and at what cost. Maintaining the collaborative relationship requires purposeful effort (Pressler & Kenner, 2012).

Historically, the lack of understanding among nurses and midwives about the role of the IHW has led to nurses and midwives preferring other health professionals for collaborative care efforts, leaving IHWs feeling neglected and under-valued. this affects the cultural safety of services for Aboriginal and Torres Strait Islander people (Ridoutt & Pilbeam, 2010) and leads to a high turnover of IHW staff, poor overall performance of health staff and inconsistencies in healthcare available and received by the community (Si et al., 2006).

IHWs identify four major barriers to their successful work with nurses and midwives: (1) insufficient training; (2) lack of clear division between their role and the roles of nurses; (3) an unstable relationship with non-Indigenous health staff; and (4) a high demand for acute care (which excludes them) (Si et al., 2006).

For successful interprofessional practice, nurses, midwives and IHWs need a partnership of mutual respect and trust. This will help to ensure optimal healthcare for Aboriginal and Torres Strait Islander patients (Eckermann et al., 2010).

Nursing and midwifery decision-making framework

In contemporary healthcare settings, nurses and midwives are responsible for making decisions about their practice. Their decision-making capacity reflects the education, competence and authorisation that the nurse or midwife has attained to assess, interpret and determine an appropriate care plan for the client, to coordinate the delivery of care and provide the supervision of associated activities (NMBA, 2020a).

Nursing and midwifery practice is supported by decision-making frameworks developed by the NMBA. In Australia, the NMBA has developed a professional practice framework consisting of standards, codes and guidelines as part of its function under relevant legislation. The NMBA Decision-making Framework for Nursing and Midwifery (DMF) is an important part of the Australian nursing and midwifery professional practice framework, developed to ensure 'consistent, safe, person/woman-centred, and evidence based' approach to decision-making (NMBA, 2020a, p. 1).

The introduction of the DMF to the discussion about IHWs aims to highlight the professional standards and guidelines that already exist to guide the development and maintenance of effective interprofessional practice relationships with IHWs. The DMF is essential to individual practice decisions; however, it can also assist in decisions associated with expanding scope of practice, and when nurses and midwives delegate aspects of their care to others, including other nurses, midwives, enrolled nurses, students and UHCW such as IHWs.

The information presented in this chapter about the application of the DMF is not conclusive, as the other elements of the Australian nursing and midwifery professional practice framework could not be captured. In practice, it is best to consider the DMF alongside the other guiding documents. Furthermore, the DMF is designed to be dynamic; however, in this chapter it will be applied to specific scenarios to assist your understanding of delegation and collaboration with an IHW.

The Decision-making Framework Summary: Nursing (Figure 10.4) and Decision-making Framework Summary: Midwifery (Figure 10.5) are essential tools for delegating nursing and midwifery activities to an IHW. While they were developed specifically for nurses and midwives making decisions associated with nursing and midwifery activities (i.e. activities that are included in the individual and professions' scope of practice), they also recognise that in some circumstances nurses and midwives must work with non-nurses (IHWs included) in order to deliver healthcare that meets the needs of patients.

Unlike other UHCWs, IHWs are able to work independently of the Registered Nurse and complete similar practices. This is enabled through education and competency opportunities, health service policies and legislation.

QUESTION FOR REFLECTION

- Read through the Decision-making Framework Summary: Nursing and Decision-making Framework Summary: Midwifery, and take note of where they reference potential delegation and collaboration with an IHW.

Decision-making framework summary: Nursing

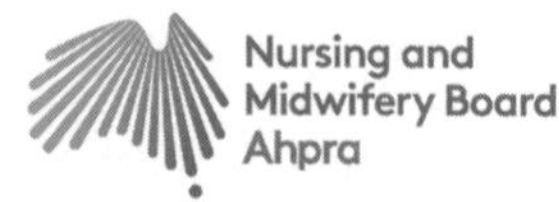

To be read in conjunction with the NMBA *Decision-making framework for nursing and midwifery (2020)*
Note: the order in which these issues are considered may vary according to context

Identify need/benefit

- Has there been a comprehensive assessment by a registered nurse to establish the person's health and cultural needs?
- Has there been appropriate consultation with, and consent by, the person receiving care?
- Is the activity in the best interests of the person receiving care?

Reflect on scope of practice and nursing practice standards

- Is this activity within the current, contemporary scope of nursing practice?
- Have Commonwealth or state/territory legislative requirements (e.g. specific qualification needed) been met?
- If authorisation by a regulatory authority is needed to perform the activity, does the registered nurse, enrolled nurse or health worker have it or can it be obtained before the activity is performed?
- Will performance comply with nursing standards for practice, codes and guidelines, as well as best available evidence?
- If other health professionals should assist, supervise or perform the activity, are they available?

Consider context of practice, governance and identification of risk

- Is this activity/practice/delegation supported by the organisation and/or by the educational institution (for students)?
- Have strategies to avoid or minimise any risk been identified and implemented?
- If organisational authorisation is needed, does the registered nurse, enrolled nurse or health worker have it or can it be obtained before performing the activity?
- Is the skill mix, model of care and staffing levels in the organisation adequate for the level of support/supervision needed to safely perform the activity/delegation?
- If this is a new practice:
  - Is there a system for ongoing education and maintenance of competence in place?
  - Have relevant parties and stakeholders been involved in planning for implementation?

Select appropriate, competent person to perform activities

(Delegation of care is made by a registered nurse)

- Have the roles and responsibilities of registered nurses, enrolled nurses and health workers been considered?
- Does the registered nurse, enrolled nurse or health worker have the necessary educational preparation, experience, capacity, competence and confidence to safely perform the activity either autonomously or with education, support and supervision?
- Are they competent and confident in performing the activity and accepting the delegation?
- Do they understand their accountability and reporting responsibilities?
- Is the required level of education, clinical supervision/support available?

Yes to all

Action

- Perform the activity, **or** delegate to a competent person who then reconfirms consent from the person receiving care, **and**
- document the decision and the actions, **and**
- regular review of the delegation providing guidance, support and clinically focused supervision, **and**
- evaluate outcome.

No to any

Action

- Reconsider decision about whether to implement practice/activity/delegation, **and**
- consult/seek advice/collaborate, **and/or**
- refer if needed to complete the action, **and**
- if appropriate, plan to enable integration/practice changes (including developing/implementing policies, gaining qualifications as needed), **and**
- document the decisions and the actions, **and**
- evaluate outcome.

Figure 10.4 Decision-making Framework Summary: Nursing

Source: NMBA (2020c).

Decision-making framework summary: Midwifery

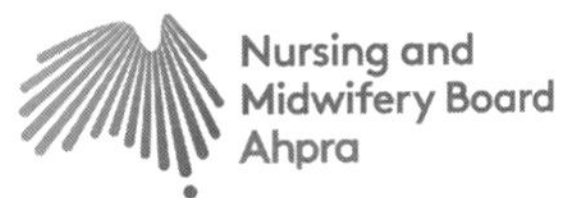

To be read in conjunction with the NMBA *Decision-making framework for nursing and midwifery (2020)*

Note: the order in which these issues are considered may vary according to context

Identify need/benefit

- Has there been a comprehensive assessment by the midwife to establish the woman or newborn's health and cultural needs?
- Has there been appropriate consultation with, and consent by, the woman?
- Is the activity in the best interests of the woman receiving care?

Reflect on scope of practice and midwifery practice standards

- Is this activity within the current, contemporary scope of midwifery practice?
- Have Commonwealth or state/territory legislative requirements (e.g. specific qualification needed) been met?
- If authorisation by a regulatory authority is needed to perform the activity, does the midwife or health worker have it or can it be obtained before the activity is performed?
- Will performance comply with midwifery standards for practice, codes and guidelines, as well as best available evidence?
- If other health professionals should assist, supervise or perform the activity, are they available?

Consider context of practice, governance and identification of risk

- Is this activity/practice/delegation supported by the organisation and/or by the educational institution (for students)?
- Have strategies to avoid or minimise any risk been identified and implemented?
- If organisational authorisation is needed, does the midwife or health worker have it or can it be obtained before performing the activity?
- Is the skill mix, model of care and staffing levels in the organisation adequate for the level of support/supervision needed to safely perform the activity/delegation?
- If this is a new practice:
  - Is there a system for ongoing education and maintenance of competence in place?
  - Have relevant parties and stakeholders been involved in planning for implementation?

Select appropriate, competent person to perform activities

(Delegation of care is made by a midwife)

- Have the roles and responsibilities of midwives and health workers been considered?
- Does the midwife or health worker have the necessary educational preparation, experience, capacity, competence and confidence to safely perform the activity either autonomously or with education, support and supervision?
- Are they competent and confident in performing the activity and accepting the delegation?
- Do they understand their accountability and reporting responsibilities?
- Is the required level of education, supervision/support available?

Yes to all

Action

- Perform the activity, **or** delegate to a competent person who then reconfirms consent from the woman receiving care, **and**
- document the decision and the actions, **and**
- regular review of the delegation providing guidance, support and clinically-focused supervision, **and**
- evaluate outcome.

No to any

Action

- Reconsider decision about whether to implement practice/activity/delegation, **and**
- consult/seek advice/collaborate, **and/or**
- refer if needed to complete the action, **and**
- if appropriate, plan to enable integration/practice changes (including developing/implementing policies, gaining qualifications as needed), **and**
- document the decisions and the actions, **and**
- evaluate outcome.

Figure 10.5 Decision-making Framework Summary: Midwifery

Source: NMBA (2020b).

CASE STUDY

Working with an Aboriginal and Torres Strait Islander health worker

Linda was a Registered Nurse employed as the Clinical Nurse on Warraber Island in the Torres Strait. This was her first time working in a Torres Strait Island community. 'A new adventure,' Linda boasted to her friends before leaving Brisbane.

On Linda's first day at Warraber Island, she met her two colleagues (the only other local health staff). Betty and Jack were both IHWs. Betty took Linda around the health centre for an orientation. There were two treatment rooms, a waiting room and a medication room.

Betty was the health centre manager and she held a Certificate IV in Aboriginal and Torres Strait Islander Primary Health Care (Practice). She explained to Linda that, while she was the operational lead, Linda would be the clinical leader. This was a new operational structure for Linda, as her operational leader had always been a Nurse Unit Manager.

Betty told her that Jack had completed his Certificate II in Aboriginal and Torres Strait Islander Primary Health Care, and was currently enrolled in a Certificate III at the Cairns TAFE. She said that Jack mostly did the cleaning, driving and follow-up with clients, while the Registered Nurse and Betty did the 'hands-on practice'.

Betty said Linda and Jack would have to go and visit some community members that morning. She said that Linda should change into a t-shirt before going out, as the spaghetti-strapped top Linda was wearing would not be acceptable for the community (Linda considered it appropriate for the weather). As it was Linda's first day, she chose to follow Betty's advice and thought she would perhaps challenge her at a later date.

Betty indicated that Linda should follow Jack to the car. Linda and Jack left the clinic, and Jack began to introduce her to the islanders. Every second house or so, Jack stopped the car to introduce Linda to some of the local people. Linda met the chairman of the island, local Elders and the priests. After some time, she became a little nervous about spending so much time away from the clinic on her first day.

For each person Linda met, Jack provided an explanation of who they were related to and how. He also briefly made mention of some of their health problems. By lunchtime, Linda was back at the clinic, where Betty was just completing the changing of a client's dressing.

QUESTIONS FOR REFLECTION

- Identify three episodes where Linda was confused or did not agree with something. Then choose one of these episodes and describe why you think Linda was confused or in disagreement. Briefly explain the reasons behind these issues.
- Identify the information in the case study that is relevant to delegating decision making using the Decision-making Framework Summary: Nursing or Decision-making Framework Summary: Midwifery.

Delegating tasks to Indigenous health workers

Delegating involves consultation between and conferring from one person to another the authority to perform some action. A delegation relationship is established when a nurse or midwife delegates an aspects of nursing or midwifery practice to another person – that is, a nurse or midwife or to another health worker (e.g. IHW). In such instances, the nurse or midwife (as the delegator) maintains **accountability** for the decision to delegate, monitor performance and evaluate outcomes. While the health professional accepting the delegation (delegate) maintains responsibility for their actions and is accountable for providing the delegated care, and cannot subdelegate (NMBA, 2020a, p. 9).

delegating In the nursing and midwifery context, the transfer of authority to a competent person to perform a specific activity in a specific context. The delegatee may be another nurse or midwife, or another health worker.

accountability In the nursing and midwifery context, this includes decisions, actions, behaviours and responsibilities associated with the nursing or midwifery role. Nurses and midwives must be able to justify their actions to others, including healthcare consumers, the nursing and midwifery regulatory authority, employers and the public. When delegating activities, nurses and midwives remain accountable for the decision to delegate, for monitoring performance of the delegate and for evaluating associated outcomes.

Delegation is an important leadership skill that will assist the student nurse and midwife to work effectively as a team member. While the student nurse and midwife must work directly under the supervision of a registered nurse or registered midwife, and has no authority to delegate, this skill may be developed through simulation experience and case studies (Nowell, 2016; Saccomano & Zipp, 2014). Poor delegation can influence the quality of care, outcomes for patients and satisfaction of both staff and patients (Hopkins et al., 2012).

Nurses and midwives are responsible for using the Decision-making Framework Summary: Nursing and Decision-making Framework Summary: Midwifery, as well as associated guidelines, to determine the most appropriate individual to undertake the delegated task. If the relevant criteria are met, the nurse or midwife may delegate tasks to an IHW. If the criteria are not met, the nurse or midwife must consider whether to delegate to a different IHW or another health professional, or to complete the task personally. Some IHWs may require direct and indirect supervision, depending on their education, competency and local policies.

CASE STUDY

Delegating nursing tasks

A client arrived at the Warraber Island Health Clinic. Mrs Sara Flora was a 70-year-old woman with diabetic ulcers on her left foot. While Linda watched Betty finish changing Sara's dressing, Sara interrogated Linda about her personal life. Linda felt a little distracted as she keenly watched Betty's technique and asked occasional questions about the types of dressings used at the clinic.

Linda had worked for some years on a surgical ward and considered herself competent with post-operative wound dressings. However, she had limited experience in caring for wounds related to chronic disease of patients in a community setting.

After completing the dressing, Betty explained to Sara that she needed to have some blood taken as well. Sara's Chronic Disease Care Plan highlighted that she was due to have her cholesterol levels checked. Linda overheard this and assumed that, as the most clinically trained health professional in the clinic, she would need to take the blood. Linda said she had not yet done her phlebotomy course, but would give it a try.

(cont.)

Betty reassured Linda that she had completed her training and was able to provide all the care Sara needed. This was bit of a shock for Linda. In her previous roles, not even nurses were able to take blood. But here was an IHW with a Certificate IV qualification stating that she could take blood!

Not wanting to be rude, but concerned about Sara's safety and Betty's lack of qualifications, Linda insisted that she was happy to try. Betty eventually turned to Linda and said, 'Nurse, I am very competent in taking blood, much like completing a complex wound dressing. If you wish to see my qualifications just say so and I will bring them in for you!'

This left both Linda and Sara a little stunned.

QUESTIONS FOR REFLECTION

- Reflecting on the Decision-making Framework Summary: Nursing and Decision-making Framework Summary: Midwifery, which of the two health professionals is competent to complete (a) the dressing and (b) blood-taking?
- While blood-taking falls within the scope of the nursing and midwifery profession, in some contexts it is not applicable and therefore not required in the scope of the individual nurse. Explain why, in this context, blood-taking would be considered a skill within the scope of local health staff.
- If Linda had already completed the phlebotomy course and was leading the care with Sara, describe how she would determine the right person to undertake this activity.

Professional boundaries and therapeutic relationships

All health professionals need to think carefully about their professional boundaries and how these influence the therapeutic relationships they establish with clients. By understanding their professional boundaries, health professionals can establish and maintain a safe and therapeutic relationship with the person receiving their care. In this relationship, the balance of power usually sways towards the care provider, because she or he or they hold personal information about the person receiving care, are members of the healthcare team, action decisions related to the patient's care, to name a few factors that influence the associated power dynamics. The care recipient is thus vulnerable to exploitation and abuse of trust. This means that it is the care provider's responsibility to ensure that professional boundaries are not breached.

The therapeutic relationship is optimised when there is no existing dual relationship – that is, when there is no additional relationship apart from that of professional care provider and care recipient. However, in remote and regional settings, dual relationships are common: it is not unusual for health professionals to care for people they know personally (NMBA, 2018, pp. 11–12).

Dual relationships refer to pre-existing non-professional relationships that may create conflicts or impair judgement. They can be a significant challenge for IHWs, as the family and community relationships and associated responsibilities may complicate the delivery of adequate healthcare to them and compromise the maintenance of professional boundaries.

Ethical and sociocultural dilemmas are often reported by IHWs, and can result in unforeseen demand on both the health service and its staff. IHWs identify that:

- They may spend more time facilitating social welfare than providing healthcare (for example, on housing, transport and money issues).
- They may be employed alongside family members, in similar roles and even in management and governance roles, which may be beneficial but may also bring challenges and ethical dilemmas.
- They may be considered as junior in a professional context (they may be working with an older relative) or a personal capacity (they may be caring for an older relative), and this can present challenges.
- Coordinating after-hours care can be challenging in remote locations with limited staff; the community's expectations may not acknowledge business hours and the after-hours roster, and this can lead to staff burnout.
- Family conflict within Aboriginal and Torres Strait Islander communities may affect local health staff and influence relationships within the health team as well as provider–recipient relationships; this can create short-term or long-term challenges for the health service.
- Breaches of professional conduct and client confidentiality have been known to occur, and may be exacerbated by the community grapevine.

(Genat, 2006; Mitchell & Hussey, 2006; Ridoutt & Pilbeam, 2010; Topp et al., 2018)

Waipuldanya, a 'barefoot doctor' from the Northern Territory, experienced this dilemma when caring for his mothers-in-law (discussed by Lockwood, 1966, p. 118). Due to marriage laws, Waipuldanya had inherited a number of mothers-in-law in addition to his other roles and responsibilities. The marriage laws informed his relationships with his mothers-in-law, and a taboo was placed upon him to never look at them or speak to them. In order for him to deliver healthcare to his mothers-in-law, Elders needed to intervene and negotiate with the mothers-in-law to lift the taboo.

The Registered Nurse may be able to assist the IHW in managing dual relationships to ensure the maintenance of the therapeutic relationship with the IHW and patients. Collaboration in the delivery of holistic care to the entire community can assist in alleviating this pressure on the IHW, and can foster effective interprofessional collaboration.

CASE STUDY

Negotiating professional boundaries

Later, during her first afternoon at work, Linda found herself spending longer than expected trying to organise access to all of the online software programs. These were essential because they allowed Linda to access patients' online care plans and look up blood-test results and other information.

(cont.)

A young woman entered the health centre, introduced herself as Anna and said that she had not been feeling well. Linda was intent on completing the task at hand, so she looked around to see whether her colleagues were busy. She found Jack in one of the treatment rooms doing readings for his course, so she asked him whether he could see a client. He said he didn't mind.

When Linda introduced Jack to Anna, they started speaking to each other in what she assumed was the local language. Linda assumed that they knew each other, so she went back to her computer work. Not long after, Linda noticed Anna leaving the health centre. She realised that it must have been a very short consultation, or not one at all. Linda assumed that Jack probably told Anna to come back later as he wanted to get back to his coursework.

Linda decided to ask Jack about the situation. She soon discovered that Anna was married to Jack's brother. Traditionally, Jack was not supposed to talk to Anna, let alone care for her.

QUESTIONS FOR REFLECTION

- Like the continuum of professional behaviour, the relationships within Aboriginal and Torres Strait Islander communities have boundaries. Knowing about the expectations of the relationship between Jack and Anna, how should Linda have managed this delegated activity? Was it appropriate to delegate?
- Cultural expectations will vary from community to community. Be mindful that IHWs are often members of the community. How would you (a) find out this information and (b) support the IHW to navigate professional and cultural expectations?

Conclusion

The work of IHWs gained prominence and importance during the policy eras of self-determination and self-management. The growth of the Aboriginal Medical Services has seen an expansion of employment opportunities for health workers. The list of tasks being shifted from nurses and midwives to IHWs is growing. While some may celebrate this as acknowledgement of the role, there is a risk that this is simply occurring for the convenience of health managers and other health professionals.

While some confusion remains about the role, the NATSIHWA (2012) Professional Practice Framework and regulation of IHPs are signs that the role is becoming more consolidated.

IHWs are valued colleagues, especially for nurses and midwives seeking to contribute to closing the gap in health outcomes and life expectancy between Indigenous and other Australians. However, while IHWs are important cultural brokers, they cannot assume the role of the cultural conduit for every case. Cultural safety remains the responsibility of all health professionals.

By practising in accordance with established nursing and midwifery professional frameworks for practice and delegation, nurses and midwives can optimise their interprofessional practice with IHWs. This will optimise the care provided to Aboriginal and Torres Strait Islander people.

Learning activities

1. Search online for some job vacancies for IHWs. What jobs are currently available? Where are they located? From the advertisements, what can you learn about the scope of the IHW's role and how the different jobs may vary?
2. Choose a client-based nursing or midwifery task that you have recently learnt about or reflected upon. If you were undertaking this task with an Aboriginal or Torres Strait Islander client, how could you involve an IHW in the task? What benefits would this bring? What challenges might it present for you?
3. Choose a client-based nursing or midwifery task that you feel confident completing. Could you delegate this task to an IHW? Why or why not? Might it be appropriate to delegate in some situations but not others?

FURTHER READING

Bond, C., Brough, M., Willis, J. ... Lewis, T. (2019). Beyond the pipeline: A critique of the discourse surrounding the development of an Indigenous primary healthcare workforce in Australia. *Australian Journal of Primary Health*, 25(5), 389–394.

NATSIHWA (2012). *The Aboriginal and Torres Strait Islander Health Worker Professional Practice Framework*. Retrieved from www.natsihwa.org.au/aboriginal-and-torres-strait-islander-health-worker-professional-practice-framework

NMBA (2020). *Frameworks*. Retrieved from www.nursingmidwiferyboard.gov.au/Codes-Guidelines-Statements/Frameworks.aspx

Topp, S.M., Edelman, M. & Taylor, S. (2018). 'We are everything to everyone': A systematic review of factors influencing the accountability relationships of Aboriginal and Torres Strait Islander health workers (AHWs) in the Australian health system. *International Journal for Equity in Health*, 17(67). doi:10.1186/s12939-018–0779-z

Visit the companion website at www.cambridge.org/highereducation/isbn/9781108794695/resources to see further online resources.

REFERENCES

AHMAC (2012). *Aboriginal and Torres Strait Islander Health Performance Framework 2012 Report*. Canberra: AHMAC.

AHMAC (2017). *Aboriginal and Torres Strait Islander Health Performance Framework 2017 Report*. Canberra: AHMAC.

AHRC (2012). *National Anti-Racism Strategy 2012*. Retrieved from www.humanrights.gov.au/sites/default/files/National%20Anti-Racism%20Strategy.pdf

ATSIHPBA (2020). Registrant data. Retrieved from www.atsihealthpracticeboard.gov.au/About/Statistics.aspx

Bond, C., Brough, M., Willis, J. ... Lewis, T. (2019). Beyond the pipeline: A critique of the discourse surrounding the development of an Indigenous primary healthcare workforce in Australia. *Australian Journal of Primary Health*, 25(5), 389–394.

Davidson, P.M., DiGiacomo, M., Abbott, P. ... Davison, J. (2008). A partnership model in the development and implementation of a collaborative, cardiovascular education program for Aboriginal health workers. *Australian Health Review*, 32(1), 139–46.

Dettwiller, P., Raines, T., Cubillo, P. & Stothers, K. (2015). Aboriginal and Torres Strait Islander health practitioner students' perspectives on an interprofessional education program. In *LIME Good Practice Case Studies, Vol. 3*. Melbourne: Onemda VicHealth Koori Health Unit, University of Melbourne

DHWA (2012). *Successful Characteristics of Community Based Maternity Services in Remote and Very Remote Australia*. Perth: DHWA.

DPMC (2020). *Closing the Gap: Prime Minister's Report 2020*. Canberra: DPMC.

Dwyer, J., Shannon, C. & Godwin, S. (2007). *Learning from Action Management of Aboriginal and Torres Strait Islander Health Services*. Darwin: Cooperative Research Centre for Aboriginal Health.

Eckermann, A.K., Dowd, T., Chong, E., Nixon, L., Gray, R. & Johnson, S. (2010). *Binan Goonj: Bridging Cultures in Aboriginal Health* (3rd edn). Sydney: Elsevier.

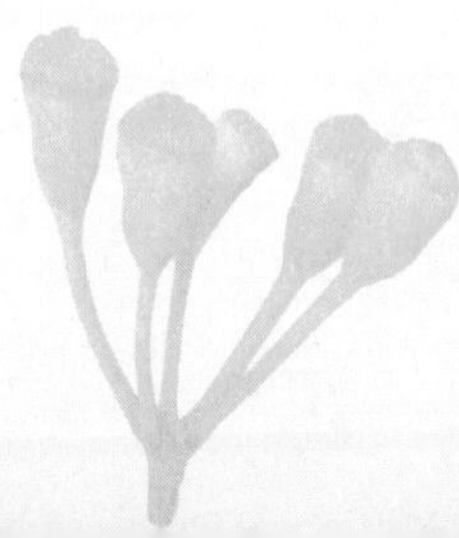

Etowa, J., Jest, C. & Vukic, A. (2011). Indigenous nurses' stories: Perspectives on the cultural context of Aboriginal health care work. *The Canadian Journal of Native Studies*, 31(2), 29–46.

Ferdinand, A., Paradies, Y. & Kelaher, M. (2013). *Mental Health Impacts of Racial Discrimination in Victorian Aboriginal Communities: The Localities Embracing and Accepting Diversity (LEAD) Experiences of Racism Survey*. Melbourne: Lowitja Institute.

Genat, B. (2006). *At the Front Line, Aboriginal Healthworker*. Perth: University of Western Australia Press.

Gwynne, K. & Lincoln, M. (2017). Developing the rural health workforce to improve Australian Aboriginal and Torres Strait Islander health outcomes: A systematic review. *Australian Health Review*, 41(2), 234–8.

Hartz, D.L., Blain, J., Caplice, S. ... Tracey, S.K. (2019). Evaluation of an Australian Aboriginal model of maternity care: The Malabar Community Midwifery Link Service. *Women and Birth*. 32(5), 427–36.

HWA (2011). *Aboriginal and Torres Strait Islander Health Worker Project Interim Report*. Adelaide: HWA.

HWA (2013). *Australia's Health Workforce Series: Health Workforce by Numbers*. Adelaide: HWA.

Hill, K.L., Harvey, N., Felton-Busch, C., Hoskins, J., Rasalam, R., Malouf, P. & Knight, S. (2017). The road to registration: Aboriginal and Torres Strait Islander health practitioner training in North Queensland. *Rural and Remote Health*. Retrieved from www.rrh.org.au/journal/article/3899

Hopkins, U., Itty, A.S., Nazario, H., Pinon, M., Slyer, J. & Singleton, J. (2012). The effectiveness of delegation interventions by the registered nurse to the unlicensed assistive personnel and their impact on quality of care, patient satisfaction, and RN staff satisfaction: A systematic review. *Joanna Briggs Institute Library of Systematic Reviews*, 10(15), 895–934.

HRSCAA (1979). *Aboriginal Health: Report*. Canberra:HRSCAA.

HREOC (1997). *Bringing Them Home: Report of the National Inquiry into the Separation of Aboriginal and Torres Strait Islander Children from their Families*. Sydney: HREOC.

ICN (2008). *Assistive Nursing Personnel*. Geneva: ICN.

Industry Reference Committee (2019). *Aboriginal and Torres Strait Islander Health Worker, Industry Reference Committee Industry Skills Forecast*. Retrieved from www.skillsiq.com.au/site/DefaultSite/filesystem/documents/Industry-Skills-Forecasts-June2017/2019%20Final%20ISFs/2019%20Industry%20Skills%20Forecast%20Aboriginal%20and%20Torres%20Strait%20Islander%20Health%20Worker%20IRC%20Web.pdf

Javanparast, S., Windle, A., Freeman, T. & Baum, F. (2018). Community health worker programs to improve healthcare access and equity: Are they only relevant to low- and middle-income countries? *International Journal of Health Policy and Management*, 7(10), 943–54.

Kildea, S., Hickey, S., Nelson, C. ... Tracy, S. (2018). Birthing on Country (in our community): A case study of engaging stakeholders and developing a best-practice Indigenous maternity service in an urban setting. *Australian Health Review*, 42(2), 230–8.

Lockwood, D. (1966). *I, the Aboriginal*. Adelaide: Rigby.

Mackean, T., Withall, E., Dwyer, J. & Wilson, A. (2020). Role of Aboriginal health workers and liaison officers in quality care in the Australian acute care setting: A systematic review. *Australian Health Review*, 44(3), 427–33.

Mitchell, M. & Hussey, L.M. (2006). The Aboriginal health worker. *Medical Journal of Australia*, 184(10), 529–30.

Murray, R.B. & Wronski, I. (2006). When the tide goes out: Health workforce in rural, remote and Indigenous communities. *Medical Journal of Australia*, 185(1), 37–8.

NAHSWP (1989). *A National Aboriginal Health Strategy*. Canberra: NAHS.

NATSIHWA (2012). *The Aboriginal and Torres Strait Islander Health Worker Professional Practice Framework*. Canberra: NATSIHWA.

NATSIHWA (2019). *The Importance of Aboriginal and Torres Strait Islander Health Workers and Health Practitioners in Australia's Health System*. Canberra: NATSIHWA.

NATSIHWA (2020). Publications – other documents.

NMBA (2018). *Code of Conduct for Nurses*. Canberra: NMBA

NMBA (2020a). *Decision-making framework for nursing and midwifery*. Canberra: NMBA.

NMBA (2020b). *Decision-making Framework Summary: Midwifery*. Canberra: NMBA.

NMBA (2020c). *Decision-making Framework Summary: Nursing*. Canberra: NMBA.

NMBA (2020d). *Professional Standards*. Retrieved from www.nursingmidwiferyboard.gov.au/Codes-Guidelines-Statements/Professional-standards.aspx

Nowell, L.S. (2016). Delegate, collaborate, or consult? A capstone simulation for senior nursing students, *Nursing Education Perspectives*, 31(1), 54–5.

Pressler, J.L. & Kenner, C.A. (2012). Interprofessional and interdisciplinary collaboration in nursing, *Nurse Educator*, 37(6), 230–2.

Queensland Consolidated Acts (2009). *Health Practitioner Regulation National Law Act 2009*. Retrieved from www.austlii.edu.au/au/legis/qld/consol_act/hprnla2009428

Queensland Health (2016). *Health (Drugs and Poisons) Regulation 1996: Drug Therapy Protocol – Indigenous Health Worker Isolated Practice Area*. Brisbane: Queensland Health.

Ramsden, I. (2002). Cultural safety and nursing education in Aotearoa and Te Waipounamu. Unpublished PhD thesis, Victoria University of Wellington.

Ridoutt, L. & Pilbeam, V. (2010). *Final Report Aboriginal Health Worker Profession Review*. Darwin: Northern Territory Department of Health and Families.

Saccomano, S.J. & Zipp, G.P. (2014). Integrating delegation into the undergraduate curriculum. *Creative Nursing*, 20(2), 106–15.

Si, D., Bailie, R.S., Togni, S.J., d'Abbs, P.H.N. & Robinson, G.W. (2006). Aboriginal health workers and diabetes care in remote community health centres: A mixed method analysis. *Medical Journal Australia*, 185(1), 40–5.

Stamp, G.E., Champion, S., Anderson, G. … Muyambi, C. (2008). Aboriginal maternal and infant care workers: Partners in caring for Aboriginal mothers and babies. *Rural and Remote Health*, 1(883), 1–12.

Topp, S.M., Edelman, A. & Taylor, S. (2018). 'We are everything to everyone': A systematic review of factors influencing the accountability relationships of Aboriginal and Torres Strait Islander health workers (AHWs) in the Australian health system. *International Journal for Equity in Health*, 17(67). doi.org/10.1186/s12939-018–0779-z

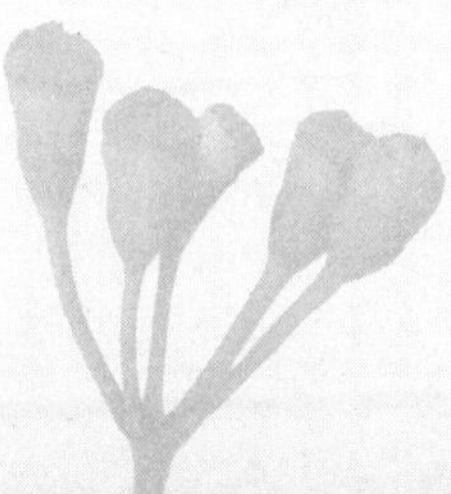

Torzillo, P. & Kerr, C. (1991). Contemporary issues in Aboriginal public health. In J. Reid & P. Trompf (eds), *The Health of Aboriginal Australia*. Sydney: Harcourt Brace Jovanovich, pp. 326–80.

WHO (1978). *Declaration of Alma-Ata*. Geneva: WHO.

WHO (2008). *Task Shifting: Rational Redistribution of Tasks among Health Workforce Teams: Global Recommendations and Guidelines*. Geneva: WHO.

Wright, A., Briscoe, K. & Lovett, R. (2019). A national profile of Aboriginal and Torres Strait Islander health workers, 2006–2016. *Australian and New Zealand Journal of Public Health*, 43(1), pp. 24–6.

Zwarenstein, M., Goldman, J. & Reeves, S. (2009). Interprofessional collaboration: Effects of practice-based interventions on professional practice and healthcare outcomes, *Cochrane Database of Systemic Reviews*, 3, CD000072. doi:10.1002/14651858.CD000072.pub2

LEGISLATION CITED

Health Practitioner Regulation National Law Act 2009 (Qld)

Practitioners and Allied Professionals Registration Act 1986 (NT)

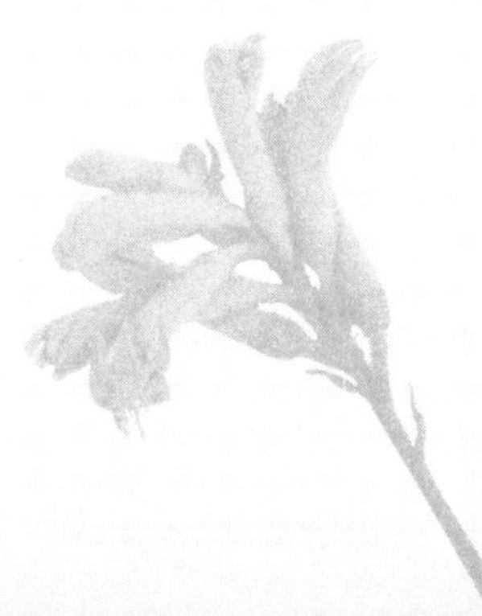

11 Indigenous-led qualitative research

Raelene Ward and Bronwyn Fredericks

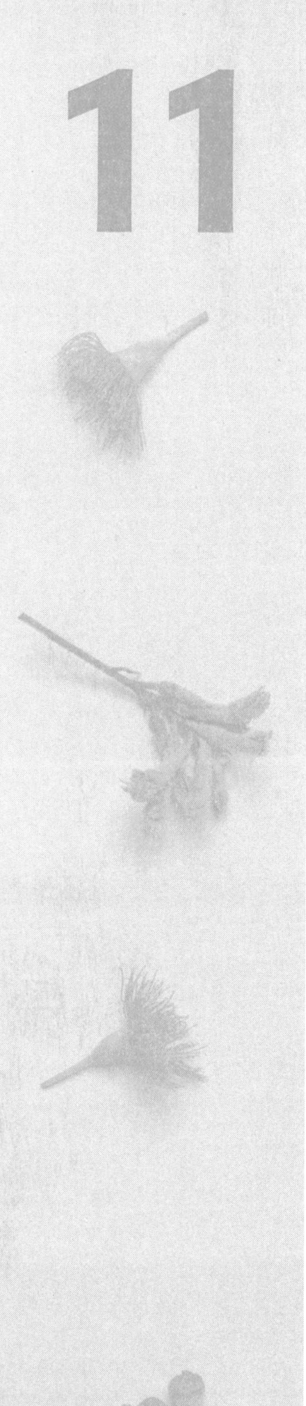

LEARNING OBJECTIVES

This chapter will help you to understand:

- The history and development of research with Aboriginal and Torres Strait Islander people and communities
- The application of cultural safety when developing and implementing research with Indigenous people and communities
- Perspectives and issues relevant to research with Aboriginal and Torres Strait Islander people and communities
- Guidelines that discuss appropriate and ethical ways to conduct research with Aboriginal and Torres Strait Islander people
- Protocols and processes in working towards being a culturally safe researcher with Aboriginal and Torres Strait Islander people and communities.
- Development and implementation of a research project with Aboriginal and Torres Strait Islander people and communities

KEY WORDS

community protocols
ethical guidelines
mixed-methods approach
qualitative research
quantitative research

Introduction

Research is vital to the health professions. It has the potential to inform and change health policy and practice and, through that change, to improve Indigenous health outcomes.

However, while research is vitally important, it is not neutral. Historically, much research has been conducted *on* rather than *with* Indigenous communities. Typically, research has been carried out by non-Indigenous researchers who want to find out about Indigenous peoples and their cultures. Research has traditionally been designed to suit the agenda and interests of the non-Indigenous people conducting research. Research of the past was often conducted in ways that did not address Indigenous priorities or benefit Indigenous communities in any way. In many cases, the research brought no benefit to the peoples being studied or was harmful and destructive for communities. As Smith (2012, p. 3) notes, 'we [Indigenous people] are the most researched people in the world'.

While research today is guided by strong codes for ethical practice, there are continuing concerns about the benefits that research can bring to the communities being studied and the extent to which Indigenous people are involved as active participants and initiators of the research that is driven and applicable to them. Memories of past inappropriate research practices contributed to why Aboriginal and Torres Strait Islander people were reluctant to participate in research. However, there is a growing desire and commitment to develop an Indigenous, responsive approach to research to encourage research conducted by, for and with Aboriginal and Torres Strait Islander people. This chapter provides an overview of past research practices, ethical considerations in research and culturally safe research, considers recent changes and provides a glimpse of future research possibilities for Aboriginal and Torres Strait Islander people.

Research on Indigenous people

Every person has experiences, values, norms and learnings that inform the ways in which they see and interpret the world. Much of our learning and practices are based in research – either formal research that we read about and study, or informal research that we gather through our interactions with others. From the earliest days of Australian colonisation, ill-formed perceptions and assumptions have guided policies and interactions with Aboriginal and Torres Strait Islander people.

History tells us that research with Aboriginal and Torres Strait Islander people has been largely carried out by non-Indigenous people: including anthropologists, archaeologists and religious leaders who have studied cultural practices and belief systems; teachers who have studied education and learning; lawyers who have studied legal practices and traditional justice; government policy advisors and consultants who have studied a wide variety of issues from a policy perspective; and nurses, doctors and other health professionals who have studied health, traditional health practices and health promotion activities.

In many cases, research conducted about Aboriginal and Torres Strait Islander people has demonstrated poor practice. For example, researchers may ask inappropriate questions that seem invasive to Aboriginal and Torres Strait Islander people and their communities. At times, researchers have not sought permission to conduct research, have not acknowledged the rights of research participants and have not given participants an opportunity to agree to take part in the research. In some situations, communities have not even been aware or fully informed that non-Indigenous people were conducting research while they were in the community. These practices are now disappearing, as robust **ethical guidelines** are in place to guide researchers.

ethical guidelines Include the right for participants to be informed about the research, the right to freely consent to take part in the research, the right to refuse or withdraw from research, the right to confidentiality and/or anonymity, and the need for researchers to maximise benefits and minimise risks.

Cruse (2001, p. 27) explains that 'many researchers have ridden roughshod over our communities, cultures, practices and beliefs, and we are now in a position to prevent this from continuing.' Aboriginal and Torres Strait Islander people are increasingly developing their research skills and capacity to lead research, are more aware of research practices and are demanding to be involved in research that focuses on their communities.

Today, it is not solely non-Indigenous researchers who conduct research in Australia. Indigenous researchers are increasingly becoming involved in research activities. There are growing numbers of people who are undertaking research within and about their communities, including Indigenous nurses and midwives. In Australia, the landscape of Aboriginal and Torres Strait Islander research has changed enormously over the past 30 years. There is a developing understanding of how to conduct appropriate and valuable research with Aboriginal and Torres Strait Islander people and how to use that research to inform changes in both policy and practice.

The push for change in research

Since the 1970s, Indigenous people all over the world have advocated for changes to the ways in which research is carried out with Indigenous people and in communities. A number of publications have explored how research with Indigenous communities should take place, what ethics processes are required and how to involve Indigenous people in research (e.g. Chilisa, 2012; Gower, 2012; Laycock et al., 2009; Smith, 2012). Historically, research practices undertaken on Indigenous people and their communities were not reciprocated back to the participants and were deemed to be inappropriate and offensive.

Over time, Indigenous people have continued to be actively engaged in determining who, what, where, when and how research may take place in their communities, and the conditions under which it should be approved (Fredericks, 2008). Of course, this does not mean that inappropriate research no longer takes place; however, inappropriate research is much less likely to occur today. For many Aboriginal and Torres Strait Islander people, research has become a big part of contemporary life, including ways to conduct it, write about it, talk about it, tell jokes about it and, as Smith (1999, p. 1) indicates, 'even write poetry' about it.

In recent years, there has been a steady increase in the numbers of Aboriginal and Torres Strait Islander people undertaking research, applying for research grants and publishing research outcomes. In the field of Aboriginal and Torres Strait Islander health, there are now several strong collaborative research teams that include both Indigenous and non-Indigenous researchers. There is also an increase in research undertaken by nurses and designed to inform nursing practice.

Several documents are available to guide research involving Aboriginal and Torres Strait Islander people. Some of the recent documents include the following:

- *National Statement on Ethical Conduct in Human Research* (NHMRC, 2007, updated 2018)
- *Ethical Conduct in Research with Aboriginal and Torres Strait Islander Peoples and Communities: Guidelines for Researchers and Stakeholders* (NHMRC, 2018a)
- *Keeping Research on Track II* (NHMRC, 2018b)
- *AIATSIS Code of Ethics for Aboriginal and Torres Strait Islander Research* (AIATSIS, 2020)
- *Developing a Set of Principles to Set a Foundation for Conducting Aboriginal Research the Right Way in SA* (SAHMRI, 2013).

In addition, several other useful documents have been produced by Indigenous organisations with an interest in research, including:

- *We Don't Like Research. But in Koori Hands it Could Make a Difference* (VicHealth KHRCDU, 2000)
- *We Can Like Research … In Koori Hands: A Community Report on Onemda VicHealth Koori Health Unit's Research Workshops in 2007* (Onemda VicHealth Koori Health Unit, 2008)
- *Research – Understanding Ethics* (KHRCDU, 2001)
- *Wardliparingga: Aboriginal Research in Aboriginal Hands* (SAHMRI, 2014)
- *Supporting Indigenous Researchers: A Practical Guide for Supervisors* (Laycock et al., 2009)
- *Researching Indigenous Health: A Practical Guide for Researchers* (Laycock et al., 2011)

The two documents produced by the VicHealth Koori Health Research and Community Development Unit (KHRCDU) were important documents when they were published, as they offered an Aboriginal perspective of research, discussed community understandings of research and research ethics, and explored how research outcomes could make a positive difference. The other documents in the list are designed to foster the growth and development of students and researchers who work in Aboriginal and Torres Strait Islander health and alongside Indigenous and non-Indigenous researchers.

Many guidelines and protocols about how to consult and engage with Aboriginal and Torres Strait Islander people (there are two separate protocols for Aboriginal and Torres Strait Islander people) and how to undertake ethical research are now freely available online. It is important to consult these guidelines when planning any research with Aboriginal and Torres Strait Islander people.

Culturally safe research

Having prior experience in working alongside Aboriginal and Torres Strait Islander peoples in research is something that not everybody can say they have been a part of. This is one of the key aspects that communities will often seek out in determining what kind of experience a researcher has and if they are someone the community can have faith in when undertaking research. To understand the main aspects of culturally safe research requires you to understand and be aware of your own cultural values and beliefs, and to acknowledge there are differences in power, recognising where you are positioned in community relationships with Aboriginal and Torres Strait Islander peoples is integral to research practices. This is supported by understanding the historical context of invasion, colonisation and the impact of policies and practices imposed on Aboriginal and Torres Strait Islander people.

Some additional factors need to be considered prior to doing research with Aboriginal and Torres Strait Islander people – for instance, stepping back and taking the time to reflect on your knowledge, experience and skillset as part of a process to recognise what your strengths and weaknesses are and to prepare to build on these as an individual and within a research team. Be mindful that 'from little things big things grow', which often starts with having a yarn – a specific type of Indigenous conversation – with other people around you within your context and your community (Bessarab & Ng'andu, 2010). This, in turn, supports the need to establish the researcher within the community. This can also be a process whereby the community learns and understands more about you as a researcher, asking questions about what kind of projects you have been involved in with Aboriginal and Torres Strait Islander people and communities. This is a form of doing quality checks by the community, checking your résumé, your connections, your relationships, your record and history, and even your publications. From an Aboriginal and Torres Strait Islander community perspective, these checks validate many questions and concerns about researchers.

Culturally safe Indigenous research

The National Collaborating Centre for Aboriginal Health (NCCAH, 2013, p. 1) in Canada identifies 'culturally safe healthcare systems and environments are established by a continuum of building blocks' as shown in Figure 11.1.

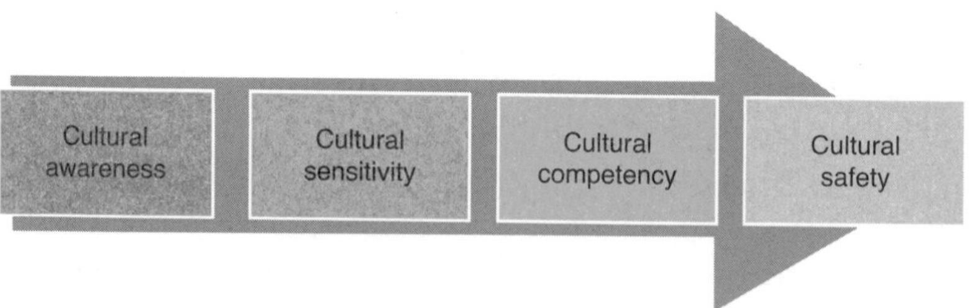

Figure 11.1 A continuum of culturally safe healthcare

Source: Reproduced from National Collaborating Centre for Aboriginal Health (NCCAH, 2013, p. 1).

Cultural safety originated from New Zealand due to the ongoing and harmful impacts of colonisation towards Māori people in major hospitals and health-related services. A widely accepted definition of cultural safety by the Nursing Council of New Zealand (NCNZ, 2011, p. 7) is:

> The effective nursing practice of a person or family from another culture … The nurse delivering the nursing service will have undertaken a process of reflection on his or her

> own cultural identity and will recognise the impact of his or her culture on his or her professional practice. Unsafe cultural practice comprises any action which diminishes, demeans or disempowers the cultural identity and wellbeing of an individual.
>
> (NCNZ, 2011, p. 7)

Within Australian healthcare systems, there is increasing recognition that continually improving cultural safety for Indigenous people on all levels increases the quality of healthcare, whereby the values and beliefs are respected and differences are acknowledged. Negative behaviours and attitudes directed towards Indigenous people also need to be acknowledged and explored with Indigenous people at the forefront (AIHW, 2019).

When developing protocols about cultural safety, consideration should be given to the 'experience of the Indigenous people, of the care they are given, their ability to access services and to raise concerns are imperative to changing behaviours' (AIHW, 2019, p. 4). Additionally, 'some of the essential features of cultural safety include an understanding of one's culture; an acknowledgment of difference, and a requirement that caregivers are actively mindful and respectful of this difference' (AHMAC, 2016, p. 18).

The presence or absence of cultural safety is determined by the experience of the recipient of care and is not denied by the caregiver (AHMAC, 2016; AIHW, 2019). For a greater understanding of cultural safety, see Chapter 3.

Beginning the research journey

Many health researchers have had little or no experience of conducting research about Aboriginal and Torres Strait Islander health. While many health professionals have some experience in working with Aboriginal and Torres Strait Islander people as clients, they have little experience in a research context. It can be difficult for researchers who have no previous experience of working with Aboriginal and Torres Strait Islander people to demonstrate that they understand how to work with Indigenous people in a research context. On the other hand, working with people in a professional context does not mean researchers are equipped to conduct research – this is applicable to both Indigenous and non-Indigenous people. Researchers who have worked with cultural groups other than their own (whether in their home countries or in Australia) may have more insight and the ability to relate. Even though our learning and experiences can support the work undertaken with different people from different backgrounds, demonstrating caution and sensitivity remains necessary: what works well in one culture may not be appropriate for people from another culture or community, or even another country.

Research is a specialised field with important contextual and ethical considerations, which requires careful planning and involvement of an experienced research team. Referring to the document *Keeping Research on Track II* (NHMRC, 2018b) will assist Aboriginal and Torres Strait Islander people and researchers to become familiar with the research journey and understand what is required at each step. This process will ensure that everyone benefits and has a shared respect for the values, diversity, priorities, needs and aspirations in the entire research journey. Aboriginal and Torres

Strait Islander people have well established values, and protocols that are separate from each other and expressed in different ways. However, collectively Aboriginal and Torres Strait Islander people share six common values regarding research (Figure 11.2): (1) spirit and integrity; (2) reciprocity; (3) respect; (4) equity; (5) cultural continuity; and (6) responsibility (NHMRC, 2018b, pp. 7–8).

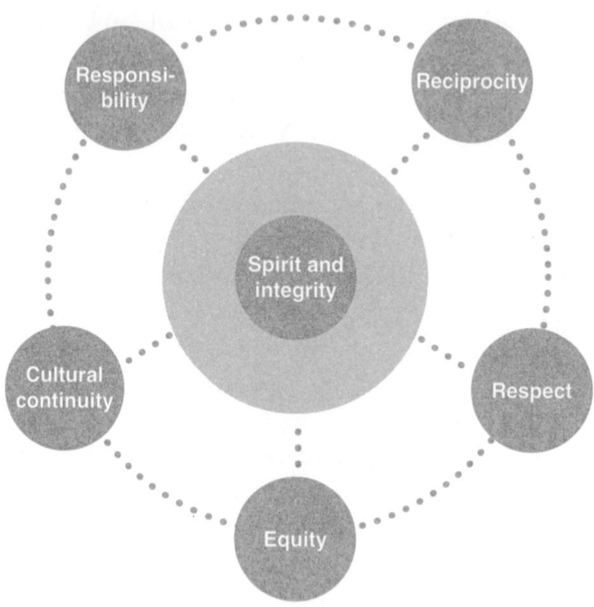

Figure 11.2 The six core values

Source: Reproduced from NHMRC (2018b, p. 7).

The nursing and midwifery workforces are increasingly mobile, and the variety of professional experiences available may include opportunities for research. Participating in research can be challenging and interesting. It can also be highly rewarding to participate in research that results in positive changes in people's health. However, it is important to remember that research must be designed in a way that is appropriate for the local community participants, and that research practices are constantly developing. What worked within one community may not translate well to other communities. What worked for a nurse twenty years ago may not work well today. Nurses and midwives who participate in research need to remain up to date on current research practices and be aware of recent publications in their field.

Nurses and midwives can be an important part of a research team. They bring to research projects a range of skills, experiences and knowledge that can help to ensure that research is well designed and successfully conducted. They also bring local, clinical and systems knowledge that will be highly valued within the research team.

Research teams may include nurses, midwives, doctors, health workers, university researchers, community researchers and community representatives. On some occasions, cultural mentors may be engaged to assist researchers (both Indigenous and non-Indigenous) in their work with a designated community or region. This is particularly likely if the research addresses sensitive matters. These types of partnerships and collaborations can benefit everyone and develop the capacity of both the researchers and the local community (NHMRC, 2018b). As much as possible, local researchers and community members should be involved in the research process – as part of the research team, not simply as participants. Nurses can play a key role here by facilitating initial interactions and offering localised advice.

There are increasing numbers of Aboriginal and Torres Strait Islander people undertaking research and working within research teams to address the poor health of Indigenous people. Organisations such as the National Indigenous Researchers and Knowledge Network (NIRAKN) can help both health professionals and researchers to contact experienced Indigenous researchers. NIRAKN also conducts master classes, critical reading groups, symposia and workshops for both Indigenous and non-Indigenous researchers. Other groups, institutes and universities also offer research developmental opportunities (for example, the University of Melbourne, which offers summer and winter residential schools in Indigenous research). See Laycock et al. (2011) for some personal stories and case studies.

Applying ethical research with Aboriginal and Torres Strait Islander peoples and communities

In Australia, the Australian Institute of Aboriginal and Torres Strait Islander Studies (AIATSIS) provides 'leadership in the field of ethics and protocols for research related to Aboriginal and Torres Strait Islander peoples and collections', under the *AIATSIS Act 1989* (AIATSIS, 2020b). The most recent guidelines are published in the *AIATSIS Code of Ethics for Aboriginal and Torres Strait Islander Research* (AIATSIS, 2020a), which ensures that research 'follows a process of meaningful engagement and reciprocity between the researcher and the individuals and/or communities involved in the research' (AIATSIS, 2020b).

The research ethics framework, as outlined in the AIATSIS Code is structured around four principles:

1. Indigenous self-determination
2. Indigenous leadership
3. impact and value
4. sustainability and accountability.

(AIATSIS, 2020a, p. 9)

Each principle gives rise to following responsibilities, elaborated in detail within the Code:

- recognition and respect
- engagement and collaboration
- informed consent
- cultural capability and learning
- Indigenous led research
- Indigenous perspectives and participation
- Indigenous knowledge and data
- benefit and reciprocity
- impact and risk

- Indigenous land and waters
- ongoing Indigenous governance
- reporting and compliance.

(AIATSIS, 2020a, p. 9)

QUESTIONS FOR REFLECTION

- Refer to the four principles above and describe in your own words why each principle is important to building strong Indigenous research.
- Identify how you would apply each principle through considered activities such as focus groups.
- Select one of the responsibilities and align it with a chosen principle, then outline how you would address this in your research project.
- Review the AIATSIS website at https://aiatsis.gov.au. Download the application form for ethics approval and attempt to complete it. Identify any questions with which you are having problems with and discuss in a group setting.
- Identify a Queensland Health Hospital Human Research Ethics Committee (HREC) and outline the process for ethics approval.

Qualitative research

qualitative research Research that involves exploring themes about 'how' and 'why' people act in particular ways, and that seeks to develop theories relevant to those people (which are not generalised to the whole community).

Qualitative research, in simple terms, is about words, meanings, interpretations, explanations, experiences and descriptions, to seek the truth from participants in order to gain a deeper understanding of participants' situations (Greenhalgh et al., 2017). It is also about ideas, opinions and perspectives regarding a problem or generating new ways of doing things (Austin & Sutton, 2014). Some examples of qualitative questions are:

1. Why do young Indigenous people have high rates of suicide?
2. Why are there fewer Indigenous people compared with non-Indigenous people attending university?
3. What are some of the reasons why Indigenous people over-present in emergency departments?

Types of qualitative research

There are several common approaches to qualitative research. *Phenomenology* is about exploring people's everyday experiences and how they understand their experiences from their own perspective. *Ethnography* is about the researcher being present in a situation through observation – or, from a cultural perspective, the researcher is embedded in the community. *Grounded theory* is a bottom-up approach where the researcher presents with no preconceived ideas and as the data are collected and analysed, themes begin to emerge. A *case study* is an in-depth look at an individual or a small group of participants – it is presented to participants with the researcher exploring the participants and their behaviour. *Narrative* occurs over a long period of time, capturing a participant's story, exploring how participants tell their story, perceive it and make sense of it (Greenhalgh et al., 2017).

Common qualitative methods

For the purpose of conducting qualitative research, data may be collected in a variety of ways, including through observation, interviews, focus groups and surveys. *Observation* involves taking detailed notes to record what has been seen, heard or encountered in the field. *Surveys* involve the collection of information through distributing questionnaires with open-ended questions. *Interviews* require the researcher to engage with participants one on one, and ask questions in conversation. *Focus groups* involve asking questions and generating discussion among a group of people. They can be a useful way to gauge the attitudes of a specific group of people, particularly when broader community consultation is not possible. They are particularly useful when the relevant interest group is relatively easy to identify and when group conversation is important. Focus groups were well suited in the example project.

CASE STUDY

Understanding your own research skills and contribution

Provided within this section is an example of a completed research project. The research project originated from the concept of an Aboriginal Registered Nurse working in an Aboriginal Medical Service (AMS). There was a need to understand why Indigenous people were over-accessing the emergency department and how this research contributes to improving Indigenous health outcomes in a major regional hospital.

Title

A comparative, quantitative study on Indigenous and non-Indigenous retrospective Emergency Department information data in rural and regional emergency departments in the Darling Downs in southern Queensland.

The aim of this study is to describe the differences (if any) between Indigenous and non-Indigenous adults who presented to emergency departments in a regional area during the calendar year 2016–17.

Study design

This study is a retrospective descriptive study comparing data recorded in the Emergency Department Information System (EDIS) with regard to differences between Indigenous and non-Indigenous adult presentations. The study is undertaken across four districts and within nineteen hospital health service sites.

Participants

All presentations to emergency departments of people aged sixteen years or over at the listed study sites will be accessed. People under the age of sixteen will be

(cont.)

excluded from this study. The sample size is approximately 200,000 (some data sets will be included in multiple episodes of care) (Kondalsamy-Chennakesavan et al., 2019).

*****

You have an opportunity to be part of a research team. You identify as a novice researcher working towards postgraduate studies in either a Master's or PhD. Other members on the team are early career researchers and experienced researchers. Think about your own situation and your nursing and research experience as you answer the questions that follow.

QUESTIONS FOR REFLECTION

- What are the key aspects of this study regarding research (processes, community protocols, ethics, cultural considerations)?
- What skills might you have to contribute to a research project about this topic with Indigenous people? How could you develop your skills?
- What are your strengths in research? What are some areas on which you need to work?
- How could this research project affect Indigenous people who participate in the research? What issues do you need to consider in planning the research?

QUESTIONS FOR REFLECTION

- Describe qualitative research.
- Look up and identify what constitutes a retrospective study.

Planning a research project

This section discusses the planning process for a research project undertaken within four Aboriginal communities in Queensland between 2007 and 2009. The project explored the health services and health issues experienced by Aboriginal people in one community. In this project, 40 per cent of the researchers were Aboriginal and/ or Torres Strait Islander people. The research team also included staff from the community health service. It is a concrete example of how university researchers can engage with Indigenous communities and health centre staff to undertake practical research that brings benefits to the local community.

Understanding Indigenous community protocols

community protocols The accepted ways of working and communicating within a community; the system of rules, either spoken or unspoken, that guide behaviour within the community

The first step in planning the research with an Aboriginal community is to thoroughly understand the relevant **community protocols**. The NHMRC (2018b) document *Keeping Research on Track II* is an excellent place to begin. The eight steps listed provide researchers with some examples of what is important to consider when undertaking the research journey. These are particularly useful in any research project.

Community engagement

The first stage of the project involved engaging with the community and undertaking a community analysis to identify the parameters of the research, get to know the community and build rapport with potential participants and the community at large. Much time was spent engaging with the partners and groups that would be working on this project.

Undertaking protocols of engagement and consultation was imperative to building a rapport with the Indigenous community members and to building and maintaining relationships (NHMRC, 2018b). The research community did not have a specific set of research protocols, but it did have an accepted way of engaging and consulting with the community. The research team needed to learn about this process and make sure it was followed: this 'way' was appropriate within this community where the research took place.

The research project was designed in close consultation with the Indigenous community. The researchers wanted to ensure that, unlike past research, the local Indigenous people had ownership of the research, contributed to the design of the methodology and participated in the entire research journey, and controlled the outcomes – including how these were disseminated. It was necessary to ensure that Indigenous people became empowered in the research by defining the problem and creating solutions. The research team sought to ensure that local Indigenous people were active and equal participants in the research (Newman et al., 1999). To achieve this, they identified and recruited Indigenous people through networking and liaising with local Indigenous services. Further interaction included liaising with mainstream services, participating in community meetings and programs, and attending events and gatherings where Indigenous people congregated and embodied their sense of community. The researchers wanted to embed the project within the community, rather than embedding the community into what the project team 'wanted' (Ward, 2019).

Ethics approval process

Research projects within an institution must be approved by a Human Research Ethics Committee (HREC) established within a university, hospital or school before any research can begin. Gaining ethics approval and identifying which HREC to approach for a research project will be dependent upon the population group and location, methodology, data collection and design of the study, to mention just some key areas. HRECs require a full plan of the project, often called a 'protocol', and a statements about how participants' safety will be ensured and that no harm will be imposed. The committee will also want to see any research templates, such as information provided to participants referred to as a participant information sheet, a consent form and any developed questionnaires, surveys or interview schedules. The project in this example was submitted to a university HREC at the end of 2008 and approved in early 2009. The HREC provided an approval number for ethical and legal purposes.

The initial phase of engaging with the Indigenous community and obtaining ethics clearance took quite some time, purely because it involved Indigenous people. Research projects are not quick: they need time, adequate consultation, informed agreements and careful data-collection techniques. Getting to know the community, developing the community's understanding of the project and reaching agreement on how to conduct the research can also be time-consuming, but be prepared to take this journey – however long it takes – when working with Indigenous people and communities. If this stage is not considered carefully, the research itself is unlikely to be successfully supported within the community. Understanding the time involved in planning and developing research is a key component of conducting research, and researchers need to plan how they will keep the research on track, maintain community relationships and ensure that the research relationships are maintained throughout the whole process, and even after the project itself is completed (Ward, 2019).

Identifying participants

Two groups of participants were involved in this research: the local Aboriginal population and the local AMS. The researchers identified the Aboriginal population through their engagement processes with the community. The researchers gathered information about local health and counselling services through desk research, such as the Commonwealth Care-link Centre database of organisations, the telephone directory, the local community directory, the local City Council Community Directory and other databases. Thirty-six services providing health and counselling services within this community. It was further identified that Indigenous people regularly used the local hospital and the AMS and in-house counselling services (Ward, 2019).

From the initial scoping and engagement with key Indigenous stakeholders, the researchers learned that Indigenous community members had little knowledge about most of the services provided within their community. There also seemed to be little understanding of how services could link to community members and connect with other services. The majority of the services found were located within the small town's main business area, while a large proportion of the Indigenous population lived on the outskirts of town, making access to services difficult due to a lack of transport services and limited finances for public transport (Ward, 2019; Ward & Gorman, 2010).

Research methods

Prior to recruiting participants and collecting data, two information sessions were provided within the community to explain the project and seek support. A central location in the community was chosen, with good access, catering, transport and child care in support of community people attending. At each of the information sessions, all aspects of the research were explained and provided on a one-page flyer for people to take away. Information included why the research was being conducted, how it would be implemented, the risks and benefits for the community, how community members could become involved and details of the ethics team to validate ethics approval or concerns regarding the research. At the end of each session, the researchers invited people to stay and discuss any questions about the presentation. The information sessions also gave the researchers an opportunity to recruit participants for the initial focus groups if they were interested (Ward, 2019; Ward & Gorman, 2010).

quantitative research Research that involves counting and measurement, and that seeks to test or support existing theories. Quantitative research may include statistical techniques to measure significance and to generalise findings across a community.

mixed-methods approach Research that uses a combination of quantitative and qualitative approaches within a research study/project.

The research study incorporated qualitative and **quantitative research** methods, within a **mixed-methods approach**. There is an increased interest in using mixed-methods approach in health research, as it allows researchers to build on the strengths and to minimise the weaknesses of other methods, and is more flexible and suitable for many topics in various communities settings (Chilisa, 2012).

The qualitative methods included face-to-face interviews, focus groups and community meetings (including attending any health promotion or education programs being held in the community) (Ward, 2010).

Recruiting participants

Approximately 500 Indigenous people lived in the community at the time of the study. To recruit participants, the researchers decided not to approach people individually, but rather invited the whole community to participate and let them decide whether to be involved, enabling community members to participate in a focus group of their choice.

Some community members were happy to participate, but only if certain people were not present in the same focus group. To account for this, the lead researcher asked each individual participant whether they had concerns with other people locally and asked the person to raise this with her separately before attending a focus group.

The researchers also conducted a focus group with community service providers. They contacted service providers by telephone to identify relevant people to invite to the group. They also asked services to identify local Indigenous people whom the researchers could approach for an interview.

When the lead researcher made contact with a potential participant, she discussed the background of the research, the person's consent to participate, a suitable time and place to meet (for interviews) or the details of the group session (for focus groups), advice on how long the process would take, information about how the data would be recorded for later transcription and analysis and information on the person's right to leave the study at any stage. She also talked about who was on the research team, how the research was being conducted, what was expected from participants, the risks and benefits of the research, how anonymity would be maintained and how the project's data would be stored safely. All this information was included on a consent form and was also discussed with participants. Participants gave their consent by signing the consent form (Ward, 2019).

Conducting the focus groups

Focus groups are often used to explore new research areas and uncover issues that require further investigation. They are often used early in a research project to help plan the rest of the research study.

Focus groups are small groups of participants who share similar interests that are relevant to the research. The groups are relatively small (often around eight to twelve people, and rarely more than twenty). Focus group participants do not represent the community as a whole. Instead, they are chosen deliberately because of the insights they can offer to the researcher. Focus groups are usually informal discussions about a topic that are led by the researcher (called the focus group moderator).

Focus groups have advantages and disadvantages that influence their value to researchers. Because participants have some knowledge of the issue under discussion, views can be explored in depth more quickly than in other consultation methods. The group's knowledge also means members often develop innovative ideas and solutions (Ward, 2010). However, the group's knowledge also brings disadvantages, because people's ideas may not represent those held by other individuals in the community. It is also possible that the group's discussion will be dominated by one person who has particularly strong views. Organising focus groups takes a lot of time and effort, and there is always a risk that participants won't turn up. Moderating a focus group successfully requires a lot of skill and experience. Because focus groups tap into participants' existing knowledge and skills, they are usually not an appropriate method for encouraging participants to deliberate on a topic and develop new ideas.

The researchers adapted the focus group method to follow the conversational flow of an Aboriginal 'yarning' process (Bessarab & Ng'andu, 2010) to encourage Aboriginal participants to come together in a supportive environment.

The focus groups were conducted in locations that were familiar and comfortable, and that suited as many people as possible. The researchers arranged each group a few weeks in advance to ensure people's availability, commitment and attendance. Prior to the focus group meeting, the lead researcher met participants informally to discuss the research, their involvement and how to arrange the groups.

The four focus groups conducted for the project were audio-recorded and transcribed for analysis. Participants were invited to review the transcripts if they wanted to and were assured that they could have full access to all information relating to the research (Ward, 2019).

Displaying the findings

The researchers shared their findings from the interviews and focus groups with graphs and illustrations, and with words that were relevant to the local Indigenous people. They wanted to make sure everyone could access the information they had gathered. Much of the qualitative information included stories that demonstrated Aboriginal community reasons, views, perceptions, beliefs, practices and interpretations of services. The researchers analysed the stories to look for descriptive themes and to find commonalities.

CASE STUDY

Research in new fields

Sometimes researchers want to conduct a study in a new field and need to work without having extensive literature and previous research to guide them. The research project itself may help to develop new understandings and form a new literature base in the field.

One project in a new field of investigation by Fredericks et al. (2013) involved a team that developed a participatory action research project to design and trial an iPad application designed to provide monitoring and self-care for Indigenous Australians who had experienced heart failure. This project focused on Indigenous people with heart failure who lived in Ipswich (in Southeast Queensland) and attended the Kambu Medical Centre, Ipswich Community Health Heart Failure Centre and West Moreton Health Service District.

The project involved health professionals, an information technology (IT) team and heart failure patients in three cycles of developing and reflecting on the iPad application. Nursing staff were extensively involved in the project by helping to choose participants and implementing the study. Only people with heart failure who were clinically stable were invited to participate in the study, and nurses provided the initial health assessments.

The research was based on community participation and ownership. It was built from evidence that IT-supported health education can decrease re-hospitalisation and improve self-management skills. All resources used for the project remained with the community health service and members of the Ipswich community, so the benefits continued after the project was completed.

The project successfully demonstrated that an iPad application can be developed to provide healthcare support for Indigenous Australian heart failure patients. A funding application was subsequently developed to expand the project to other communities in Queensland and South Australia. Clinicians and researchers in New Zealand became interested in adapting the project for their communities.

QUESTIONS FOR REFLECTION

- What steps would have been involved in designing and implementing this project?
- Identify some of the problems and concerns that may have surfaced during the project and suggest how the team might have resolved them.
- What things must the team consider if they wish to translate the project to other communities?
- What have you learned from this process that you can apply in future research?

Conclusion

Traditionally, Aboriginal and Torres Strait Islander people have been seen as passive subjects and recipients of research. Research was typically conducted by non-Indigenous people, and conducted *on* Indigenous people, not *with* them. Much of this research brought little or no benefit to the Aboriginal and Torres Strait Islander people who participated in it. Many Indigenous people continue to remember the effects of poorly conducted and inappropriate research.

Today, health research is guided by strong ethical statements and guidelines for practice. What lies ahead is a future in which Indigenous and non-Indigenous people can work together in research to bring about improved health outcomes. While some of this research will be specific to Indigenous people and individual communities, other research will focus on whole-of-population problems. Health research in Australia has a dynamic future and the capacity to make real changes to people's health and wellbeing.

Learning activities

Imagine that you are a Registered Nurse working in a multidisciplinary clinic in an Aboriginal and Torres Strait Islander community controlled health service (CCHS) in a regional community. You have been contacted by a nurse who works in community health – someone you know. The nurse said that she wants to 'get up a research project on Aboriginal people with diabetes' and wants to do it with 'some people from a university'. It will be part of her postgraduate degree studies. She wants you to be involved and she wants the research team to have access to data from your health service.

Complete the following tasks:

1. Read some background material about conducting research with Aboriginal and Torres Strait Islander people, communities and organisations. Choose at least two sources from the lists presented earlier in this chapter (one from each list). Make some notes about the issues you will need to consider if you decide to participate in this study.
2. Identify what the research project might mean for you (in your work in the health service and under a community-based board and CEO). (See Chapter 6 for more information about the structure of CCHSs.)
3. Identify the steps that you might need to take in order to move forward with this project. What do you need to learn about? What are the possible benefits for your service? What are the possible risks?
4. Identify the planning and approval steps for the nurse who contacted you and the research team from the university. What do you need to check that they successfully complete?
5. How could you participate in this project in a way that helps to build the research capacity among your colleagues in the health service? How could you participate in a way that brings benefit to your service?

FURTHER READING

AIATSIS (2020a). *AIATSIS Code of Ethics for Aboriginal and Torres Strait Islander Research.* Canberra: AIATSIS. Retrieved from https://aiatsis.gov.au/sites/default/files/2020-10/aiatsis-code-ethics.pdf

Fredericks, B., Clark, R.A., Adams, M., Atherton, J., Taylor-Johnson, S., Wu, C-J. & Buitendyk, N. (2013). Using participatory action research to assist in heart failure self-care amongst Indigenous Australians: A pilot study. *Action Learning Action Research Journal*, 19(2), 40–60.

Jamieson, L., Paradies, Y., Eades, S., Chong, A., Maple-Brown, L., Morris, P. & Brown, A. (2012). Ten principles relevant to health research among Indigenous Australian populations. *The Medical Journal of Australia*, 197(1), 16.

Kowal, E. & Anderson, I. (2012). *Genetic Research in Aboriginal and Torres Strait Islander Communities: Continuing the Conversation. Discussion paper from the second Lowitja Institute Roundtable on Genetic Research in Aboriginal and Torres Strait Islander Communities.* Melbourne: Lowitja Institute and University of Melbourne.

NHMRC (2020). Comparison table between AIATSIS and NHMRC ethics guidelines. Retrieved from www.nhmrc.gov.au/sites/default/files/documents/Indigenous%20guidelines/Comparison-table-AIATSISandNHMRC-ethics-guidelines.pdf

Visit the companion website at www.cambridge.org/highereducation/isbn/9781108794695/resources to see further online resources.

REFERENCES

AHMAC, National Aboriginal and Torres Strait Islander Health Standing Committee. (2016). *The Cultural Respect Framework for Aboriginal and Torres Strait Islander Health 2016–2026.* Canberra: AHMC.

AIATSIS (2020a). *AIATSIS Code of Ethics for Aboriginal and Torres Strait Islander Research.* Canberra: AIATSIS. Retrieved from https://aiatsis.gov.au/sites/default/files/2020–10/aiatsis-code-ethics.pdf

AIATSIS (2020b). *Ethical Research.* Retrieved from https://aiatsis.gov.au/research/ethical-research

AIHW (2019). *Cultural Safety in Health Care for Indigenous Australians: Monitoring Framework.* Canberra: AIHW. Retrieved from www.aihw.gov.au/reports/indigenous-australians/cultural-safety-healthcare-framework

Austin, Z. & Sutton, J. (2014). Qualitative research: Getting started. *The Canadian Journal of Hospital Pharmacy*, 67(6), 436–40.

Bessarab, D. & Ng'andu, B. (2010). Yarning about yarning as a legitimate method in Indigenous research. *International Journal of Critical Indigenous Studies*, 3(1), 37–51.

Chilisa, B. (2012). *Indigenous Research Methodologies.* Thousand Oaks, CA: Sage.

Cruse, S. (2001). Encouraging research guidelines to be put into practice: An Aboriginal Health Research Ethics Committee in action. *Kaurna Higher Education Journal*, 7, 23–7.

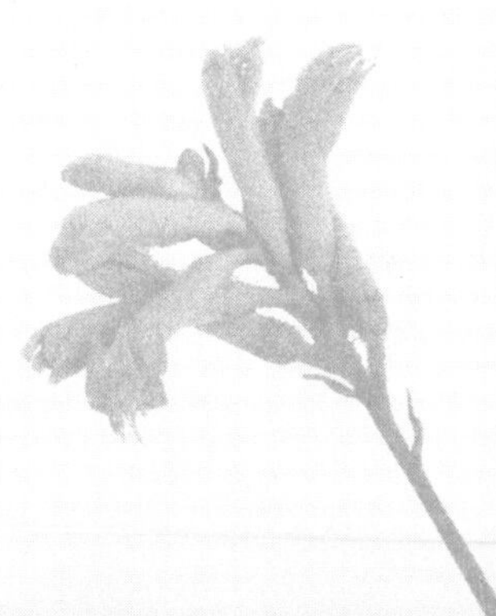

Fredericks, B. (2008). Making an impact researching with Australian Aboriginal and Torres Strait Islander peoples. *Evaluation, Innovation and Development*, 5(1), 24–35.

Fredericks, B., Clark, R.A., Adams, M., Atherton, J., Taylor-Johnson, S., Wu, C-J. & Buitendyk, N. (2013). Using participatory action research to assist in heart failure self-care amongst Indigenous Australians: A pilot study. *Action Learning Action Research Journal*, 19(2), 40–60.

Gower, G. (2012). Ethical research in Indigenous Australian contexts and its practical implementation. Retrieved from https://ro.ecu.edu.au/ecuworks2012/131

Greenhalgh, T.M., Bidewell, J., Crisp, E., Lambros, A and Warland, J. (2017). *Understanding Research Methods for Evidence-based Practice in Health.* Brisbane: John Wiley & Sons.

Kondalsamy-Chennakesavan, S., King, A., King, H., Ward, R and Rahman, M. (2019). *Differences Between Indigenous and Non-Indigenous Adults Presenting to Emergency Departments Within Darling Downs Hospital Health Service Hospitals.* Brisbane: University of Queensland and Queensland Health.

Koori Health Research and Community Development Unit (KHRCDU) (2000). *We Don't Like Research. But in Koori Hands it Could Make a Difference.* Melbourne: VicHealth Koori Health Research and Community Development Unit.

Koori Health Research and Community Development Unit (KHRCDU) (2001). *Research: Understanding Ethics.* Melbourne: VicHealth Koori Health Research and Community Development Unit.

Laycock, A. with Walker, D., Harrison, N. & Brands, J. (2009). *Supporting Indigenous Researchers: A Practical Guide for Supervisors.* Darwin: Cooperative Research Centre for Aboriginal Health.

Laycock, A. with Walker, D., Harrison, N. & Brands, J. (2011). *Researching Indigenous Health: A Practical Guide for Researchers.* Melbourne: Lowitja Institute.

NCCAH (2013). *Towards Cultural Safety for Métis: An Introduction for Heath Care Providers.* Canada: University of Northern British Columbia.

NCNZ (2011). *Guidelines for Cultural Safety, and the Treaty of Waitangi and Māori Health in Nursing Education and Practice* (2nd edn). Wellington: NCNZ.

Newman, J., Acklin, F., Trindall, A., Arbon, V., Brock, K., Bermingham, M. & Thompson, C. (1999). Story-telling: Aboriginal Indigenous women's means of health promotion. *Aboriginal and Islander Health Worker Journal*, 23(4), 18–21.

NHMRC (2007). *National Statement on Ethical Conduct in Human Research* 2007. Canberra: NHMRC, Australian Research Council and Universities Australia. Retrieved from www.nhmrc.gov.au/about-us/publications/national-statement-ethical-conduct-human-research-2007-updated-2018#block-views-block-file-attachments-content-block-1

NHMRC (2018a). *Ethical Conduct in Research with Aboriginal and Torres Strait Islander Peoples and Communities: Guidelines for Researchers and Stakeholders.* Canberra: NHMRC. Retrieved from www.nhmrc.gov.au/about-us/resources/ethical-conduct-research-aboriginal-and-torres-strait-islander-peoples-and-communities

NHMRC (2018b). *Keeping Research on Track II.* Canberra: NHMRC. Retrieved from www.nhmrc.gov.au/about-us/resources/keeping-research-track-ii

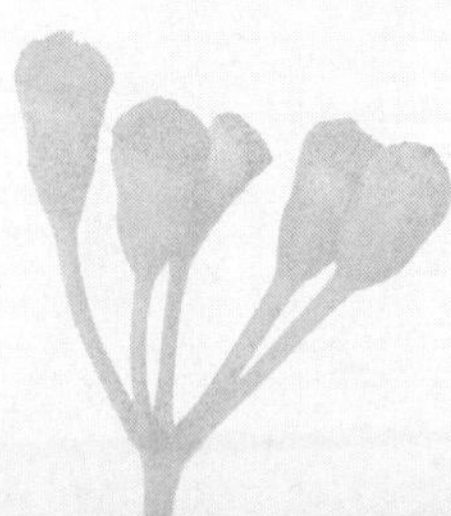

Onemda VicHealth Koori Health Unit (2008). *We Can Like Research … in Koori Hands: A Community Report on Onemda VicHealth Koori Health Unit's Research Workshops in 2007*. Melbourne: Onemda VicHealth Koori Health Unit, University of Melbourne.

SAHMRI (2013). Developing a set of principles to set a foundation for conducting Aboriginal research the right way in SA. *SAHMRI Newsletter*, 3.

SAHMRI (2014). *Wardliparingga: Aboriginal Research in Aboriginal Hands*. Adelaide: SAHMRI. Retrieved from www.sahmri.org/m/downloads/Wardliparingga_Accord_companion_document.pdf

Smith, L.T. (1999). *Decolonising Methodologies: Research and Indigenous Peoples*. London: Zed Books.

Smith, L.T. (2012). *Decolonizing Methodologies: Research and Indigenous Peoples* (2nd edn). London: Zed Books.

Ward, R. (2010). In the event of a crisis: What services are accessed and available to the Aboriginal community of Dalby who have been affected by suicide and/or self-harm. Unpublished Master's thesis, University of Southern Queensland.

Ward, R. (2019). Suicide prevention: Exploring Aboriginal understandings of suicide from a social and emotional wellbeing framework. Unpublished PhD thesis, University of Southern Queensland.

Ward, R. & Gorman, D. (2010). Racism, discrimination and health services to Aboriginal people in south west Queensland. *Aboriginal and Islander Health Worker*, 34(6), 3–5.

LEGISLATION CITED

AIATSIS Act 1989 (Cth)

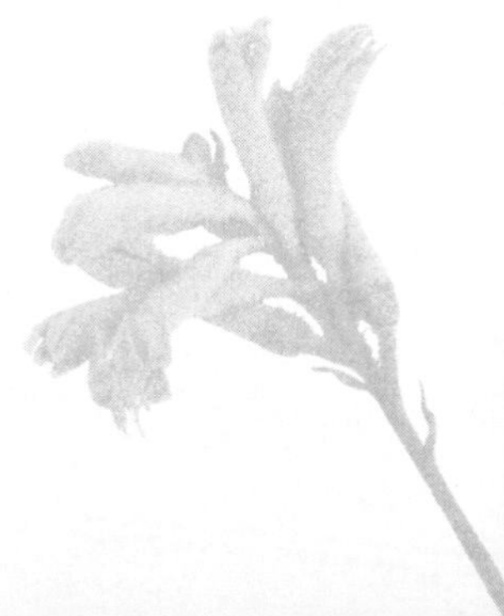

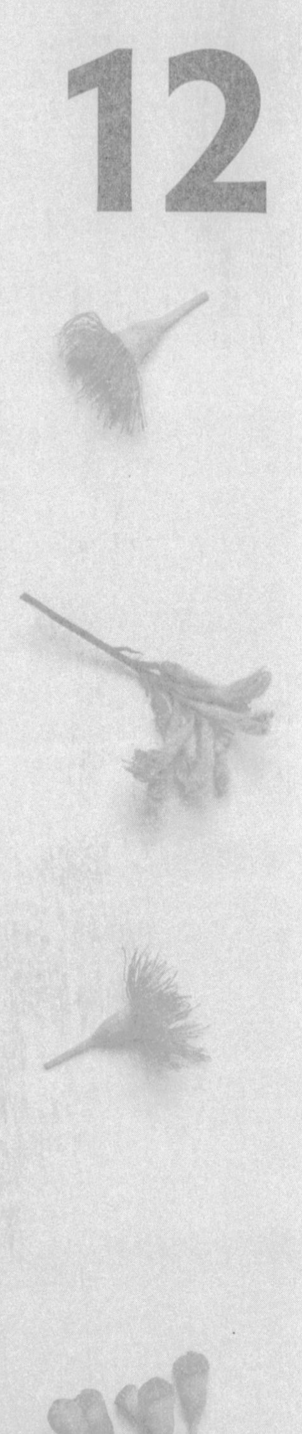

12 Aboriginal and Torres Strait Islander quantitative research

Ray Lovett, Makayla-May Brinckley and Roxanne Jones

LEARNING OBJECTIVES

This chapter will help you to understand:

- Quantitative research and Aboriginal and Torres Strait Islander peoples in context
- Key terms and definitions associated with research
- What constitutes an Indigenous methodology
- How to incorporate appropriate quantitative methods in research involving Aboriginal and Torres Strait Islander peoples

KEY WORDS

chi-squared test
confidence interval
descriptive statistics
exposure variable
hypothesis
Indigenous methodology
inferential statistics
methodology
method
outcome variable
research
variable

Introduction

Research is important in the creation of new knowledge or as a way of understanding phenomena. This chapter primarily concerns quantitative research. The chapter begins with a discussion about quantitative research and Indigenous people in context to provide an overview of the vexed discussion on methodological approaches advocated in Indigenous research. This is followed by an overview of Indigenous quantitative research in the Aboriginal and Torres Strait Islander context, including what is defined as research and the key differences between research methodology and methods. The authors then introduce concepts of Indigenous quantitative research practices and include a case study on the Yawuru wellbeing framework to illuminate how methodology affects research and therefore understanding.

The final section of the chapter describes participatory action research as a methodology that is appropriate when conducting research with Aboriginal and Torres Strait Islander peoples in Australia and looks at how appropriate quantitative methods can contribute to new knowledge and understanding through the case study of an Aboriginal Ranger study in Central Australia.

Quantitative research and Indigenous peoples in context

There is a commonly held view in research involving Indigenous peoples worldwide that quantitative research methods are inherently less appropriate than qualitative methods (Blackstock, 2009). If we examine this assumption closely, we can come to understand how this view has arisen and inform ourselves about what this view actually means.

One reason for this view is that Indigenous peoples are portrayed at storytellers, primarily through verbal or ceremonial means, and that understanding and interpreting these practices lend themselves to qualitative research approaches (Blackstock, 2009) (see Chapter 11). It can thus be theorised that qualitative approaches dominate the creation of new knowledge and the ways in which phenomena come to be understood within the Indigenous world.

A second reason for qualitative approaches being a dominant research methodology in Indigenous research is the very limited recognition of Indigenous scientific knowledge informing Western science. Western research designs are investigations or experiments that aim to discover and interpret facts. The Western research methodology tends to generalise or homogenise experiences to find 'universal truths' (Saini, 2012). It is a systematic approach to collecting, analysing and creating new knowledge that involves strict protocols and methods in order that the research is transparent enough for other researchers to replicate the study (Saini, 2012). The Western view of research regards science, research and the subsequent knowledge production as the best way to construct 'truth' through testable hypotheses.

This limited recognition of Indigenous scientific knowledge in Western science is evident in a historical lack of attribution (and even biopiracy) of knowledge developed by Indigenous peoples, particularly in the areas of pharmacopeia and medicine (see

Chapter 2). For example, willow bark was used in traditional medicine as a pain reliever and antipyretic for more than 3500 years. The active ingredient derived from willow bark, salicin, was subsequently refined throughout the 1800s, and eventually led to the development of aspirin, one of the world's most widely available drugs. A recent historical review on the development of aspirin does not credit discovery from ancient or historical knowledge, but instead attributes the claim of 'discovery' to Western institutions and their methods (Desborough & Keeling, 2017).

Western science imposed onto Indigenous communities leaves them as objects of study for Western agendas and privileges non-Indigenous ways of knowing, being and doing (Rigney, 2001). Western research has a history of being – and often continues to be – unethical, exploitative, harmful and intrusive for Indigenous communities generally, and Aboriginal and Torres Strait Islander communities specifically (Saini, 2012). It has therefore been criticised as having negative consequences for Aboriginal and Torres Strait Islander communities, including unethical practices, questionable data outcomes and the silencing of Aboriginal and Torres Strait Islander voices (Kite & Davy, 2015).

Additionally, the Western research methodology has been criticised as assisting in the colonisation and oppression of Aboriginal and Torres Strait Islander peoples (Wilson, 2008). Research is a way of regulating and realising colonialism through the rules and institutions of scholarly disciplines (Saini, 2012). These research methodologies are largely controlled by non-Indigenous researchers, who are motivated by the needs of non-Indigenous society (Bainbridge et al., 2015; Wilson, 2008). Non-Indigenous Australians are thus privileged in the research environment as they are the dominant culture and in a normative position of power. This can make it difficult for Aboriginal and Torres Strait Islander researchers to break through the dominant Western control, power and ownership of research conduct and research findings. As non-Indigenous people own the research environment, this therefore means that Western epistemologies and ontologies are shaping public discourse, government policy and models of care (Ryder et al., 2019).

QUESTIONS FOR REFLECTION

- Who benefits from research?
- How can Aboriginal and Torres Strait Islander knowledge/s be included in the research process?
- How are Aboriginal and Torres Strait Islander epistemologies and ontologies included in the research design?

Subject to and the subject of research

The predominance of qualitative approaches in Indigenous research is also a consequence of the history of damage attributed to quantitative methods applied to Indigenous peoples worldwide. Indigenous peoples have experienced quantitative 'scientific' research based on disproven racial theories, including the work of Samuel George Morton and the pseudo-science at the time of craniometry (Morton, 1839). While these studies were conducted almost 200 years ago, this unscientific, unethical and extractive quantitative research continues to cast a long shadow (see Chapter 2). In addition, the results of Morton's study and others quantitative research have been used to subjugate and control Indigenous lives by reinforcing colonial superiority through notions of civilisation and the need to 'civilise the natives'. The scientific method and resultant knowledge production have been used on numerous occasions to justify laws and policies such as that resulting in the Stolen Generations in Australia (Wilson & Dodson, 1997).

Globally, Indigenous communities have unique histories, but there is a commonality of Indigenous communities being inappropriately researched, with little to no cultural respect and without corresponding improvements in their health (Walker et al., 2014). The Western research methodology has always excluded Aboriginal and Torres Strait Islander voices and knowledges, and has created circumstances where Aboriginal and Torres Strait Islander people have been among the most inappropriately researched groups in history (Rigney, 1999; Ryder et al., 2019). For decades, research has measured, tested and investigated Aboriginal and Torres Strait Islander people under the guise of better understanding their cultures. However, this is research that 'has neither been asked for, nor has it any relevance for the communities being studied' (Wilson, 2008, p. 15). This type of research is done '*of* and *on* (but never *by*)' Aboriginal and Torres Strait Islander people (Wilson, 2008, p. 49). This leaves Aboriginal and Torres Strait Islander people, communities, and Country exploited for research done without consent or collaboration.

The Western research methodology is neither benefiting Aboriginal and Torres Strait Islander communities nor improving their health outcomes. In some instances, this research approach is worsening health outcomes and has led to Aboriginal and Torres Strait Islander people and communities distrusting researchers (Munns et al., 2017). The dominant Western research methodology is also critiqued by Aboriginal and Torres Strait Islander people as being too focused on describing health problems without aiming to solve them and producing harmful and exploitative research that perpetuates damaging stereotypes about Aboriginal and Torres Strait Islander people (Bainbridge et al., 2015).

By accepting Western science as the only valid and reliable way to understand our reality and privileging it as the authority in constructing 'truth', this simultaneously upholds power structures of dominant cultures and illegitimatises other knowledge systems. As Rigney (2001, p. 3), a researcher and educator from the Narungga, Kaurna and Ngarrindjeri nations, argues:

> The notion that science is 'authoritative', 'neutral' and 'universal' privileges science. It gives science the status of a standard measure against which all other 'realities' may be evaluated and judged to be either 'rational' or otherwise. If science indicates to us that there is no such thing as Indigenous Dreaming, then the Indigenous Australians whose realities are informed by the logics of Dreaming are therefore deemed irrational.

QUESTIONS FOR REFLECTION

- How is power distributed in the research relationship?
- How will Aboriginal and Torres Strait Islander people benefit from the research?

There are some key aspects in which Western research activities and methodologies differ from Aboriginal and Torres Strait Islander cultures, including beliefs about knowledge, knowledge ownership and data sovereignty, how knowledge is transmitted, and the purpose and benefits of the research (Gorman & Toombs, 2009). Using only a Western research methodology excludes Indigenous peoples from the process of knowledge construction. It leaves the Indigenous base as devalued and less valid under Western scientific notions of acceptable research standards and homogenises all Indigenous peoples (Saini, 2012).

For Indigenous populations around the world, this has meant that research, and particularly quantitative research, should be treated with much suspicion. But is quantitative research the problem? Or does the problem lie with who is doing it, including their underlying beliefs, which then influence how they conduct the research and what (or who) they are doing the research for?

In the first text dedicated to Indigenous statistics as a methodology, Walter and Andersen (2013) address the issues described above by discussing three premises for quantitative research:

1. The culture of the producer of statistics has influence in their work (and therefore their work is never unbiased), and thus the cultural framework of the researcher influences the representation of the Indigenous statistics they are producing.
2. *Methodologies*, not methods, shape what research is produced (see next section).
3. There is a need to understand how non-academic knowledge is taken and translated within the academy, given the power dynamics on which this system is built (which applies to both qualitative and quantitative research).

Defining research

research 'the creation of new knowledge and/or the use of existing knowledge in a new and creative way so as to generate new concepts, methodologies and understandings' (DIISRTE, 2012, p. 7).

variable Any attribute, phenomenon, or event that can have different values (Porta, 2008).

hypothesis The theory that a scientist has about the result of an experiment. It is what the scientist thinks will happen, based on previous experiments, literature or research (Smithson, 2000).

confidence interval A 'range of values containing a specified percentage of the sampling distribution of [a] statistic' (Smithson, 2000, p. 148). A confidence interval tells us how likely it is that our result from the sample is a true representative result of the whole population.

Research has been occurring across the globe for millennia. If we think about the concept of research and what this means, it is the manner in which we understand the world around us. The word itself contains clues to its meaning, re(search) is about searching and seeking; we are exploring and observing, or sometimes both. When we explore or observe we tend to establish connections between different events or observations that help provide us with the explanations and interpretations of connections or relationships. This process creates a complex collection of data and information.

Over time, humans have developed ways of systematically collecting, organising and processing that information to help us understand sometimes complex phenomena. These systems of knowledge creation and understanding are what is understood as research.

Research also uses specific words and definitions. It is important to be aware and to begin to understand these terms. In the research process, researchers typically start by deciding which **variables** to test. Once variables have been defined, a **hypothesis** can be formulated.

Once a hypothesis is stated, it must be tested. To test a hypothesis, researchers take a random sample of the population and run the experiment. When testing a hypothesis, it is unlikely that a true, real result can be 100 per cent certain, because no experiment can fully replicate real life. Researchers therefore use a **confidence interval** to say how sure they are that the result from the test is true.

Many statistical tools can be used to test a hypothesis. One of the most commonly used statistical tools to assess an association between two categorical variables (common categorical variables include gender, age groups, disease status) is the **chi-squared test**. This is a procedure for testing whether two categorical variables are related (or not) in a population. The chi-squared test calculates a chi-squared value, which is then used to assess the probability of that value being due to chance. If the chi-squared value falls below the 'chance threshold' (usually set at less than 5 per cent), then the result is said to be statistically significant (Liamputtong, 2016).

chi-squared test A statistical test to assess whether two categorical variables are associated – that is, one affects the other.

Methodology and methods

This section describes the distinction between research methodology and research methods.

Methodology

A **methodology** is a general research strategy that outlines how the research is to be undertaken. The methodology should consist of a rationale for the research approach and identifies the lens through which the analysis occurs (Howell, 2013). The methodology influences the method(s) selected to generate the data.

methodology The overarching strategy and rationale of a research project, including methods, theories and principles (Neuman, 2011).

A single methodological approach can include multiple methods to create understanding and knowledge. Examples of methodologies include:

- phenomenology – the philosophical study of 'lived experience'
- ethnography – observes the social world and describes people's cultures, customs, beliefs and behaviours
- participatory – an approach that views the participants and community as active researchers with equal power and influence in the research process
- grounded theory – assumes a blank slate and constructs theories by using an inductive approach (see also Chapter 11).

The scientific methodology consists of

> a question and suggested explanation (hypothesis) based on observation, followed by the careful design and execution of controlled experiments, and finally validation, refinement or rejection of this hypothesis.
>
> (*Nature Methods*, 2009, p. 237)

Methodology is the worldview/lens through which research is designed, conducted, and understood (Walter & Andersen, 2013). It includes the

- axiology
- ontology
- epistemology
- sociocultural position
- theoretical/philosophical framework
- research method.

Walter and Anderson (2013) highlight that we need to understand what informs our research methodologies and research frameworks, because without this understanding our research can be affected in various ways and our research practice and outcomes can be undermined.

QUESTION FOR REFLECTION

- Look up each term in the bullet list above and write down your interpretation of its meaning.

Methods

method The process of gathering, testing, analysing and drawing conclusions from data in order to test a hypothesis.

Methods describe how researchers will collect data.

In quantitative research, common methods include:

- *Surveys.* These comprise a set of questions that gather information about a research objective and hypothesis. Surveys typically include some demographic information (for example, age, sex and geographical location of the participant). They then ask a set of questions on the research topic that will help the researcher either prove or disprove their research hypothesis.
- *Experiments.* A process whereby a researcher uses a set of variables to either prove or disprove a hypothesis. Simple experiments involve two variables: one variable which stays the same throughout the experiment (the dependent or outcome variable), and another variable that is manipulated (or changed) in the experiment (the independent or exposure variable). The goal is to see whether the manipulation of the independent variable changes the dependent variable. Some complex experiments can use more than two variables.
- *Analysis of secondary data.* Secondary data are data that have already been collected by someone other than the person who will be using or analysing the data. Examples include census or government department data, or literature in public libraries or educational institutions.

The quantitative research approach typically sees numerical data gathered, generalised through analysis and subdivided into smaller pieces of information so the research can be better understood (Almalki, 2016).

In qualitative research, common methods include:

- interviews
- focus groups
- field notes
- observation.

The focus of this chapter is on quantitative research methods, so students are encouraged to look up these qualitative methods independently (see Chapter 11).

Indigenous methodologies in Australia

Indigenous methodology An overarching strategy and rationale of research that centres on the needs and wants of Aboriginal and Torres Strait Islander communities throughout the whole research process, from research inception through its implementation until completion.

This section highlights the elements of an Indigenous approach to research in Australia and concludes with a case study where Indigenous research contrasts with Western research methodologies.

For the purposes of this chapter, **Indigenous methodology** is referred to as research related specifically to Aboriginal and Torres Strait Islander peoples. Indigenous research is 'research by Indigenous Australians whose primary informants are Indigenous Australians and whose goals are to serve and inform the Indigenous struggle for self-determination' (Rigney, 1999, p. 116). Indigenous methodologies are focused on the *why* of the topic and approach, the *conception* and definition of the issue being researched, the *how* of measurement and instruments development/use and the *who* in decision making. The approach comes from an Indigenous lens or worldview.

During the decades from the 1960s to the 1980s, Aboriginal and Torres Strait Islander people began to study in and graduate from higher education, which saw the beginning of the inclusion of Indigenous perspectives in research. From the mid-1990s, Aboriginal and Torres Strait Islander people were heavily critiquing Western research and calling for the introduction of more progressive methodologies (Rigney, 2001). During this time, however, Aboriginal and Torres Strait Islander people were still overwhelmingly being *researched* instead of being the *researchers* (Wilson, 2008). From the 1990s to the 2000s, we began to see Aboriginal and Torres Strait Islander scholars asserting their power and developing their own research knowledge systems and ways of doing research (Rigney, 2001).

Aboriginal and Torres Strait Islander people then began conducting their own research, which 'emanates from, honours and illuminates their worldviews' (Wilson, 2008). It was clear that adapting the dominant Western methodology in Indigenous research would not be enough to overcome the negative research history in Aboriginal and Torres Strait Islander communities. The underlying beliefs, tools and systems of the Western methodology cannot be fully removed, so instead a new Indigenous methodology needed to be developed. By using an Indigenous research methodology, Aboriginal and Torres Strait Islander people don't have to justify themselves or validate themselves to the dominant culture, but instead decide for themselves how research will be conducted, analysed and presented (Wilson, 2008).

Elements of an Indigenous research methodology

An Indigenous research methodology conducts research in collaboration with communities, on their terms, with their research agendas placed front and centre. Overall, Indigenous research methodologies are an ethical, respectful, beneficial and relevant process of research for Aboriginal and Torres Strait Islander peoples.

Researchers using an Indigenous research methodology are often Aboriginal and Torres Strait Islander people who share the same worldviews as the research participants – which helps to ensure congruency between the concept being studied and the tools developed to measure it (Kite & Davy, 2015). However, you do not have to be an Aboriginal or Torres Strait Islander researcher to use an Indigenous research methodology. Non-Indigenous researchers using Indigenous research methodologies in partnership with Aboriginal and Torres Strait Islander communities are an essential component of the overall health and wellbeing research field.

The following questions provide a good guide for both Aboriginal and Torres Strait Islander researchers and non-Indigenous researchers to conduct research using an Indigenous research methodology:

1. *Why are you researching this topic?* Research questions should be driven by the Aboriginal and Torres Strait Islander community within which you are doing the

research. This will make the research meaningful and relevant, and the results more likely to effect change.

2. *How is the topic defined?* Aboriginal and Torres Strait Islander communities must be involved in defining the research topic and concepts used in the research. As the researcher, you should work in partnership with the community to define these concepts within the community's worldview.
3. *How are you developing the measure/instrument used to assess the topic?* You must work with Aboriginal and Torres Strait Islander communities to develop ways to accurately measure research concepts. In an Indigenous research methodology, the methods, data collection and data analysis should all make sense from an Aboriginal or Torres Strait Islander worldview – no matter what method is being used (surveys, focus groups, etc.).
4. *Who is making these decisions about how to conduct the research?* If the answer is not the Aboriginal and Torres Strait Islander people that are being researched, then the methodology is not an Indigenous methodology. In an Indigenous research methodology, the Aboriginal and Torres Strait Islander people are active, decision-making participants throughout the whole research process.

Crucially, an Indigenous research methodology does not homogenise Aboriginal and Torres Strait Islander people, cultures or experiences. It respects cultural and historical differences and works with communities to meet their needs. Researchers working to improve Aboriginal and Torres Strait Islander health must address the needs of communities in ways that are relevant and appropriate to the community's frame of reference and worldview (Gorman & Toombs, 2009). This means that the application of an Indigenous research methodology will change according to the needs and cultures of each Aboriginal and Torres Strait Islander community. An Indigenous research methodology must be flexible in its design and implementation, as each Aboriginal and Torres Strait Islander community has its own cultures, research agendas and community capacity that need to be respected and adjusted for accordingly.

There are, however, some key aspects to an Indigenous research methodology that are universal to all Aboriginal and Torres Strait Islander communities. These are:

- active partnerships with Aboriginal and Torres Strait Islander communities
- Aboriginal and Torres Strait Islander worldviews (ways of knowing, being, and doing)
- political integrity (resistance and intellectual sovereignty).

Active partnerships with Aboriginal and Torres Strait Islander communities

Indigenous methodologies place Aboriginal and Torres Strait Islander people as active participants in the research process (Moreton-Robinson & Walter, 2009). It is essential for researchers to develop active partnerships with the Aboriginal and/or Torres Strait Islander communities in which they are working. A key element of research success is ensuring this active involvement from Aboriginal and Torres Strait Islander communities in the planning, conduct, evaluation and publication of the research (Saini, 2012). Utilising Indigenous research methodologies while undertaking quantitative research can occur in a number of ways, including through the use of methodologies in the form of participatory action research (PAR) (demonstrated in the two case studies in the following section). PAR is a 'participatory, democratic process concerned with developing practical knowing in the pursuit of worthwhile human purposes, grounded in a participatory worldview' (Reason & Bradbury, 2001, p. 201). There are important elements to PAR that align with Indigenous research methodologies. PAR values building long-term, collaborative relationships between communities and researchers (Munns et al., 2017). The power is shared in such a relationship, allowing community voices to be privileged and acknowledged throughout all aspects of the research project.

Aboriginal and Torres Strait Islander worldviews: Ways of knowing, being and doing

A comparison approach is common in Western research methodologies. This is where the dominant culture is rated over another culture (Wilson, 2008). We see this occurring in Australia when the dominant Western culture is researching Aboriginal and Torres Strait Islander cultures and comparative results are made – for example, in reporting the prevalence of tobacco use in Australia. When we focus on comparisons, we see that Aboriginal and Torres Strait Islander people smoke at much higher rates than non-Indigenous Australians. In 2018–19, Aboriginal and Torres Strait Islander people aged 15 years and over were almost three times as likely as other Australians to be daily smokers (van der Sterren et al., 2020). However, when we only focus on Aboriginal and Torres Strait Islander smoking trends, we see a decrease over time in the prevalence of daily smoking of almost 13 per cent, from 50 per cent of Aboriginal and Torres Strait Islander people smoking daily in 2004–05 to just 37 per cent in 2018–19. We also see that rates over time have lowered for both Aboriginal and Torres Strait Islander men and women, and the proportion of daily smokers is lowest for the youngest age group, aged between 15 and 17 years (van der Sterren et al., 2020). These represent great improvements for the health of Aboriginal and Torres Strait Islander people that can be overlooked when using a comparative approach. The comparative approach used in Western research methodologies can be harmful to Aboriginal and Torres Strait Islander communities, as it results in an under-estimation of improvements in smoking rates for Aboriginal and Torres Strait Islander people. Instead of focusing on strengths, it also falls into a deficit model. By utilising Aboriginal and Torres Strait Islander worldviews and ways of knowing, being and doing, the comparison approach is left behind, and we can focus on ways of improving community health that are culturally safe and strengths based.

Political integrity: Resistance and intellectual sovereignty

Employing an Indigenous research methodology involves resistance against the dominant system and reimagining how research is understood and defined in Australia. It is an act of self-determination for Aboriginal and Torres Strait Islander people, as it privileges Aboriginal and Torres Strait Islander voices, histories, and knowledge (Kite & Davy, 2015). Resisting the dominant research approaches to instead use an Indigenous research methodology produces research that engages with the Australian history of genocide, survival and resistance to oppression. It 'seeks to uncover and protest' oppressive powers and support the personal, community, cultural and political struggles of Aboriginal and Torres Strait Islander people (Rigney, 1999, p. 117). It is clear that it is not enough to simply use the current dominant system – Aboriginal and Torres Strait Islander people must develop and employ their own research frameworks and methodologies. Without doing this, it is simply Western research done by Aboriginal and Torres Strait Islander people (Martin & Mirraboopa, 2003).

In an Indigenous research methodology, Aboriginal and Torres Strait Islander people are active participants in the research. This helps to connect Aboriginal and Torres Strait Islander communities' political struggles, lived and historical experiences, traditions and community interests with the research to enact change, meet community needs and provide a holistic approach to the research (Kite & Davy, 2015; Rigney, 1999). These community interests are often research areas that are not commonly researched within a Western research methodology (Bainbridge et al., 2015). This can include culture, spirituality, connection to Country and racism research. In this sense, an Indigenous research methodology is inherently political, as it privileges Aboriginal and Torres Strait Islander worldviews, knowledge and realities, and emphasises the social, historical and political contexts that shape communities today (Martin & Mirraboopa, 2003).

Sovereignty is the right of all peoples to have full ownership, governance and control over their own matters. Conceptually similar to self-determination, sovereignty is about the ability of people to decide their own political, economic, social and cultural development. Intellectual sovereignty is the right to have ownership and control over your thoughts, ideas and intellectual data. Using an Indigenous research methodology means pushing boundaries 'in order to make intellectual space for Indigenous cultural knowledge systems that were denied in the past' (Rigney, 2001, p. 9). In an Indigenous research methodology, intellectual sovereignty means that the participants of a study have input into the study question and design, transparency in the analysis and conclusions drawn from their data, and ownership of the data they provide for the study. If intellectual sovereignty is embedded in an Indigenous research methodology, this means Aboriginal and Torres Strait Islander participants in a study have agency throughout the research process. They have input and ownership in the study and over the data they provide.

Indigenous quantitative research

Indigenous quantitative research methodologies do not merely involve an Aboriginal or Torres Strait Islander researcher conducting quantitative research. Rather, they assume that the research is framed, developed and undertaken from an Indigenous worldview, considering Indigenous epistemological, ontological and axiological methodologies (Moreton-Robinson & Walter, 2009).

Indigenous quantitative research is underpinned by a cultural framework or approach. This section highlights two case studies where Indigenous quantitative research was undertaken. Like all research, quantitative research uses specific language, so throughout this section we spend some time defining key terms and providing examples.

Quantitative research is any research conducted with numerical data. Quantitative methods in research utilise a numerical system of variables to measure and then analyse data. There are two types of variables – an **outcome variable** and an **exposure variable**.

outcome variable (can also be called a dependent variable) An outcome whose variation we seek to explain (or account for) by the influence of exposure variable(s) (Porta, 2008).

exposure variable (can also be called an independent or explanatory variable) A characteristic observed or measured that is thought to influence an outcome within the defined area of relationships under study (Porta, 2008).

For example, we might be interested in the relationship between smoking status (exposure variable) and being diagnosed with lung cancer (outcome variable). The exposure always precedes (comes before) the outcome (Figure 12.1).

Figure 12.1 Example of the relationship between an exposure variable and an outcome variable

In this example, the exposure variable is smoking status, which varies by the following categories: non-smoker, ex-smoker and current smoker, with each category of exposure thought to influence the outcome according to the level of exposure to smoking.

Generally, variables can be classified in two ways, as either categorical or continuous (Table 12.1).

Table 12.1 Classification of variables

Types of variable			
Categorical			
Binary	Categories	Ordinal	
Only two response options	More than two responses and does not always require an order	Increases or decreases in equal increments	Measurable numeric value
For example:	For example:	For example:	For example:
Yes or no 0 or 1	No, yes, maybe Education level	1, 2, 3, 4, 5, 6, 7 Low, medium, high	A person's age in years
Analysis methods used for each variable type			
Descriptive analysis			
Percentage or number	Percentage or number	Percentage or number	Mean, median, range
Inferential analysis			
Chi-squared, logistic regression	Chi-squared	Chi-squared, ordinal regression	T-test, linear regression

Quantitative data are used to describe the outcome and exposures (descriptive analysis) and may also be used to quantify a relationship between two variables or more than two variables (inferential analysis). In the examples in this chapter, we will focus on **descriptive statistics** and **inferential statistics** for categorical variables.

Descriptive statistics are useful in all types of research, as they provide the reader with a sense of what the data 'look like' in their simplest form.

descriptive statistics Explain the frequency, characteristics and overview of a sample of data, analysing one variable at a time (univariate analysis). Commonly, descriptive analysis is shown in the form of frequency tables in the form of absolute numbers, percentages and frequencies.

inferential statistics These 'take data from a sample and make inferences about the larger population from which the sample was drawn' (Frost, 2020).

This section demonstrates how Indigenous methodologies can be applied to quantitative research. Two case studies are provided. The first concerns the wellbeing of Yawuru and the second concerns the wellbeing of Aboriginal Rangers in Central Australia. They are both intended to be applied examples.

Applying an Indigenous quantitative research methodology for wellbeing: descriptive and inferential statistics

CASE STUDY

Yawuru wellbeing

Wellbeing is a misunderstood concept with little agreement about its meaning. It is often used interchangeably with notions of health, quality of life or happiness. Wellbeing is therefore often poorly defined in research. For Aboriginal and Torres Strait Islander people generally, wellbeing is understood to be the holistic social, emotional and cultural wellbeing of a person, their family, community and land. However, each Aboriginal and Torres Strait Islander tribe has its own unique culture and history, which further define their people's understanding of wellbeing.

A 2016 study utilised an Indigenous research methodology to uncover and measure wellbeing in the Yawuru people, the native title holders of Broome in Western Australia (Yap & Yu, 2016b). The Yawuru people are the first Aboriginal community to have taken control of their own data collection in this area. The aim of this study was to identify and define a set of wellbeing indicators that are 'grounded in the lived experiences' of the Yawuru people (Yap & Yu, 2016b, p. 315).

Developing wellbeing frameworks is only useful and relevant if they incorporate Aboriginal and Torres Strait Islander worldviews. In this study, the Yawuru are active participants in the design, implementation, and control of the study in order to centre the Yawuru worldview at every stage.

Why are the Yawuru people researching and measuring wellbeing?

Wellbeing was identified by the Yawuru people as an area important to their community that needed to be measured and understood. The community selected a steering committee of Yawuru men and women who worked in partnership with the two researchers: one non-Indigenous researcher and one Yawuru researcher. The work was also carried out as a PhD research project. This work was driven by the Yawuru people's desire to better understand their wellbeing so they could live a good life. Yawuru worldviews shaped the development of the wellbeing indicators.

How is wellbeing conceptualised?

Focus groups were facilitated by the research team to define the elements of a concept called *mabu liyan*, which is the centre of Yawuru being and emotions; it forms wellbeing, keeps people grounded in their identity and connections to Country, family and community, and links to how people care for themselves (McKenna & Anderson, 2011). Good *liyan* comes from 'touching, eating, feeling, being and doing. *Liyan* is also about how one relates to others, to the surroundings, and to the environment' (Yap & Yu, 2016b, p. 324). Wellbeing is thus conceptualised through the concept of *liyan*. Using a cultural concept enables this work to be culturally safe, relevant to the community and grounded in its members' understanding of the world and their wellbeing.

How did the Yawuru people develop the wellbeing measure?

Wellbeing indicators were derived and developed by Yawuru people through semi-structured interviews and focus groups. These interviews and focus groups gave the researchers a large breadth of information about what wellbeing is. These initial indicators were then brought back to the community, where Yawuru people, in focus groups, were able to select and group together the wellbeing indicators that were relevant and meaningful to them and their wellbeing. This information was collated, and the Yawuru were again invited to focus groups to discuss and finalise the wellbeing indicators.

Who makes these decisions?

The Yawuru people were at the centre of this research project. Participatory action research is a method where participants play an active role in the research process, from its beginning to the end. This method was used to measure Yawuru wellbeing: partnerships were made between the community and researchers to enable shared decision-making, and the Yawuru had control over and ownership of the research process and the final data outcomes.

Outcome of the study

The Yawuru people developed a set of wellbeing indicators based on the Yawuru worldview and culture. Indicators include family, identity and relatedness; community; connection to Country; connection to culture; and safety and respect. These indicators were refined into questions and the questions were put into a survey (method) with the intent of the survey being used to monitor and measure wellbeing in the Yawuru community over time. Utilising an Indigenous research methodology to define and measure Yawuru wellbeing results in research that is ethical, mutually beneficial and relevant to the Yawuru people.

QUESTIONS FOR REFLECTION

- This study uses an Indigenous worldview, the Yawuru concept of *liyan*, to conceptualise wellbeing. How would using a Western worldview affect the research process and study outcomes?
- Why is it important that the Yawuru people are actively involved in the development of the wellbeing indicators?
- What do you anticipate would happen if Yawuru weren't involved in the development of the wellbeing indicators?

Descriptive statistics from the Yawuru wellbeing survey results *describe* an outcome variable – here, life satisfaction – in relation to demographic information – here, age groups. Table 12.2 is reproduced from the study report and provides an example of descriptive analysis.

Table 12.2 Yawuru reporting of life satisfaction by age group (%)

	Very dissatisfied	Dissatisfied	Neutral	Satisfied	Very satisfied
18–28 years	2.2	0.0	28.3	32.6	37.0
29–44 years	3.7	5.6	29.6	40.7	20.4
45+ years	0.0	1.9	9.6	44.2	44.2

Source: Adapted from Yap & Yu (2016a, p. 95).

The data show us the differences in life satisfaction of Yawuru people in different age groups. They indicate that the 29–44-year-old group have the highest rate of life dissatisfaction, at 3.7 per cent very dissatisfied and 5.6 per cent dissatisfied, and an additional 29.6 per cent of people in this group report 'neutral' life satisfaction. These data give the Yawuru people an idea of a key target demographic where community wellbeing programs may be useful for improving life satisfaction. Additionally, we can see that most Yawuru people across all groups are satisfied or very satisfied with their lives.

These data are important as the Yawuru people have found that life satisfaction is a good indicator of the wellbeing of their people. Assessing health and wellbeing in terms relevant to their community produces data that are culturally relevant and beneficial to the Yawuru. They can then use these data to target key demographics and key wellbeing outcomes to improve the lives of their community members in ways that align with their cultural values.

Descriptive statistics are also useful to provide a summary of the phenomena under study, such as access to Country – a fundamental wellbeing attribute for Yawuru.

Figure 12.2 indicates that over a quarter of the youngest Yawuru group feel unable to access Country for fishing and hunting. As the Yawuru people designed their study

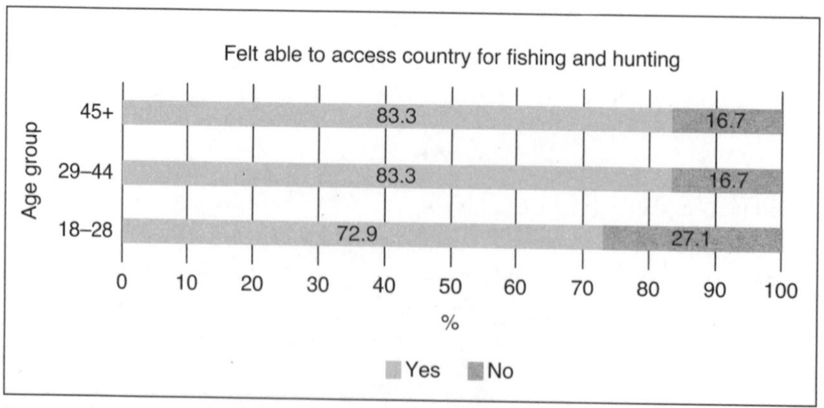

Figure 12.2 Yawuru reporting of access to Country by age

Source: Adapted from Yap & Yu (2016a, p. 66).

with cultural indicators that are important to their community, they can now use these data to target cultural programs at people aged 18–28 years to improve their cultural and Country connections.

CASE STUDY

Family and other wellbeing benefits of being an Aboriginal Ranger in Central Australia

The description of the following case study and associated results are adapted from Jones et al. (2018a).

For Aboriginal Rangers, working on country provides employment and income. The Rangers wanted to know whether there were additional wellbeing benefits (in addition to employment). Therefore, they wanted to study the association between being a Ranger or not, and health and wellbeing outcomes.

Our 2017 study utilised an Indigenous research methodology to measure and understand the association between being an Aboriginal Ranger and wellbeing (Jones et al., 2018a). The Rangers were interested in broader concepts of wellbeing beyond the individual and were also interested in family wellbeing. Rangers are looked up to in many communities, and this was considered in the survey design and analysis phases.

In this study, the Rangers were active participants in the design, implementation and control of the study in order to centre the Rangers as the focal point of the research.

The study was conducted in partnership with the Central Land Council (CLC), which employs and supports Ranger groups to care for their lands. The CLC was interested in evaluating the multiple benefits of its Ranger program, including wellbeing benefits. Synergies were identified with the research team's work in developing and testing quantitative measures of cultural engagement, expression and practice with a diversity of Aboriginal and Torres Strait Islander groups across the country as part of the development of a national longitudinal study.

How is wellbeing conceptualised?

Focus groups were conducted by the research team to define the elements of culture and wellbeing. Using cultural concepts enables this work to be culturally safe, relevant to the community and grounded in members' understanding of the world and their wellbeing.

How did they develop the wellbeing measures?

Wellbeing was assessed through four measures: life satisfaction, general health, psychological wellbeing and family wellbeing. The life satisfaction and general health measures are commonly used in both the general Australian and Aboriginal and Torres Strait Islander populations, with good uptake in both populations. Through the study

(cont.)

consultation and development phase, the Rangers did not identify a need to modify or adapt these two measures. Psychological distress was measured using a culturally modified, five-item Kessler Psychological Distress Scale (K5). The K5 was developed to remove potentially offensive items and improve cultural appropriateness in the Aboriginal and Torres Strait Islander population (AIHW, 2009). It was further refined during study development, with clarifying descriptors added to improve conceptual understanding of participants. Family wellbeing was measured using the Western Australian Aboriginal Child Health Survey family functioning scale (Silburn et al., 2006) and was modified during the study development process.

Modifying health and wellbeing measures that are used in the general population helps to improve the cultural acceptability and safety of Aboriginal and Torres Strait Islander participants when measures developed for use in Aboriginal and Torres Strait Islander populations do not yet exist. Work is currently underway to assess the validity of the measures used in this study.

Who makes these decisions?

The CLC and Rangers were at the centre of this research project. Participatory action research is a method whereby participants play an active role in the research process, from its beginning to the end. A strength of the Ranger study is the participatory research approach and the ongoing community engagement and feedback with participants. The research team ensured a two-way collaboration with the Ranger group in the establishment, implementation and reporting of the research. The reciprocal nature of this relationship allowed for joint seminars and presentations to be undertaken to disseminate the research.

Outcomes of the study

This study provided evidence about the broader benefits of Ranger programs and provided novel quantitative evidence of the potential health and wellbeing benefits of participation in a Ranger program. This study adds strength to ongoing assertions from community, Aboriginal organisations and conservation groups that working on country through Ranger programs is contributing towards closing gaps in health, employment and education.

QUESTIONS FOR REFLECTION

- This study uses an Indigenous worldview that gives equal weight to money and wellbeing. How do you think using a Western worldview would affect the research process and study outcomes?
- Why is it important that the Rangers are actively involved in the development of the wellbeing indicators?
- What do you anticipate would happen if Rangers weren't involved in the development of the study?

The Ranger case study provides a real-life example of how research can be developed in consultation (and collaboration) with community members. Continuing to use the Ranger case study as an example, we will now demonstrate how descriptive and inferential analysis methods were used.

In Table 12.3, the sociodemographic characteristics of the Ranger group are presented in a frequency table. Percentages are reported for each sociodemographic characteristic. The N represents the total number of people who reported each characteristic. This is known as a descriptive analysis.

Table 12.3 Sociodemographic factors, by Ranger status

	Rangers (N = 43)		Non-Rangers (N = 160)	
Sociodemographic factors	**%**	**n**	**%**	**n**
Gender				
Male	60	26	31	50
Female	28	12	65	104
Missing	12	≤5	5	6
Age group (years)				
16–24	≤11	≤5	17	27
25–34	33	14	29	47
35–44	16	7	17	27
>45	30	13	26	42
Missing	≤11	≤5	11	17
Education				
Year 10 or less	44	19	54	87
Year 12 and above	44	19	31	49
Missing	12	≤5	15	24
Employment				
Not employed	0	0	59	95
Employed	100	43	33	52
Missing	0	0	8	13
Financial status				
Low	37	16	54	86
High	42	18	31	49
Missing	21	9	16	25

Note: the ≤ sign is utilised to ensure the data presented remain deidentified. If for instance only one female participated in the study, someone may recognise her data when presented in that way and thus be identifiable.

Source: Reproduced from Jones et al. (2018a, p. 6).

Another way to present the results from Table 12.3, is to write out the description, which might look like this:

> A total of 43 Rangers and 160 non-Rangers participated in the study; 60% (n = 26) and 31% (n = 50) of participants were male, respectively. Participants ranged from 16 to 77 years in age, with a mean age of 37 years. All Rangers were employed whereas only 33% (n = 52) of non-Rangers were employed. Forty-two percent (n = 18) of Rangers reported high financial status compared to 31% (n = 49) of non-Rangers.
>
> (Jones et al., 2018a, p. 6)

An alternate way of presenting data is a graph, although a graph is more appropriate when presenting one aspect of the data – for example, the percentage in each category of financial status.

Inferential statistics and analysis are used to compare two or more variables in a dataset and can be used to determine whether one variable (the exposure variable) changes the outcome (or outcomes variable). Inferential analysis utilises confidence intervals and/or statistical significance to determine the strength and level of the relationship between the outcome and exposure variables.

Measures of independence between two or more categorical data are analysed with 2 × 2 tables and a statistical test called the chi-squared test for independence. To assess independence, we need a binary outcome variable and an exposure variable.

Our exposure variable in this example is Ranger: Yes/No.

Our outcome variable or the thing we are interested in is High Family wellbeing: Yes/No.

Our first step is to state our hypotheses: 'Ranger status is independent (is not linked) to high family wellbeing.'

To assess whether Ranger status is independent, we need to calculate the probability that Ranger status is independent of high family wellbeing. To do this, we use a chi-squared test for independence with a probability value (p-value) that indicates how confident we can be about the level of independence. In statistics, a p-value of less than 0.05 (or a one in 20 chance) is generally considered the threshold. To calculate the p-value, we lay out the data we have on Rangers and high family wellbeing in a 2 × 2 table (Table 12.4).

Table 12.4 Ranger status by high family wellbeing (observed values)

		High family wellbeing		
		No	Yes	Total
Ranger	No	72	70	142
	Yes	10	26	36
	Total	82	96	178

Chi-squared tests rely on the difference between the observed and expected numbers in each cell. We next need to calculate 'expected value' for each cell (Table 12.5).

Table 12.5 Formula for calculation for expected values

		High family wellbeing		
		No	Yes	Total
Ranger	No	$\frac{82 \times 142}{178}$	$\frac{96 \times 142}{178}$	142
	Yes	$\frac{36 \times 82}{178}$	$\frac{96 \times 36}{178}$	36
	Total	82	96	178

Expected values are therefore as shown in Table 12.6.

Table 12.6 Calculated expected values

		High family wellbeing		
		No	Yes	Total
Ranger	No	65.42	76.58	142
	Yes	16.58	19.42	36
	Total	82	96	178

To calculate the chi-squared value, subtract the expected values in each cell from the observed values (Table 12.4), square the total then divide by expected value (Table 12.7).

Table 12.7 Formula for calculation for chi squared values

		High family wellbeing		
		No	Yes	Total
Ranger	No	$\frac{(65.42 - 72)^2}{65.42}$	$\frac{(76.58 - 70)^2}{76.58}$	142
	Yes	$\frac{(16.58 - 10)^2}{16.58}$	$\frac{(19.42 - 26)^2}{19.42}$	36
	Total	82	96	178

This gives you the chi-squared values, shown in Table 12.8.

Table 12.8 Chi-squared values

		High family wellbeing		
		No	Yes	Total
Ranger	No	0.66	0.56	142
	Yes	2.61	2.23	36
	Total	82	96	178

We then sum the calculated values: 0.66 + 0.56 + 2.61 + 2.23 = 6.07 after rounding.

Our chi-squared statistic = 6.07

To get from chi-squared to a p-value we also need to also calculate the degrees of freedom.

Degrees of Freedom = (rows − 1) × (columns − 1)

In this example we have 2 rows and 2 columns, so DF = (2 − 1) (2 − 1) = 1 × 1 = 1

Degrees of freedom = 1

After consulting a chi-squared table (these are freely available online and included in statistics publications), we can see that our p-value is 0.01375. meaning the result is unlikely due to chance as the p-value is below the threshold of 0.05.

Remember that our hypothesis is: 'Ranger status is independent (not linked) to high family wellbeing.' We therefore reject the hypothesis and conclude that Ranger status is linked to high family wellbeing.

Further statistical analysis can be performed to indicate how much being a Ranger contributes to high levels of family wellbeing using additional statistical tools such as regression (Jones et al., 2018a).

There are online calculators that can be used conduct these tests. For further information, see www.socscistatistics.com/tests/chisquare2/default2.aspx. Numerous texts are also available on the subject (Neuman, 2011).

Conclusion

Research is typically conducted within a Western framework or methodology. When a Western framework is used in research on Aboriginal and Torres Strait Islander people, this has often resulted in data that neither benefit communities nor produce positive health outcomes. An Indigenous research methodology uses Aboriginal and Torres Strait Islander ways of knowing, being and doing to frame the overarching rationale and strategy of a research project. It is informed by Aboriginal and Torres Strait Islander research questions, methods and approaches, and produces work that centres the needs and wants of Aboriginal and Torres Strait Islander people. Communities are empowered to participate in research that is of priority to them, leading to a shared research agenda. Importantly, the methods of analysis in quantitative research can be used in the same fashion as all other research, without losing sight of the lens through which interpretation of the results occurs. Conducting research within an Indigenous research methodology results in research that is culturally safe, relevant and applicable to Aboriginal and Torres Strait Islander people, and is more likely to result in health improvements.

Case studies including the Yawuru Wellbeing study and the Aboriginal Rangers study demonstrate how an Indigenous research methodology can be implemented to produce data needed by Aboriginal and Torres Strait Islander communities. Indigenous quantitative research can and should be done within an Indigenous research methodology to form ethical partnerships and beneficial results for Aboriginal and Torres Strait Islander communities.

Learning activities

1. Investigate how Indigenous organisations are conducting research with Aboriginal and Torres Strait Islander communities. How does the traditional Western research methodology differ from an Indigenous research methodology? (Visit the website of the Lowitja Institute: www.lowitja.org.au.)
2. Read the Guidelines for Ethical Research in Australian Indigenous Studies (AIATSIS, 2012). Choose one principle and explore how you would implement this principle as a nurse or midwife treating a patient. (The Guidelines can be viewed at https://aiatsis.gov.au/sites/default/files/2020–09/gerais.pdf.)
3. Read the *Mayi Kuwayu* (Jones, 2018b) study protocol paper. Revisit the chapter section 'Elements of an Indigenous Research Methodology' and answer the four questions proposed using this protocol paper. Does the *Mayi Kuwayu* study adequately address all four questions?

FURTHER READING

Research, and particularly quantitative research, has a vexed history in relation to Indigenous people and populations. Increasing use of Indigenous methodologies in the area, including in quantitative approaches, is now occurring thanks to Indigenous trailblazers such as the following:

Kovach, M. (2009). *Indigenous Methodologies: Characteristics, Conversations, and Contexts*. Toronto: University of Toronto Press.

Rigney, L.-I. (1999). Internationalization of an Indigenous anticolonial cultural critique of research methodologies: A guide to Indigenist research methodology and its principles. *Emergent Ideas in Native American Studies*, 14(2), 109–21.

Tuhiwai Smith, L. (2012). *Decolonizing Methodologies: Research and Indigenous Peoples*. London: Zed Books.

Walter, M. & Andersen, C. (2013). *Indigenous Statistics: A Quantitative Research Methodology*. London: Routledge.

Wilson, S. (2008). *Research is Ceremony: Indigenous Research Methods*. Halifax, NS: Fernwood Publishing.

Visit the companion website at www.cambridge.org/highereducation/isbn/9781108794695/resources to see further online resources.

REFERENCES

AIATSIS (2012). *Guidelines for Ethical Research in Australian Indigenous Studies*. Canberra: AIATSIS. Retrieved from https://aiatsis.gov.au/sites/default/files/2020–09/gerais.pdf

AIHW (2009). *Measuring the Social and Emotional Wellbeing of Aboriginal and Torres Strait Islander Peoples*. Canberra: AIATSIS.

Almalki, S. (2016). Integrating quantitative and qualitative data in mixed methods research: Challenges and benefits. *Journal of Education and Learning*, *5*(3). doi:10.5539/jel.v5n3p288

Bainbridge, R., Tsey, K., McCalman, J.A .... Lawson, K. (2015). No one's discussing the elephant in the room: Contemplating questions of research impact and benefit in Aboriginal and Torres Strait Islander Australian health research. *BMC Public Health*, 15(696). doi:10.1186/s12889-015–2052-3

Blackstock, C. (2009). First Nation children count: Enveloping quantitative research in an Indigenous envelope. *First Peoples Child & Family Review*, 4(2), 135–43.

Desborough, M.J.R. & Keeling, D.M. (2017). The aspirin story – from willow to wonder drug. *British Journal of Haematology*, 177(5), 674–83.

DIISRTE (2012). *Higher Education Research Data Collection: Specifications for the Collection of 2011 Data*. Canberra: Australian Government.

Frost, J. (2020). Difference between descriptive and inferential statistics. Retrieved from https://statisticsbyjim.com/basics/descriptive-inferential-statistics

Gorman, D. & Toombs, M. (2009). Matching research methodology to Australian Indigenous culture. *Aboriginal & Islander Health Worker Journal*, 33(3), 4–7.

Howell, K. (2013). *An Introduction to the Philosophy of Methodology*. Thousand Oaks, CA: Sage.

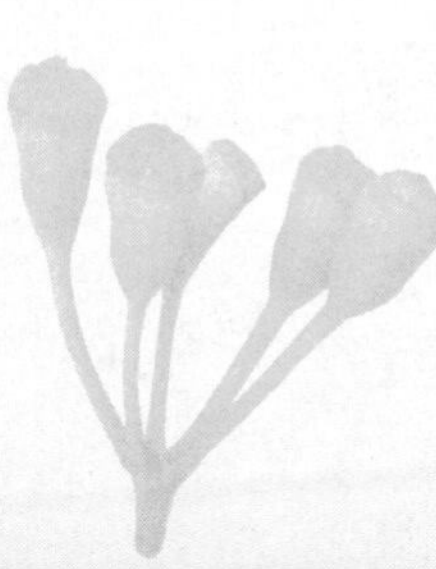

Jones, R. Thurber, K.A. Chapman, J. … Lovett, R. (2018a). Associations between participation in a Ranger Program and health and wellbeing outcomes among Aboriginal and Torres Strait Islander people in Central Australia: A proof of concept study. *International Journal of Environmental Research and Public Health*, 15(7), 1478.

Jones, R., Thurber, K.A., Chapman, J. … Lovett, R. (2018b). Study protocol: *Our Cultures Count*, the Mayi Kuwayu study, a national longitudinal study of Aboriginal and Torres Strait Islander wellbeing. *BMJ Open 2018*(8): e023861.

Kite, E. & Davy, C. (2015). Using Indigenist and Indigenous methodologies to connect to deeper understandings of Aboriginal and Torres Strait Islander peoples' quality of life. *Health Promotion Journal of Australia*, 26(3), 191–4.

Liamputtong, P. (ed.) (2016). *Research Methods in Health: Foundations for Evidence-Based Practice* (3rd edn). Melbourne: Oxford University Press.

Martin, K. & Mirraboopa, B. (2003). Ways of knowing, being and doing: A theoretical framework and methods for Indigenous and indigenist research. *Journal of Australian Studies*, 27(76), 203–14.

McKenna, V. & Anderson, K. (2011). *Kimberley Dreaming: Old Law, New Ways: Finding New Meaning*. Sydney: World Congress for Psychotherapy.

Moreton-Robinson, A. & Walter, M. (2009). Indigenous Methodologies in Social Research. In M. Walter (ed.), *Social Research Methods* (2nd edn). Melbourne: Oxford University Press, Ch. 22.

Morton, S. (1839). *Comparative View of the Skulls of Various Aboriginal Nations of North and South America*. Philadelphia, PA: J. Dobson.

Munns, A., Toye, C., Hegney, D., Kickett, M., Marriott, R. and Walker, R. (2017). Peer-led Aboriginal parent support: Program development for vulnerable populations with participatory action research. *Contemporary Nurse*, 53(5), 558–75.

Nature Methods (2009). Defining the scientific method. *Nature Methods*, 6(4), 237.

Neuman, L. (2011). *Social Research Methods: Qualitative and Quantitative Approaches* (7th edn). Boston: Allyn and Bacon.

Porta, M. (2008). *Dictionary of Epidemiology*. Oxford: Oxford University Press.

Reason, P. & Bradbury, H. (2001). *Handbook of Action Research: Participative Inquiry and Practice*. London: Sage.

Rigney, L.-I. (1999). Internationalization of an Indigenous anticolonial cultural critique of research methodologies: A guide to indigenist research methodology and its principles. *Emergent Ideas in Native American Studies*, 14(2), 109–21.

Rigney, L.-I. (2001). A first perspective of Indigenous Australian Participation in Science: Framing Indigenous research towards Indigenous Australian intellectual sovereignty. *Kaurna Higher Education Journal*, 7, 1–13.

Ryder, C., Mackean, T., Coombs, J.U. , Williams, H. , Hunter, K., Holland, A.J.A. & Ivers, R.Q. (2019). Indigenous research methodology – weaving a research interface. *International Journal of Social Research Methodology*, 23(3), 255–67.

Saini, M. (2012). *A Systematic Review of Western and Aboriginal Research Designs: Assessing Cross-Validation to Explore Compatibility and Convergence*. Prince George, BC: National Collaborating Centre for Aboriginal Health.

Silburn, S., Zubrick, S., DeMaio, J. … Pearson, G. (2006). *The Western Australian Aboriginal Child Health Survey: Strengthening the Capacity of Aboriginal Children, Families and Communities*. Perth: Curtin University of Technology and Telethon Institute for Child Health Research.

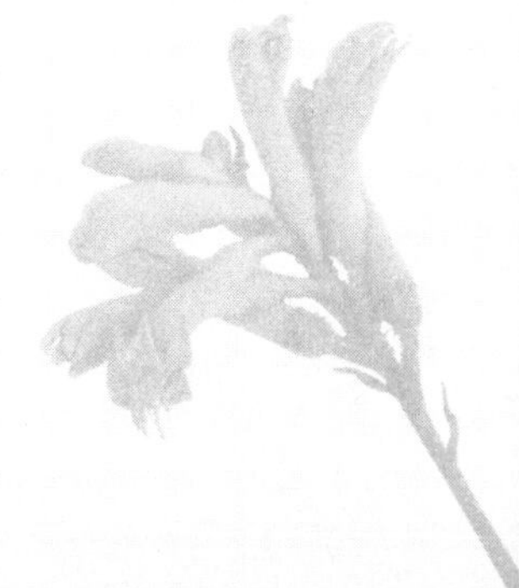

Smithson, M. (2000). *Statistics with Confidence.* Thousand Oaks, CA: Sage.

van der Sterren, A., Greenhalgh, E., Hanley-Jones, S., Knoche, D. & Winstanley, M. (2020). Prevalence of tobacco use among Aboriginal and Torres Strait Islander peoples. In E. Greenhalgh, M. Scollo & M. Winstanley (eds), *Tobacco in Australia: Facts and Issues:* Melbourne: Cancer Council Victoria.

Walker, M., Fredericks, B., Mills, K. & Anderson, D. (2014). 'Yarning' as a method for community-based health research with Indigenous women: The Indigenous Women's Wellness Research Program. *Health Care for Women International,* 35(10), 1216–26.

Walter, M. & Andersen, C. (2013). *Indigenous Statistics: A Quantitative Research Methodology.* London: Routledge.

Wilson, R. & Dodson, M. (1997). *Bringing Them Home: Report of the National Inquiry into the Separation of Aboriginal and Torres Strait Islander Children from Their Families.* Canberra: Commonwealth of Australia.

Wilson, S. (2008). *Research is Ceremony: Indigenous Research Methods.* Halifax, NS: Fernwood Publishing.

Yap, M. & Yu, E. (2016a). *Community wellbeing from the ground up: A Yawuru example.* Perth: Bankwest Curtin Economics Centre. Retrieved from www.curtin.edu.au/local/docs/bcec-community-wellbeing-from-the-ground-up-a-yawuru-example.pdf

Yap, M. & Yu, E. (2016b). Operationalising the capability approach: Developing culturally relevant indicators of indigenous wellbeing – an Australian example. *Oxford Development Studies,* 44(3): 315–31.

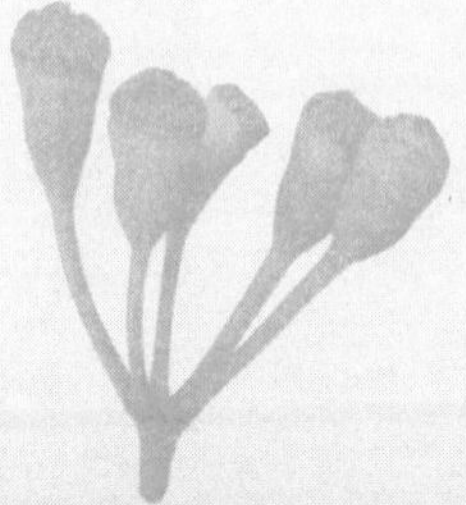

Navigating First Nations social and emotional wellbeing in mainstream mental health services

Rhonda L. Wilson and Kristin Waqanaviti

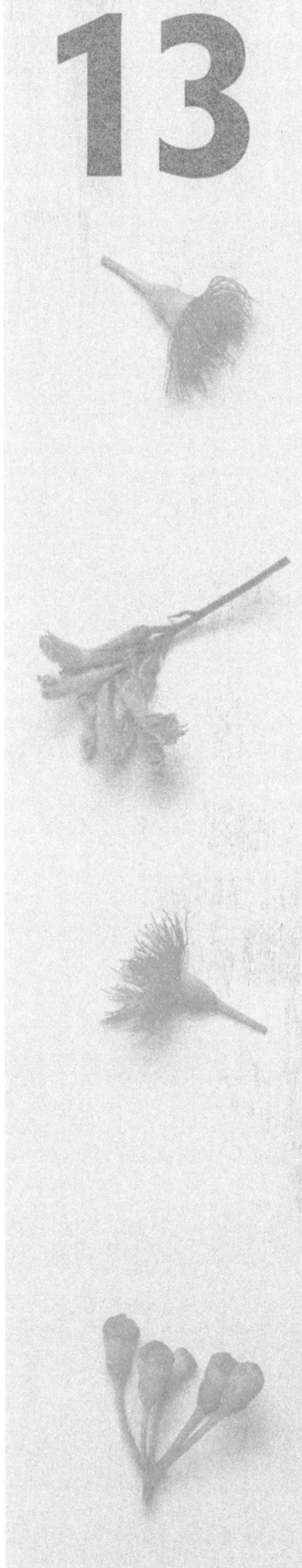

LEARNING OBJECTIVES

This chapter will help you to:

- Identify some of the determinants of social and emotional wellbeing (SEWB)
- Recognise the nature of relationships for First Nations people in relation to SEWB
- Identify SEWB strengths derived from First Nations Peoples' cultural practices
- Discuss mainstream mental health service capacity to incorporate elements of SEWB to support First Nations People
- Explore some of the contemporary threats to SEWB of First Nations Peoples
- Describe some of the strategies that nurses can implement to enhance the SEWB of First Nations Peoples within mainstream mental health settings

KEY WORDS

mental health
trauma-informed care

Introduction

This chapter aims to guide the reader to learn about providing nursing care for First Nations people with regard to culturally safe social and emotional wellbeing (SEWB). The first thing you will notice is that we use the term 'social and emotional wellbeing' instead of the dominant health culture terminology 'mental health'. We are not attempting to be controversial in doing so; rather, we are adopting a First Nations standpoint (Moreton-Robinson, 2013) to help us to understand and discuss mental health and mental illness in a relevant context for First Nations people. In doing so, we will also suggest that it is not a case of simply translating *mental health* as an alternative terminology; instead, it is necessary to understand *social and emotional wellbeing* as a phenomenon in itself that is particular to First Nations people, and then to explore mental health from that perspective. The standpoint we use is important because from a theoretical perspective it helps us to understand how we interpret the social and emotional health, and mental health, of people generally. Indigenous standpoint theory is one way to understand and privilege the unique understanding embedded in the ways of being, doing and knowing for First Nations people, and to apply culturally safe assumptions to this knowledge to make meaning in relation to mental health generally.

Mainstream or dominant culture ideas about mental health, or health more generally, usually adopt a biomedical standpoint, thereby privileging the notion of a medicalised perception of health, with disease and dysfunction codes as the main reference points for interpreting individual psychological distress (Hocking, 2017). In contrast, SEWB is concerned with more than the individual experiences of distress and dysfunction: it considers the social, emotional and cultural wellbeing of the whole community as well, while harmonising these interests with the interactions between mental, physical, cultural, spiritual health and relationship with land (Calma, Dudgeon & Bray, 2017; Commonwealth of Australia, 2017; Hocking, 2017; Salmon et al., 2019). Cultural wellbeing is made up of a range of elements, including but not limited to spiritual, environmental, ideological, social, economic, mental and physical factors (Calma et al., 2017; Commonwealth of Australia, 2017; Salmon et al., 2019). Experiences of trauma or disruption in any of these domains can interrupt SEWB for individuals and communities, and when seen in this light, and as a consequence of colonisation and the traumas associated with it, it is unsurprising that a legacy of intergenerational compromise to wellbeing is experienced by many First Nations people and communities. However, it is also no surprise that First Nations people have also demonstrated an innate capacity to thrive despite such adverse conditions. Harnessing the inherent strengths within the collective experience of intergenerational resilience that constitutes success, demonstrated by the achievement of the longest enduring and continuing culture in the world (Hocking, 2017), is likely to improve SEWB and mental health outcomes for First Nations people (Commonwealth of Australia, 2017). Mental health interventions that are able to draw from these strengths and amplify success are particularly well aligned to enhance SEWB outcomes for individuals and communities (Commonwealth of Australia, 2017). In the context of the negative narratives and stereotypes that often dominate discourse associated with First Nations people within the mainstream biomedical perception of mental illness, it is very important to consider the consolidation of cultural strengths that are inherent and that offer protection and mitigation of mental illness when they are adopted as part of a holistic recovery plan.

After reading and thinking about the content of this chapter, you will be able to describe some of the determinants of SEWB for First Nations people, and recognise the fundamental cultural and spiritual connections to people, place and culture that are strong attributes of many First Nations people. Readers will also be able to identify the strengths that are inherent in positive expressions of SEWB and how they can be derived from connections to culture and nature (environment and place). Students will be able to identify some of the ways in which mainstream mental health service can integrate SEWB concepts to enhance the recovery of First Nations people, and explore some of the barriers and threats that exist for enhancing and supporting SEWB. Lastly, students will be able to describe some of the strategies that nurses can implement to enhance the SEWB of First Nations people within mainstream, mental health settings.

The attributes and determinants of social and emotional wellbeing

Conceptualising First Nations people's health and wellbeing differs from the dominant culture in Australia in that it is not limited to either a physical or mental expression of health or wellbeing as confined to a single person (Salmon et al., 2019). In previous chapters of this book, you have had the opportunity to explore holistic concepts of health and wellbeing that include the need to consider wellbeing on a whole-of-community scale, in addition to individual needs, combined with the connectivity between the individual person and the community. Here, we build on these concepts and further explore the social, political and cultural determinants related specifically to SEWB for First Nations people. This has particular implications and relevance for nursing practice in the mental health setting (Geia et al., 2020). For example, the ways in which First Nations people are included (or not) in mental health research, and the extent to which this inclusion or absence informs clinical nursing practice – such as point-of-care processes for the treatment of mental illness and subsequent rehabilitation in the community setting – is fundamental to achieving SEWB outcomes (Tsey et al., 2007). More specifically, understanding the nature of these determinants assists in recognising the harmful effects of exposure to racism, trauma and inequality, which act to erode the integrity of positive individual, intergenerational and community SEWB, and can result in a deterioration of mental health, leading to mental illness for some First Nations people.

Contributing factors to the deterioration of SEWB can include determinants such as:

- poor general health
- inadequate housing
- loss of spiritual connection to Country
- dispossession of traditional lands

- Australia's history of colonisation
- dislocation
- disparity (socioeconomic)
- substance misuse
- over-representation of incarcerated First Nations people
- under-representation of First Nations people in the paid workforce
- failure by mainstream mental health service to recognise Indigenous knowledge and how First Nations people interpret or make meaning of the world around them.

Meanwhile, some principles that contribute to positive SEWB for First Nations people in the mainstream mental health setting include:

- cultural safety (that is, the absence of racism in any form)
- trauma-informed care
- recognition and respect of cultural and spiritual norms of First Nations people and the meaningful accommodation and support of these in the mainstream mental health setting
- holistic frameworks of care and recovery that include community wellbeing
- access to appropriate mental healthcare that maintains links to Country and culture
- respect for First Nations Elders and culture, demonstrated in terms of hospitality, kindness, welcome and physical environment
- the adoption of mental health assessment tools validated for use with First Nations people
- the inclusion of culturally safe interventions within mental health recovery plans
- a mental health workforce that includes First Nations people as clinicians
- advocacy and action to Close the Gap of disparity between First Nations people and other Australians
- self-determination and leadership
- safe and thriving families.

(Commonwealth of Australia, 2017; Hocking, 2017; Salmon et al., 2019; Wilson, 2016)

Defining social and emotional wellbeing

To First Nations people, SEWB is an expression of cultural and spiritual being and doing, rather than a limitation of an explicitly set of actions or attributes. There is no singular explanation of the nature of SEWB that adequately describes the depth of this complexity. It is incorporated within a way of being in the world that is explicitly connected with Indigeneity as individual and communal sets of lived experiences, entwined with innate respect for land, sea, ancestry, spirituality, flora and fauna. SEWB is experienced as an internalised sensation that is felt within the core of a person's humanity and is outwardly expressed through relationships between culture and lore in a continuous cycle of life and death.

The physical, spiritual and emotional feeling brought about from First Nations people's Indigeneity resonates through important cultural practices such as dance, song, language preservation and storytelling because these practices stem from survival, identifying the uniqueness of self and the functionality of self in the individual and communal socio-political constructs (Bello-Bravo, 2019). 'Indigeneity' is the term used to ethically depict the actual right of Indigenous people to claim their identity and be recognised as such by their specific community due to their inherent and undeniable relation to the geographical region, wealth of naturally occurring resources, and their specific essentiality to the life-cycle of the surrounding ecosystem and space (Bello-Bravo, 2019).

To attempt to define SEWB from Indigenous perspectives, and as a starting point, it is imperative that recognition is given to Elders, past, present and emerging. This is important because culturally these people have particular responsibility as keepers of sacred practices, which preserve the existential longevity and safety of the individual who lives within a community and is a member of a recognised family network in the traditional tribal, kinship or clan systems (Le Grande et al., 2017). This recognition of cultural Elders is an important sign of respect and is often used to demarcate the sovereignty of the people and the land on which events, and the provision of services, occur. It is therefore appropriate to acknowledge the land's Traditional Owners. These cultural practices are intrinsic components of cultural determinants of SEWB, yet they are often comprehended in biomedically orientated mainstream health services without adequate consultation with Indigenous people, or proper consideration of the Elder system. This can undermine the cultural safety of First Nations people and the effectiveness of SEWB outcomes generally (Tsey et al., 2007). Thus, in order to understand SEWB adequately, it is necessary to learn the relevance of the determinants and cultural practices from a First Nations standpoint in order to engage respectfully and to implement mental healthcare that reinforces positive SEWB.

Developing a shared understanding of social and emotional wellbeing

Public services in Australia have a limited track record in successfully engaging with First Nations people to enhance their mental health and wellbeing. The disparity gap continues to widen (Closing the Gap in Partnership, 2020). The literature is swollen with examples of Commonwealth and state failures to adequately provide care for First Nations people, and various Royal Commissions have highlighted the neglect and adversity generally – for example, the Royal Commissions into deaths in custody (Johnston, 1991), the Stolen Generations (HREOC, 1997) and incarceration rates for Indigenous people (ALRC, 2017). This circumstance is perpetuated through poorly designed research and data collection that fails to incorporate the Indigenous standpoint, methodologies and knowledges, and relies heavily on Western methodologies, assumptions and constructs. This leads to interpretations and recommendations that do not adequately represent an Indigenous standpoint, and thereby compromise the validity and reliability of the findings (Tsey et al., 2007). It is unsurprising that where this occurs, the translation of the research into practice environments leads to inadequacies in supporting the SEWB of First Nations people.

Traditionally, public policy in Australia has adopted Westernised rather than Indigenous ways of knowing in relation to the production of research to inform practice. We are seeing some change in this regard as more First Nations people are graduating from universities across health and social care disciplines. As a First Nations researcher workforce develops and proliferates, we are starting to see an incorporation of Indigenous research methodologies utilised. For example, Elvidge et al. (2020) recently validated a scale to help public health services understand and respond to the experience of cultural safety of Aboriginal people when they are hospitalised. Cultural safety is associated with SEWB, so it stands to reason that if First Nations people feel culturally safe when they are in hospital, their health outcomes will improve (Elvidge et al., 2020).

Another longitudinal study (Macedo et al., 2019) explored the experience of racism on children's SEWB, revealing findings associating the experience of racism with hyperactivity and conduct disorders. Again, we see that the experience of racism erodes SEWB and is associated with mental illness. It is thus extremely important to ensure that young people are supported in an environment that nurtures cultural safety as a protective factor, with a view to reduce the risk of developing more disruptive mental health conditions at a critical time of development and growth.

In another example, Tsey et al. (2007) conducted a study that explored the use of collaborative initiatives between Aboriginal and Torres Strait Islander people who had endured trauma, such as the survivors of the Stolen Generations. Aboriginal corporations and tertiary research experts worked together to understand the mechanisms of resilience, and how these should drive the conduct of culturally safe research about, and with, First Nations people. This collaborative mode of research engaged people at the grass roots with lived experience and involved them as partners in the research so that the real-world study findings would have relevancy and significance to First Nations people (Tsey et al., 2007). The importance of this study was amplified because it had a strategic focus to work in partnership over a ten-year sustained period. First Nations people and academic researchers committed to working together to illuminate real-world applied understandings related to SEWB and to understand ways in which local Indigenous corporations could enable First Nations people to facilitate their own SEWB journeys towards mental health recovery through self-determination, and to maintain individual and collective resilience in the future (Tsey et al., 2007).

The findings of studies such as the three examples mentioned here are increasingly being incorporated and implemented to influence SEWB practice and policy, but this change is slow. However, it has started to illuminate the structural and institutional elements of racism that continue to influence health service delivery in Australia. Significant progress has been made in dismantling these elements, but reform will continue to take considerable time, and will require courageous discussions and the incorporation of new Indigenous graduate attributes within health and nursing curricula, together with a willingness to build cultural safety within all our practices going forward (Geia et al., 2020).

Stigma and identity

A further factor that needs to be considered with regard to SEWB is that of stigma and identity. As readers will be aware from previous chapters in this book, Australia has a complex political history and relationship with First Nations people: one of colonisation and assimilation, which continues and is expressed as intergenerational trauma, and where associated consequences are drawn forward to the present time.

Volumes have been written, stories told and sung, and oral narratives recounted and passed from generation to generation about the real-world experiences of what it is to be a First Nations person in all variants – and, conversely, to be cast by powerful dominant-culture narrators in negative, derogatory and discriminatory discourses and practices. For many people, identifying as a First Nations person is explicit. For others, identification is less straightforward, with a range of variants to identification possible. A culturally relevant creative regeneration of what it means to identify as a contemporary First Nations person in the twenty-first century is increasingly helpful to foster positive SEWB generally (Carlson, 2016).

The legacy of the past continues to cause existential confusion, Sorry Business, grief and loss for many people who were impacted by these practices, and this continues to undermine SEWB for many – for example, those First Nations people who were removed from their families as members of the Stolen Generations, and their families.

Intergenerational culture, courage and identity: Rhonda's story

For Rhonda Wilson, the politics of Aboriginal identity is a powerful personal narrative of intergenerational SEWB recovery and cultural restoration.

I am the descendant of a married English immigrant farming selector and a Wiradjuri woman (the nature of the relationship is not possible to ascertain now, but typically history suggests that these types of encounters were often non-consenting, and frequently abusive). Their son was raised with cultural cognisance, and when grown was sent away to work building the railway, far removed from his culture/s and homeland. He retained the stories of his mother to pass forward, shared with his own child, my fair-skinned Aboriginal grandmother, with her own complicated history. She was born off Country, and grew to womanhood during an era when to identify as an Aboriginal woman was to concede to a non-human existence, and to live in the shadows with whatever aliases and narratives that others imagined for her as a 'truth' perhaps facilitated her survival. The tensions between hearing stories passed down the family line, the maintenance of hushed secrets and rigorous adherence to acceptable behaviours that must demonstrably 'pass' as 'white' so that a legacy of hope and success for the future is enabled for those who come after must have been a heavy and isolating burden to bear.

There is a Dreamtime Wiradjuri story about the origins of the Murrumbidgee River. Part of the story tells about the courage of a young woman who had to go on a journey by herself to find a new sources of water for her husband and family. She was cautioned by some women who said she would be exposed to the risk of coming to harm by Wahn the Crow (Green and Community of Wagga Wagga, 2002). The story resonates strongly with me, particularly the courage of a woman separated from her family with a mission to bring much-needed help to her people; the resilience to press through personal discomforts for the greater good of others; and the warning to be mindful of harm along the way. My courageous grandmother drew strength from this story, and passed it on to us: she would often declare when she saw or heard a crow lurking nearby, 'You are not coming for me now!', while shaking her finger furiously at it. In doing so, she taught us to heed the cultural and spiritual warnings, and to be strong, bolstering our SEWB.

The self-sacrifice, resilience and tenacity demonstrated by my grandmother and great-grandfather are indicative of the strengths inherent within First Nations people well before, during and after colonisation. It was important to my grandmother that her grand-daughters would 'pass', no doubt to protect us from the indignities that she must have encountered. We were encouraged to do all we could ensure our skin colour was blemish free, without darkness or even freckles; we were advised to avoid too much sun so as not to darken our skin; and I recall lemon juice and babies' wet nappies applied to my skin as a child to remove any dark pigmentation.

Later, my grandmother saved money from her pension to send me to June Daly Watkins Grooming and Deportment classes to ensure I would be acceptable in society (particularly common for Aboriginal girls of my era). For birthdays and Christmas, she would give gifts such as tableware napery – beautifully embroidered afternoon tea cloths so we could hold tea parties for societal dignitaries, should our (hoped for by her) circumstance allow. She had ambitious hopes for our future successes.

At that time, dominant culture societal pressures and incentives suggested that any hint of Aboriginality was undesirable, and that if it was possible to 'pass' as white, then this was important to achieve. This was a time when racism was overt and discrimination actively employed. A grandmother's hope for her legacy was surely that her family should have more opportunity than she had, that her sacrifice should bring freedom to those who came after her, and that concealment of identity and maintaining family secrets – denial of self – was critical to the endeavour of success. With the rise of cultural safety, a courage emerges to identify and to reclaim and restore culture that had been mourned, and concealed with the restrictive measures associated with past Commonwealth- and state-enforced discrimination.

Intergenerational trauma disrupts social and emotional wellbeing

This is not an unusual pattern for a great many First Nations families, and it is fraught with tensions and frustrations – even anger. Some people arise from it fortified with the intergenerational resilience of 65,000+ years of strength and enduring SEWB, but others succumb to the vulnerability and struggle to thrive and experience a compromise to their SEWB. The reasons for these differences are not yet fully understood, but we are beginning to understand the phenomenon more as we seek to understand the experiences of First Nations people and as we discover ways to build resilience and positive SEWB in the midst of enduring human and cultural pain.

Sometimes the political oppressions are reinforced by First Nations people and communities themselves as all parties come to terms with recovering from the restrictive measures of past policy and practice (Carlson, 2016). Society required my ancestors to deny their identity and culture, yet they managed to pass forward a cultural cognisance that defies the odds, and the intergenerational grief and loss associated with this endures in my family to this day. Yet spiritual connection to culture and connection to Land, and respect for Elders past remain inherent as a SEWB strength. As Carlson (2016, p. 1) notes, a general societal assumption was that to 'be Aboriginal must not be a good thing' and that 'any reference to being Aboriginal was an insult'. My own personal variants of family history concur.

Bronwyn Carlson (2016) and I are not particularly unusual in this regard: many other First Nations people will have had similar experiences and have worked hard to rectify the cultural damage, and to repair their crushed spirits by drawing on intergenerational cultural strengths. It is little wonder, given the complexity of Australia's relatively recent colonised past, that trauma continues to disrupt the SEWB of First Nations people, and that the expression of the distress that emerges will manifest from time to time as mental illness and distress, behavioural disturbances and even suicide for some people. This is the fact and legacy that Australia must continue to address, and mainstream mental health services are instrumental in supporting recovery for First Nations people; however, the magnitude of the recovery before us is profoundly challenging.

It is apparent that the term 'SEWB' is far more encompassing than merely an alternate term to describe 'mental health' and for the management of ill-health. SEWB from a First Nations perspective must include a shared response that holistically unifies meanings as they pertain to individual, family and community. Attempts to define SEWB have been considered across a number of themes: spiritual, racism (Calma et al., 2017; Paradies, 2016), cultural identity, kinship, trauma, connectedness to natural surroundings (living and passed), grief and loss. With historical implications (Le Grande et al., 2017, NACCHO, 1989), many of these themes have formed from a holistic social sciences approach, free from the clinical or biomedically based inferences that are usually linked to contemporary mental health diagnoses related to SEWB matters (Le Grand et al., 2017, Paradies, 2016). The complexity related to adequately defining SEWB is a work in progress, at odds with the taximetrics principles of the biomedical world. Yet enough is known to demonstrate that SEWB considerations are necessary when considering the mental health and wellbeing of First Nations people. The main theme for this section has been to assist readers to make meaning of the significant differences in SEWB when considering mental health in relation to First Nations people (Bourke et al., 2018) and to present a First Nations perspective. The ideas presented here prompt the reader to challenge any *pre-existing assumptions* about clinical and medical notions of diagnoses and the treatment of illnesses that continue to perpetuate the marginalisation of First Nations health experiences. We hope we have been able to invite the consideration of some relevant Indigenous philosophies and explanations about the influence of SEWB for First Nations people from a First Nations standpoint.

CASE STUDY

Dulcie seeks help in the emergency department

Dulcie presents to the emergency department lethargic, diaphoretic and fatigued. She explains that she feels like she has been 'sung', and believes she and her children are in danger. Dulcie presents as well dressed, physically fit, highly educated and able to communicate in English with ease. Dulcie is asking for the doctor to make contact

(cont.)

with a specific, well-known local Aboriginal Elder for help; this confuses her allocated nurse because Dulcie presents as a tall, thin woman with red hair, brown eyes and a fair complexion. Dulcie's nurse assumes that Dulcie is of Caucasian descent and continues her assessments without contacting the Aboriginal Elder identified earlier by Dulcie. Dulcie's mental state appears stable alongside her physical observations, yet Dulcie continues to demand to see this Aboriginal Elder. She remains lethargic and diaphoretic, and is becoming increasingly agitated. Dulcie states that she has no immediate family to help her and begins to shout in Arrernte tongue, which is identified by one of the hospital's Indigenous Health Workers (IHWs), who happens to pass by Dulcie's room.

QUESTION FOR REFLECTION

- What critical assumptions were made about Dulcie without consultation with her?

QUESTIONS FOR REFLECTION

- Think back to a time when your beliefs and values have been misunderstood by another person, when others have made assumptions based on their perspectives about what they think is in your best interests, but where the outcome of these assumptions has resulted in actions or repercussions that are not aligned to your truth, or are undesirable or unfavourable in your view. List some of the emotions and feelings that you can recall from your experience.
- Next (perhaps with your student nurse peers), discuss the emotional responses that arise for you, and suggest ways that initial assumptions might have been challenged and dealt with at an earlier point to bring about a more favourable outcome.
- Expand your discussion to consider how it might be for a First Nations person when assumptions are made about identity based on appearance. How might assumptions reinforce interpersonal or institutional racism, leading to adverse mental health or SEWB outcomes for that person?
- Explore what actions you can reasonably take as a nurse to enhance the SEWB of First Nations people.

Meaningful cultural connection to people and place

Cultural determinants are essential for building a foundational knowledge in a health professional's journey towards person-centred care that is evidence based and translational to the needs of each individual. Cultural determinants can dictate the efficacy of service delivery and the effectiveness of the outcomes for the person receiving treatment (Bourke et al., 2018; Kelly et al., 2009). As a result of research conducted with Indigenous Australians residing in rural and remote communities who utilise SEWB services, Carey (2013) has shown that mental health is a significant issue in these regions, but that the determinants of health are not meaningfully prioritised and categorised using the biomedical principles that usually dominate mainstream mental health service. Rather, First Nations people experience an amplification of factors that are better encapsulated by a cultural and spiritual framework that enables meaningful inclusion of elements and requirements necessary to maintain important notions such as connectedness, tradition, language, custom and social cohesion (Carey, 2013). A core principle of connection to people and place underpins positive SEWB for many First Nations people, and this needs to be considered, prioritised and accommodated within strategies and services that seek to support the mental health of First Nations people.

CASE STUDY

Werker is transferred to hospital

Werker is a young woman who was transferred to a large regional hospital via the Royal Flying Doctor Service (RFDS) from a remote community in Far North Queensland.

Werker was first brought to a remote community hospital by her aunt, who was concerned for her wellbeing. Werker's Aunty Nora reported to health professionals that Werker had been living at Nora's home for the past two weeks. She stated that Werker tended to lead an itinerate lifestyle when she was smoking marijuana, despite her family's efforts to provide her with stable living conditions.

Aunty Nora has noticed that since Werker has arrived at her home, she has experienced severe mood swings, had minimal sleep and has some scars on her arms from possible self-harming events.

Werker identifies as both Aboriginal and Torres Strait Islander. She is twenty years old and this is the first time she has been separated from her tight-knit family and community.

Werker had to travel alone due to her family being unable to afford to accompany her, and this frightened her further into silence since her departure from her remote community. Werker has a mobile phone with her family's contact details in it and a small overnight bag of clothing.

As a nurse from the Acute Care Team, you are allocated to Werker and begin your intake assessment process in conjunction with the on-call psychiatric registrar.

Werker has remained silent throughout your assessment, and more information is required to probe for possible mental illness and substance use, and to understand the biopsychosocial issues that have led to this referral.

(cont.)

QUESTIONS FOR REFLECTION

- Imagine that you have never travelled further than a radius of 200 kilometres from your family and community of origin, and that you have never flown in a small plane. What are some of the worries and concerns that you might have about where you are going, and what you have left behind? How will you find your way back to your home and people?
- People with emerging mental illness sometimes experience cognitive dysfunction, emotional dysregulation and perceptual alterations. This can make it difficult to think clearly, make personal decisions and trust others, especially in unfamiliar surroundings. The confusion can be exacerbated by substance use or misuse. Among your peers, discuss how you might implement cultural safety and SEWB strategies to support the development of a therapeutic relationship with Werker and ease her possible discomfort related to her physical separation from her people and place.

Connections to culture and the natural environment

Connection to Country is intrinsically aligned with SEWB for many First Nations people and this has been shown to support mental health wellbeing for many people (Commonwealth of Australia, 2017; Salmon et al., 2019). A positive connection to Country is characterised by strong emotional attachment to land, the natural environment, cultural practice and spirituality (Salmon et al., 2019). For example, a connection to the natural environment can been associated with a deep sense of connection to the life–death–life cycle, and characterised by a sense of 'welcome' or perhaps 'caution' or 'warning' derived from a spiritual awareness of the links between culture, spirituality and the person. Cultural and spiritual attunement to the natural world is further enhanced as people practise their culture, and cultural practice enhances care for Country entwined with the reciprocal nature of caring and sharing for and with others (Salmon et al., 2019). The loss of cultural connection to Country is a risk factor for poorer SEWB and other health outcomes.

A loss of this connection can arise:

- as a result of birthing and living 'off Country'
- as a result of experiencing less physical proximity with traditional lands and kinship.
- due to forced removal from Country and kin (e.g. through child removal, as part of the Stolen Generations, for mental health treatment, during incarceration)
- from urbanisation – and relocation/s where access to shared cultural practice is limited
- through dispossession of traditional lands – for example, disrespect shown to cultural sacred sites.

(Hepburn, 2020; Salmon et al., 2019)

All these types of events can be interpreted as a cultural and spiritual traumatisation/s that can expose First Nations people to SEWB vulnerability. Such exposures should therefore be considered during a comprehensive mental health assessment. The erosion of resilience through these types of events demonstrates a public mental health need to ensure that mental health promotion and primary care strategies include elements that authentically seek to enhance and foster the practice of culture among First Nations people to prevent the deterioration of SEWB generally and to reduce the mental illness burden for First Nations people.

QUESTION FOR REFLECTION

- Mindfulness is a useful strategy to assist with developing an appreciation of the linkages between culture and Country and in this case, to assist people to mindfully ground with the First Nations land they are presently on, and to pay attention to the deep history of Country, and allow this attention to transcend past and present, bringing poignance and connection to the present moment.
- Listen to the 10-minute audio clip, *Back to Country: A Guided Reflection on Sovereignty* (https://backto.country). Take note of the sensations and emotions you experience and consider how mindful connection to culture might be able to be incorporated into your nursing practice – for example, as a self-care strategy and/or as a mechanism to enhance your capacity for therapeutic agency as you provide mental healthcare and support for First Nations people in the future.

Social and emotional wellbeing in mainstream mental healthcare

Trauma-informed care

One useful model for assessing SEWB and treating mental health conditions in the mainstream mental health setting is the adoption of **trauma-informed care** (Commonwealth of Australia, 2017). Mental health nursing care responds to people in distress by rendering person-centred trauma-informed care interventions. For example, a person who has acquired a soft tissue injury (trauma) may have bruising and swelling, and they may experience pain (distress) that restricts their usual range of ability (movement range) and functioning. In one sense, the same can be said of psychological or cultural stresses. Distress is one possible human response to trauma and, in a similar way, it can alter a person's capacity to interact and function with a normal range of ability, adaptability, resilience and flexibility. Trauma causes distress, and at some point in life everyone experiences trauma of some kind – for example, personal, communal, racism, social, environmental, family, grief ... the list could go on. The principle is that humans experience trauma, and it is a typical life occurrence that can occur within a normal range of life experiences, with a low level of disruption. These life experiences vary in their intensity, and occasionally they require us to seek help or support from others. Nurses frequently are called upon to help at these times.

trauma-informed care A form of care that assumes that the help-seeking person is seeking help to address an episode of distress that is the result of some experience of trauma (Procter et al., 2017b).

A nurse's role is to assess the trauma experience and to respond in a way that reduces the distress associated with the trauma – that is, to provide an intervention that promotes comfort and eases pain.

Trauma-informed care is operationalised in the way that mainstream service providers, in our case nurses who work in mental healthcare settings (in-patient or community), make one initial assumption when they first meet a service-seeking person in mental distress – that is, that the person they are meeting and with whom they are beginning to develop a therapeutic rapport will have had exposure to some form of trauma (Procter et al., 2017b). The distress is a likely symptom of an underlying trauma, intergenerational trauma or multiple traumas, and could be organic or inorganic in nature (Commonwealth of Australia, 2017). When a nurse engages with a patient in this way, it enables a narrative that acknowledges a wide breadth of possibility that trauma has occurred at some point, and this standpoint extinguishes any counter-narrative of shame, embarrassment and the need to conceal. It opens the possibility of talking freely about sensitive, complex and difficult human experiences and painfulness. It also creates an alliance that positions the help-seeking person (or community) as an equal in the therapeutic relationship, and an authentic fully involved partner in the co-design of a recovery plan (Douglas et al., 2019). In this way, the nurse practises person-centredness by being with the person (or people) in distress, and by creating a SEWB environment in which they can authentically share information and decide together how they will act to reduce the pain and work towards a planned recovery (Commonwealth of Australia, 2017).

Promoting resilience

mental health The ability to cope with adversity, and the common daily stressors associated with living a regular life, while drawing from life meaningfully and with satisfying social and cultural engagement and positive community contributions (Procter et al., 2017a).

The vocabulary we use to describe mental health and mental illness is often counter-intuitive. Often, society uses the term '**mental health**' when what they mean to convey is either mental health problems (pre-diagnostic) or diagnostic categories of mental illness. This is frequently cause for confusion (Happell et al., 2013).

Resilience can be defined as the ability to bounce back and cope positively with adversity, and to draw forward the capacity for mental health and wellbeing (Foster et al., 2019). Mental health problems usually precede a formal diagnostic categorisation, and can be thought of as the mild to moderate conditions that emerge as a result of trauma and that manifest with varying degrees of distress. Often at this early stage, if a mental health problem can be identified and is followed up with implementation of suitable strategies, we can anticipate that recovery can be achieved to ameliorate the distress experienced by the person (Wilson, Wilson & Usher, 2015). For example, implementing mental health promotion and prevention strategies is ideal, as is the use of self-help or guided help strategies as a scaffolding for building early-stage resilience. These strategies are particularly suited to lessening the impact of conditions such as mild to moderate anxiety and/or depression, which are experienced by many people as a response to stressful trauma and can be triggered early in life, with many people experiencing a first episode of mild anxiety or depression between the ages of fourteen and 24 years (Murray et al., 2012). The development of healthful relationships that foster, social and environmental connection, respect and authenticity acts to promote resilience and personal agency to cope positively with stress and adversity, rather than being negatively overwhelmed by them (Stokols, Lejano & Hipp, 2013). The formation of resilience helps to mitigate the effects of trauma characterised by distress (Commonwealth of Australia, 2017). Person-centred health-promotion strategies enable an early opportunity to formulate and maintain personal resilience, and to promote wellbeing and/or recovery (Commonwealth of Australia, 2017).

Mental health nurses who are able to harness the capacity of person-centred mental healthcare while maintaining their own therapeutic agency to draw alongside others, and invest their emotional intelligence into the therapeutic relationship, will demonstrate the prerequisite professional competency that enables shared decision-making aligned with resilience-forming therapeutic outcomes within the care-delivery environment.

Strengths-based approaches: A social ecological perspective

Fundamentally, it is important to keep in mind that patients generally are equipped with an assortment of strengths – that is, the acquisition of positive personal attributes that can be extrapolated for advantage as a meaningful contribution to recovery planning. In the midst of the intensity (or absence) of emotion or distress that accompanies episodes of mental health deterioration, the repertoire of strength accumulation may need to be reinvoked and invigorated. Reframing techniques that attempt to denote the future positively and with optimism can act to instil hopefulness, not by manufacturing false hope, but by authentically interrogating the capacity for future success based on the accumulation of past successes and combined with the attributes for building new or renewed resilience.

A strengths-based approach actively looks for these personal qualities and includes them as respectfully and authentically as possible, reinforcing them and denoting them positively. A positively denoted narrative invites a help-seeker and health-provider discourse that is able to contribute to a hope-infused recovery narrative and demonstrates to the person being helped the enabling resilience that is inherently and authentically represented within them. Guiding the person to connect, or reconnect, with their internalised self-worth, value and capacity helps them to scaffold the resources within themselves, in combination with other assistive interventions, to co-design recovery with the mental health nurse as facilitator.

This collection of strengths can be seen from a social ecological perspective and describes the way that people interact and transact with each other and within the community or landscape where they experience their internal and external lives (Bronfenbrenner, 2005). Broadly speaking, an assessment of strengths can be formulated and described as the layers of personal and social capital that one has across a number of domains: first, a recognition of the *individual* and their current level of physiological and psychological fitness; second, the positive attributes and enabling supports associated with their *microsystem* of close family, friends and culture; third, the helpful characteristics and capacity contained within the person's *mesosystem* – for example, with work colleagues, community neighbourhoods, personal interest and/or sporting clubs, and social and cultural organisations; and lastly, an audit of the enablers for strength and safety in the wider *mesosystem* characterised by policies, public services and legal frameworks to support public good (Bronfenbrenner, 2005). The ecological principles that underlie strength-based approached to person-centred care require us to pay attention to the person, and their relationships (interactions and transactions) in the context of the environmental conditions and/or constraints that influence the capacity for a person to thrive with an aptitude for resilience (Wilson 2016; Wilson et al., 2015). Care needs to be taken to identify any traumatic threat/s to robust and resilient mental health that might result in a failure to develop and maintain sufficient personal mental health capital (resilience) for a person's mental health to thrive (Wilson et al., 2015). A strengths-based person-centred approach to mental healthcare requires that nurses develop a wide range of skills in assessing the mental health of a person who presents seeking help in the context of a distressing response to trauma/s. However, working with that person through to the recovery phases requires the nurse to be able to identify a wide range of factors that impact the patient's wellbeing and adaptive capacity, culminating in implementing a plan of care that harnesses the inherent strengths associated with that person and/or community, culture at that particular time and place.

Threats to social and emotional wellbeing

There are many ways in which racial discrimination, whether internalised (unconscious), interpersonal or institutional, acts individually or collectively to threaten the integrity of SEWB for First Nations people (Kelaher et al., 2018). For example, one survey revealed that Australian school students who had experienced direct or vicarious racial discrimination also experienced higher levels of socioemotional and sleep problems (Priest et al., 2020). Another study was able to draw on Australia Bureau of Statistics (ABS) data about experiences of racial discrimination and found that older First Nations people who have experienced racism are likely to actively avoid situations where they have experienced racism in the future (Temple, Kelaher & Paradies, 2020). This avoidance reinforces disadvantage and limits access to services, leading to psychological distress and poorer SEWB and worse mental health for older First Nations people (Temple et al., 2020). It is notable that racial discrimination, as seen in these two examples, appears to have adverse outcomes for SEWB for First Nations people across the lifespan. As stated by Temple et al. (2020, p. 189), 'discrimination, including racism … is a violation of human rights and should be prevented in any reasonable society'.

Sorry Business and Sad News (Torres Strait Islander): Grief and loss

For First Nations people, death and dying have strong cultural significance, with Sorry Business (Aboriginal) and Sad News (Torres Strait Islander) protocol and ceremony important aspects of the mourning process (NSLHD, 2015; Queensland Health, 2015). Family will gather together, and frequently in large numbers; the reciprocal caring and sharing during this time is a particular feature of First Nations cultural practice. For some, these practices will assist in supporting cultural proximity by connecting the person and community to their Country at a time where they may be physically distant from their Land. Sometimes cultural lore requires smoking ceremonies, and other protocols, such as not speaking the name of the deceased for a long time, among other practices (NSLHD, 2015). Nurses have a role in facilitating and supporting Sorry Business wherever possible – for example, arranging space for people to gather, showing meaningful respect and using open disclosure communication to support the SEWB of the community.

First Nations people throughout Australia experience disproportionate and prolonged grieving, and while there are many reasons for this (for example, health disparity, dispossession of land and colonisation, intergenerational trauma, high numbers of deaths in custody), it is particularly relevant in this chapter that we also acknowledge that suicides in Australia (whole of population) have previously exceeded 3000 people per year with prevalence for Aboriginal and Torres Strait Islander peoples at twice the rate of the general population (Salmon et al., 2019; Wright et al., 2020). The cumulative impact of such extensive exposure to Sorry Business leads to prolonged and complex grieving, and this can be recognised as an antecedent for deterioration in SEWB and mental illness.

Prison

Throughout Australia's colonised past, and persisting to this day, First Nations people have been over-represented in prison, dealt with mercilessly, with whole prisons and even whole islands dedicated to the incarceration of First Nations people (Weatherburn, 2014). Well before the Royal Commission into Aboriginal Deaths in Custody (Johnston, 1991), Eggleston (1976) set out to understand the nature of First Nations experiences with the judicial system. She considered two possible explanations for the large number of First Nations people in prisons: either that Aboriginal people have great levels of criminality or that the system is discriminatory. It is important to rigorously explore the possibilities. Could it be that Aboriginal people commit more crimes? Is that why they are over-represented in prisons? And if so, what could be the possible explanations for this occurrence? Or is a counter explanation that an institutional bias exists, and this circumstance makes it more likely for judicial process of First Nations offenders in a sequence that makes a particular course of action more likely. For example, if a young person commits an offence and comes to the attention of the police early, and then a subsequent event occurs within a 'warning' timeframe, an escalation of response is achieved whereas, if offences are spread out across a larger time span, they may be dealt with using a less restrictive frame of consequences. This possibility might explain a representational difference (Weatherburn, 2014).

There is a significant over-representation of incarcerated First Nations people in Australian (ALRC, 2017). First Nations adults make up 2 per cent of the whole Australian adult population, but constitute 27 per cent of all incarcerated adults in Australian prisons (ALRC, 2017, p. 40). Meanwhile, First Nations people make up 5 per cent of the 10–17-year-old age group in Australia, but this cohort makes up half of the juvenile population under correctional supervision every day (AIHW, 2020). Esteemed leaders at the First Nations Convention in 2017 responded in a statement:

> Proportionally, we are the most incarcerated people on the planet. We are not an innately criminal people. Our children are aliened from their families at unprecedented

> rates. This cannot be because we have no love for them. And our youth languish in detention in obscene numbers. They should be our hope for the future.
>
> These dimensions of our crisis tell plainly the structural nature of our problem. *This is the torment of our powerlessness.*
>
> (https://ulurustatement.org)

It seems explicit that a systemic discriminatory bias exists within our judicial institutions, and this creates a circumstance whereby First Nations are more likely to be charged, rather than to receive a warning, and incarcerated as a consequence of process. By extension, it is logical to suggest that sense of hopelessness and powerlessness might exist for First Nations individuals and communities exposed to an institutional bias that results in the profoundly perverse over-representation of First Nations people in detention and prison in Australia. A lack of hope for the future is well recognised as a threat to resilience, SEWB and mental health, and is a significant factor in suicidality. It is imperative that action is taken to dismantle racism in all forms to improve the SEWB of First Nations people (Geia et al., 2020)

CASE STUDY

Donna – Indigenous Health Worker

Donna is an Indigenous Health Worker (IHW) employed in a public health community health team in a rural community. She works in a collaborative care team and often alongside nurses, psychologists, social workers and doctors. She is referred to as 'Aunty Donna' by many of the Aboriginal young people who are clients of the mental health service. This is not only a recognition of kinship, but also of respect for Donna's position as an esteemed member of the local Aboriginal community. While the Aboriginal community holds her in high regard, it is not always the case that her health colleagues respect her in the same way. As a health service staff member, she has little authority, power or influence, with other clinicians making decisions about diagnoses, treatment plans and issuing instructions about their implementation to staff such as Donna, who are expected to comply without question. The health service has a governance structure that reinforces institutional power and uses a diagnostic biomedical model to assess and admit patients for access to health services. Cultural safety is difficult to achieve in such an environment, for both First Nations patients and staff. Donna has worked on and off as an IHW for many years. She finds the social and emotional toll on her own health overwhelming at times, and as a result resigns from her position. However, after a period of time she returns to a new position in the health service. Her line managers find it inconvenient to have these disruptions to their staff recruitment and retention workforce dynamics, and label the behaviour 'unreliable'. Donna finds it difficult to align her social, cultural and professional worlds, and feels powerless to change the circumstances. She recounts the experience of working with mental health staff who provide mental health 'care' to Aboriginal young people:

> I listened to a mental health worker tell an Aboriginal mother that her son with a mental health condition is better off in gaol, because access to treatment is better there. Do you know what they do? (Emotion welling in her tone) After they send a kid to gaol? They buy morning tea. Chocolate cake! And celebrate … the mental health staff (in a loud anger-filled tone). Yep. An orange cake today? Or a tea cake?
>
> The mental health workers said to me, 'Are you coming? Are you coming to have cake? To celebrate? He is GONE, he is off our hands.'
>
> … All those kids have SO many problems and SO many issues, and the mental health staff don't know how to address them. I think they are just leaving them down there (in gaol) to get them out of the way … they are getting sent (quiver in her voice) for so long, that by the time they get out, the next generation is coming through. And it is just going to go on like a cycle.
>
> But, how could they buy morning tea? (Disgust in her tone) … and celebrate when a kid goes to gaol?
>
> Mmmmmm sad … (a long silent reflective pause). There is a BIG gap between the mental health workers and the client.
>
> (Wilson, 2009)

The child to whom Donna is referring in this account is her nephew.

QUESTIONS FOR REFLECTION

- The promotion of SEWB and cultural safety in the multidisciplinary mental health setting workplace is important for promoting staff wellbeing. As a future nursing professional, can you suggest some ways that you might contribute to the SEWB and cultural safety of your First Nations colleagues? Discuss them with your student peers.
- Donna claims a gap exists between mental health workers and their First Nations clients. Based on your readings in the chapter, suggest some practical steps you can implement to generate therapeutic rapport and agency with First Nations people who require mental healthcare.

Promotion of social and emotional wellbeing

As raised earlier in this chapter, personal identification as a First Nations person is a determinant that has been associated with SEWB. While the practice of culture is beneficial to SEWB generally, the racism associated with identification can be detrimental to SEWB. Intra-racial exclusion and 'colourism' have been identified as factors impacting the SEWB and mental health of some First Nations people (Doyle, Hungerford & Cleary, 2017). Indigeneity is not determined by skin colour in Australia, but rather by an individual's heritage, their acceptance by a First Nations community and their participation in Indigenous community life (Carlson, 2016; Maddison, 2013). Doyle et al. (2017) have identified some ways in which mental health nurses might be able to support the SEWB for people who identify as Indigenous when they access mental health services. The following questions are a useful guide and can inform appropriate referral to Indigenous Mental Health Workers (IMHWs) and treatment planning:

- Are you living on-country or off-country?
- Are you a new move-in to this location? If so, how has that affected the way you are feeling?
- Do you know your Indigenous family?
- Did you grow up knowing you were Indigenous?

(Doyle et al., 2017)

Promoting men's social and emotional wellbeing

Supporting SEWB for First Nations men can be promoted by understanding the cultural strengths and sharing their story. A negative discourse about First Nations men often dominates popular media. A practical example that is useful for promoting SEWB is noted in a project that promoted men's health whereby older men teach, support and nurture younger men in cultural practices with benefits that extend to helping to foster resilience within communities. Some esteemed First Nations men (Adams & Collard, 2020) captured stories in communities that countered the negative discourse, replacing it with a positive narrative about cultural strengths and in sharing stories and knowledge about the strengths of First Nations young men and supporting the role they play, and aspire to play, in their relationships, families and communities (Adams & Collard, 2020). These types of activities instil hope and develop resilience and capability; they also contribute an important buffer for adversity.

CASE STUDY

Kai and Betti

Kai is an eighteen-year-old man who was recently released from a Youth Detention Centre and has returned home to live with his mother, Betti.

Kai has been experiencing difficulties with getting his life back on track and is currently a jobseeker.

Kai is the eldest son in the family and is the eldest male out of all of his cousins, so there is a lot of pressure on him to take up significant cultural responsibilities; however, Kai is focused on enjoying his youth and is often out socialising for several days at a time.

Betti is worried about Kai because she had discovered over time some troubling messages on his mobile from a teenage woman about a rocky relationship and the woman's request for Kai to stop drinking to solve his deeper issues.

Betti discovered Kai had made preparations to hang himself in the morning instead of attending men's business with his uncles.

Betti wants to handle this situation with her family in a culturally safe manner, and reports this to you. Betti states, 'Kai hates seeing doctors about anything. If I pull him up, he will run away. Kai is traumatised from a childhood experience with health services'.

As you are Betti's 'Hospital in the Home' nurse, you are responsible for her wound care but you cannot ignore the situation that Betti is facing with Kai.

QUESTION FOR REFLECTION

- From a holistic perspective, discuss in a small group with your peers some suggestions to promote SEWB for Betti and Kai that you can take from what you have learned reading this chapter.

Conclusion

This chapter has only been able to offer some introductory concepts and examples about SEWB for First Nations people in a mainstream mental health context. We have examined some of the determinants of SEWB. The chapter has explored some of the relationships First Nations people have with each other, the natural environment, and Country and culture, and identified where some SEWB strengths can be harnessed. We have contextualised SEWB in mainstream mental health service-delivery models and used some case studies to enhance our discussion. We have looked at some of the threats to SEWB integrity for First Nations people, and identified some ways in which nurses can support the SEWB of First Nations people in their care. We have identified that there is a pressing need in Australia for mental health nursing to work towards continuing to dismantle internalised (unconscious), interpersonal and institutional racism in healthcare institutions and processes (Kelaher et al. 2018), and the need to continue in the development of nursing expertise, cultural awareness and sensitivity to the improve the promotion of SEWB for First Nations people (Geia et al., 2020; Hunt et al., 2015; Molloy et al., 2019).

Learning activities

Read the *Guidelines for Best Practice Psychosocial Assessment of Aboriginal and Torres Strait Islander People Presenting to Hospital with Self-harm and Suicidal Thoughts* (Leckning et al., 2019).

1. Revise the case studies provided in the chapter and draft some questions you would like to ask the people represented in the case studies to explore aspects of psychological risk as described in the Guidelines. Page 19 in particular will be helpful for this learning activity.

2. With a learning partner, either in person or online in your study groups, role-play asking and critiquing the questions you have devised.
3. 'Culture or culturally based interventions are known to improve SEWB' (Bourke et al., 2018). Discuss this statement in a small group, or as an individual journal/ blog writing exercise, or in an online class forum.
4. As a future professional Registered Nurse, you will be required to meet the Registered Nurse Standards for Practice in Australia (NMBA, 2020). Thinking about what you have learnt in this chapter, consider the following:

   Standard 1: Thinks critically and analyses nursing practice. 1.3: respects all cultures and experiences, which includes responding to the role of family and community that underpin the health of Aboriginal and Torres Strait Islander peoples and people of other cultures.

   Using this as your basis, write a short letter to your future RN self that outlines your top three priorities for the promises you intend to keep when caring for First Nations people who require nursing care in the mainstream mental health setting.

FURTHER READING

Andersen, K., Henderson, J., Howarth, E., Williamson, D., Crompton, D. & Emmerson B. (2015). Way forward: An Indigenous approach to well-being. *Australasian Psychiatry*, 23(6), 609–13.

Commonwealth of Australia (2017). *National Strategic Framework for Aboriginal and Torres Strait Islander Peoples' Mental Health and Social and Emotional Wellbeing*. Canberra: DPMC. Retrieved from www.niaa.gov.au/sites/default/files/publications/mhsewb-framework_0.pdf

Dudgeon, P., Milroy, H. & Walker, R. (2014) (eds). *Working Together: Aboriginal and Torres Strait Islander Mental Health and Wellbeing Principles and Practice*. Canberra: Commonwealth of Australia.

Leckning, B., Ringbauer, A., Robinson, G., Carey, T. A., Hirvonen, T. & Armstrong, G. (2019). *Guidelines for Best Practice Psychosocial Assessment of Aboriginal and Torres Strait Islander People Presenting to Hospital with Self-harm and Suicidal Thoughts*. Darwin: Menzies School of Health Research.

Visit the companion website at www.cambridge.org/highereducation/isbn/9781108794695/resources to see further online resources.

REFERENCES

Adams, M. & Collard, L. (2020). *Valuing Aboriginal and Torres Strait Islander Young Men*. Video. Retrieved from https://youtu.be/vpRXhN5IfJY

AIHW (2020). *Youth Justice*. Canberra: AIHW. Retrieved from www.aihw.gov.au/reports/australias-welfare/youth-justice

ALRC (2017). *Pathways to Justice: An Inquiry into the Incarceration Rate of Aboriginal and Torres Strait Islander Peoples: Summary Report*. Retrieved from www.alrc.gov.au/publication/pathways-to-justice-inquiry-into-the-incarceration-rate-of-aboriginal-and-torres-strait-islander-peoples-alrc-133-summary.

Bello-Bravo, J. (2019). When is indigeneity: Closing a legal and sociocultural gap in a contested domestic/international term. *AlterNative: An International Journal of Indigenous Peoples*, 15(2), 111–20.

Bourke, S., Wright, A., Guthrie, J., Russell, L., Dunbar, T. &Lovett, R. (2018). Evidence review of Indigenous culture for health and wellbeing. *The International Journal of Health, Wellness, and Society*, 8(4), 11–27.

Bronfenbrenner, U. (2005). Ecological systems theory. In U. Bronfenbrenner (ed.), *Making Human Beings Human: Bioecological Perspectives on Human Development*. Thousand Oaks, CA: Sage, pp. 106–73.

Calma, T., Dudgeon, P. & Bray, A. (2017). Aboriginal and Torres Strait Islander social and emotional wellbeing and mental health. *Australian Psychologist*, 52(4), 255–60.

Carey, T.A. (2013). A qualitative study of a social and emotional well-being service for a remote Indigenous Australian community: implications for access, effectiveness, and sustainability. *BMC Health Services Research*, 13(1), 80.

Carlson, B. (2016). *Politics of Identity: Who Counts as Aboriginal Today?* Canberra: Aboriginal Studies Press.

Closing the Gap in Partnership (2020). *National Agreement on Closing the Gap*. Retrieved from www.closingthegap.gov.au/sites/default/files/files/national-agreement-ctg.pdf

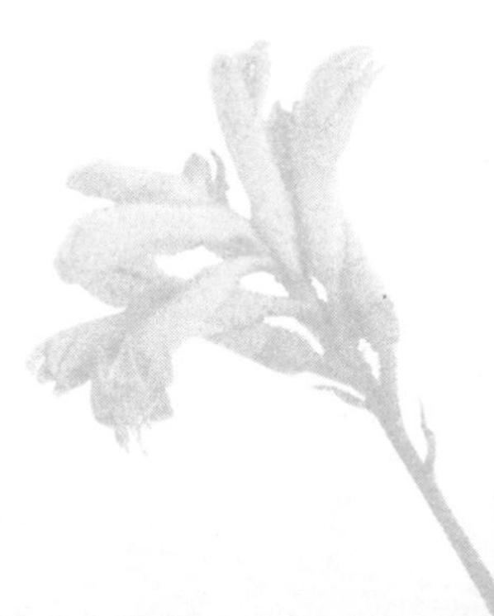

Commonwealth of Australia (2017). *National Strategic Framework for Aboriginal and Torres Strait Islander Peoples' Mental Health and Social and Emotional Wellbeing.* Canberra: DPMC. Retrieved from www.niaa.gov.au/sites/default/files/publications/mhsewb-framework_0.pdf

Douglas, L., Jackson, D., Woods, C. & Usher, K. (2019). Rewriting stories of trauma through peer-to-peer mentoring for and by at-risk young people. *International Journal of Mental Health Nursing*, 28, 744–56 doi:10.1111/inm.12579

Doyle, K., Hungerford, C. & Cleary, M. (2017). Study of intra-racial exclusion within Australian Indigenous communities using eco-maps. *International Journal of Mental Health Nursing, 26*, 129–141.

Eggleston, E. (1976). *Fear, Favour or Affection: Aborigines and the Criminal Law in Victoria, South Australia and Western Australia.* Canberra: ANU Press.

Elvidge, E., Paradies, Y., Aldrich, R. & Holder, C. (2020). Cultural safety in hospitals: Validating an empirical measurement tool to capture the Aboriginal patient experience. *Australian Health Review*, 44, 205–11.

Foster, K., Roche, M., Delgado, C., Cuzzillo, C., Giandinoto, J.-A. & Furness, T. (2019). Resilience and mental health nursing: An integrative review of international literature. *International Journal of Mental Health Nursing*, 28(1), 71–85.

Geia, L., Baird, K., Bail, K., ... Wynn, R. (2020). A unified call to action from Australian nursing and midwifery leaders: Ensuring that Black Lives Matter. *Contemporary Nurse.* doi:10.1080/10376178.2020.1809107

Green, D. and Community of Wagga Wagga (2002). *Wiradjuri Heritage Study for the Wagga Wagga Local Government Area of New South Wales.* Wagga Wagga: Wagga Wagga City Council. Retrieved from https://issuu.com/riversidewaggawagga/docs/wiradjuri_heritage_studyp?e=1541488%2F5197255

Happell, B., Cowin, L., Roper, C., Lakeman, R. & Cox, L. (2013). Mental health and illness assessment. In *Introducing Mental Health Nursing: A Service User-oriented Approach.* (2nd edn). Sydney: Allen & Unwin, pp. 265–92.

Hepburn, S. (2020). Rio Tinto just blasted away an ancient Aboriginal site. Here's why that was allowed. *The Conversation.* 27 May. Retrieved from https://theconversation.com/rio-tinto-just-blasted-away-an-ancient-aboriginal-site-heres-why-that-was-allowed-139466

Hocking, D. (2017). The social and emotional well-being of Aboriginal Australians and the collaborative consumer narrative. In N. Procter, H. Hamer, D. McGarry, R.L. Wilson & T. Froggatt (eds), *Mental Health: A Person Centred Approach.* Melbourne: Cambridge University Press, pp. 73–92.

HREOC (1997). *Bringing Them Home: Report of the National Inquiry into the Separation of Aboriginal and Torres Strait Islander Children from their Families.* Canberra: Commonwealth Government. Retrieved from https://humanrights.gov.au/our-work/bringing-them-home-report-1997

Hunt, L., Ramjan, L., McDonald, G., Koch, J., Baird, D. & Salamonson, Y. (2015). Nursing students' perspective of the health and healthcare issues of Australian Indigenous people. *Nurse Education Today*, 35, 461–7.

Johnston, E. (1991). *Royal Commission into Aboriginal Deaths in Custody, National Report*, 5 vols. Canberra: Australian Government Publishing Service. Retrieved from www.austlii.edu.au/au/other/IndigLRes/rciadic.

Kelaher, M., Ferdinand, A.S., Paradies, Y. & Warr, D. (2018). Exploring the mental health benefits of participation in an Australian anti-racism intervention. *Health Promotion International*, 33, 107–14.

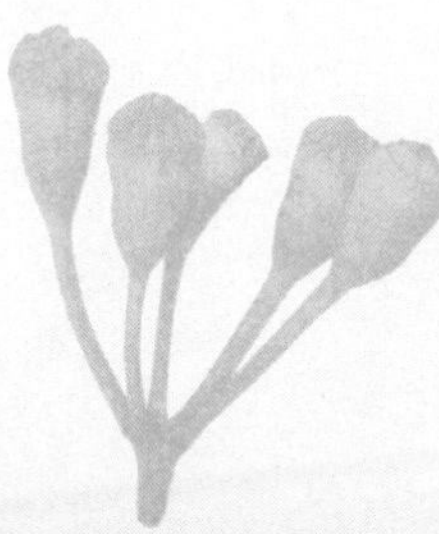

Kelly, K., Dudgeon, P., Gee, G. & Glaskin, B. (2009). *Living on the Edge: Social and Emotional Wellbeing and Risk and Protective Factors for Serious Psychological Distress among Aboriginal and Torres Strait Islander People.* Darwin: Cooperative Research Centre for Aboriginal Health.

Le Grande, M., Ski, C.F., Thompson, D.R., Scuffham, P., Kularatna, S., Jackson, A.C. & Brown, A. (2017). Social and emotional wellbeing assessment instruments for use with Indigenous Australians: A critical review. *Social Science & Medicine*, 187, 164–73.

Leckning, B., Ringbauer, A., Robinson, G., Carey, T. A., Hirvonen, T. & Armstrong, G. (2019). *Guidelines for Best Practice Psychosocial Assessment of Aboriginal and Torres Strait Islander People Presenting to Hospital with Self-harm and Suicidal Thoughts.* Darwin: Menzies School of Health Research.

Macedo, D.M., Smithers, L.G., Roberts, R.M., Haag, D.G., Paradies, Y. & Jamieson, L.M. (2019). Does ethnic-racial identity modify the effects of racism on the social and emotional wellbeing of Aboriginal Australian children? *PLoS One*, 14(8), 1–16.

Maddison, S. (2013). Indigenous identity, 'authenticity' and the structural violence of settler colonialism. *Identities*, 20, 288–303.

Molloy, L., Walker, K., Lakeman, R. & Lees, D. (2019). Encounters with difference: Mental health nurses and Indigenous Australian users of mental health services. *International Journal of Mental Health Nursing*, 28(4), 922–9.

Moreton-Robinson, A. (2013). Towards an Australian Indigenous women's standpoint theory. *Australian Feminist Studies*, 28(78), 331–47.

Murray, C.J.L., Vos, T., Lozano, R. … Lopez, A.D. (2012). Disability-adjusted life years (DALYs) for 291 diseases and injuries in 21 regions, 1990–2010: A systematic analysis for the Global Burden of Disease Study 2010. *Lancet*, 380, 2197–223.

NACCHO (1989). *National Aboriginal Community Controlled Health Organisation Submission to: Committee Secretary Senate Select Committee on Men's Health April 1989.*

NMBA (2020). *Registered Nurse Standards for Practice.* Retrieved from www.nursingmidwiferyboard.gov.au/documents/default.aspx?record=WD16%2f19524&dbid=AP&chksum=R5Pkrn8yVpb9bJvtpTRe8w%3d%3d

NSLHD (2015). *Death and Dying in Aboriginal and Torres Strait Islander (Sorry Business): A Framework for Supporting Aboriginal and Torres Strait Islander Peoples Through Sad News and Sorry Business.* Retrieved from: www.nslhd.health.nsw.gov.au/Services/Directory/Documents/Death%20and%20Dying%20in%20Aboriginal%20and%20Torres%20Strait%20Islander%20Culture_Sorry%20Business.pdf

Paradies, Y. (2016). Colonisation, racism and indigenous health. *Journal of Population Research*, 33, 83e96.

Priest, N., Chong, S., Truong, M. … Kavanagh, A. (2020). Racial discrimination and socioemotional and sleep problems in a cross-sectional survey of Australia school students. *BMJ Open.* doi:10.1136/archdischild-2020–318875

Procter, N., Baker, A., Baker, K., Hodge, L. & Ferguson, M. (2017a). Introduction to mental health and mental illness: Human connectedness and the collaborative consumer narrative. In In N. Procter, H. Hamer, D. McGarry, R.L. Wilson & T. Froggatt (eds), *Mental Health: A Person Centred Approach.* Melbourne: Cambridge University Press, pp. 1–25.

Procter, N., Hamer, H., McGarry, D., Wilson, R. L. & Froggatt, T. (2017b). *Mental Health: A person-centred approach* (2nd edn). Melbourne:Cambridge University Press.

Queensland Health (2015). *Sad News, Sorry Business: Guidelines for Caring for Aboriginal and Torres Strait Islander People Through Death and Dying.* Brisbane: Queensland Health. Retrieved from https://www.health.qld.gov.au/__data/assets/pdf_file/0023/151736/sorry_business.pdf

Salmon, M., Doery, K., Dance, P., Chapman, J., Gilbert, R., Williams, R. & Lovett, R. (2019). *Defining the Indefinable: Descriptors of Aboriginal and Torres Strait Islander Peoples' Cultures and Their Links to Health and Wellbeing.* Canberra: Research School of Population Health, Australian National University.

Stokols, D., Lejano, R.P. & Hipp, J. (2013). Enhancing the resilience of human-environment systems: A social ecological perspective. *Ecology and Society,* 18(1), 7.

Temple, J.B., Kelaher, M. & Paradies, Y. (2020). Experiences of racism among older Aboriginal and Torres Strait Islander People: Prevalence, sources, and association with mental health. *Canadian Journal on Aging,* 39(2), 178–89.

Tsey, K., Wilson, A., Haswell-Elkins, M., Whiteside, M., McCalman, J., Cadet-James, Y. & Wenitong, M. (2007). Empowerment-based research methods: A 10-year approach to enhancing Indigenous social and emotional wellbeing. *Australasian Psychiatry,* 15(supp. 1), S34–38.

Uluru Statement (2017) *The Uluru Statement from the Heart.* Retrieved from https://ulurustatement.org/the-statement

Weatherburn, D. (2014). *Arresting Incarceration: Pathways Out of Indigenous Imprisonment.* Canberra: Aboriginal Studies Press.

Wilson, R.L. (2009). Barriers to the early identification and intervention of early psychosis among young rural males. Unpublished Master's thesis, University of New England.

Wilson, R.L. (2016). An Aboriginal perspective on 'Closing the Gap' from the rural front line. *Rural and Remote Health,* 16. Retrieved from: www.rrh.org.au/articles/subviewnew.asp?ArticleID=3693

Wilson, R. L., Wilson, G.G. & Usher, K. (2015). Rural mental health ecology: A framework for engaging with mental health social capital in rural communities. *EcoHealth,* 12(3): 412–20.

Wright, M., Crisp, N., Newnham, E., Flavell, H. & Lin, A. (2020). Addressing mental health in Aboriginal young people in Australia. *The Lancet Psychiatry.* doi:10.1016/S2215-0366(19)30515–2

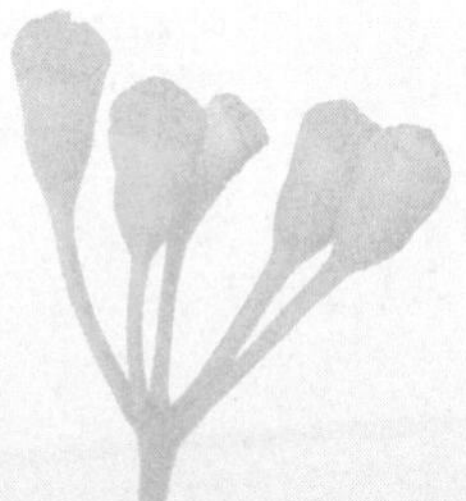

Cultural understandings of Aboriginal suicide from a social and emotional wellbeing perspective

Raelene Ward

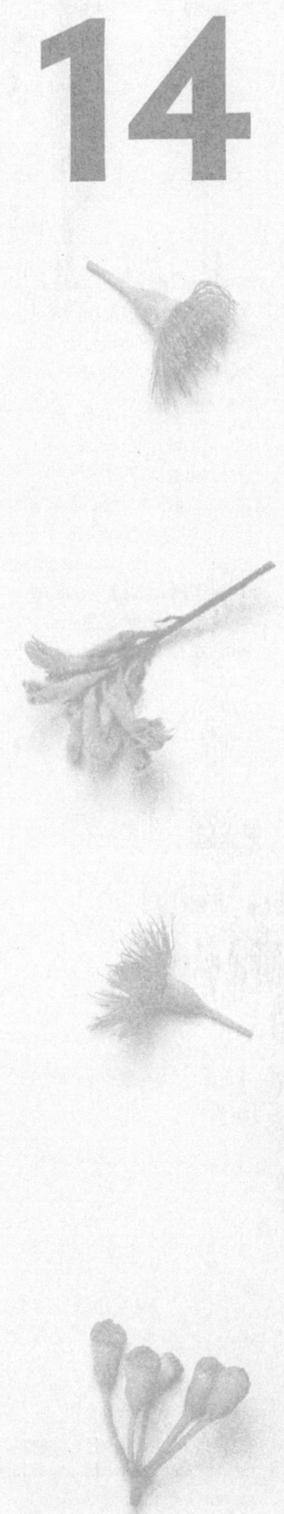

LEARNING OBJECTIVES

This chapter will help you to understand:

- Factors contributing to the rate of suicides and intentional self-harm by Indigenous peoples
- Why suicides are higher in the Aboriginal population than in the general population and how they impact Aboriginal people and communities
- The differences between mental health and social and emotional wellbeing (SEWB)
- Contemporary Indigenous perspectives of SEWB
- The importance of cultural safety in health service provision

KEY WORDS

Aboriginal suicide and/or intentional self-harm
cluster suicides
mental health
psychological distress
social and emotional wellbeing (SEWB)

Introduction

This chapter is written from the perspective of the author's PhD research, which was conducted in four Aboriginal communities (Ward, 2019). This research explores Aboriginal understandings of suicide, including the cultural, behavioural and social aspects of rural, remote, semi-urban and urban Aboriginal communities across the Darling Downs and Southwest Queensland. The chapter will provide the reader with background information on the historical and contemporary understandings of **Aboriginal suicide and/or intentional self-harm** from within a **social and emotional wellbeing (SEWB)** framework. Culturally, suicide has a considerable impact on the family and the wider community, disrupting SEWB and the mental health of Aboriginal and Torres Strait Islander people. SEWB from the Aboriginal or Torres Strait Islander perspective is not completely recognised or valued within the broader healthcare system. Historically in Australia, suicide and self-harm were not evident in traditional Aboriginal and Torres Strait Islander societies before the 1960s (Cantor et al., 1998; Hunter & Milroy, 2006; Parker, 2010, 2012; Ward, 2019). Hence, in today's society, we understand Indigenous suicide as a national catastrophe of significant concern that is gaining momentum as a serious public health issue that is not simple to fix; statistics are likely to under-estimate the true scale of the problem (ATSISPEP, 2015; Georgatos, 2015; MHCNSW, 2013).

Aboriginal suicide and/or intentional self-harm When an Aboriginal person acts on their intention of ending their own life or harming themselves.

social and emotional wellbeing (SEWB) A holistic view of wellness that incorporates individual and community responses to non-medical aspects of health, such as spiritual strength, overall happiness, a sense of purpose and hope for the future.

Understanding Australian Indigenous suicides

For Indigenous people, the history of invasion and colonisation since 1788 has not been a dignified progression, nor one that is encouraging or supportive of SEWB; rather, the costs to people and communities have been catastrophic. Aboriginal and Torres Strait Islander peoples' 'contact history has been one of ignominy and the mood has been miserable for the most part ... and these experiences have had profound implications for the collective and the individual' (Tatz, 2011, p. 1) and their poor SEWB has been linked to past effects of colonisation and government policies, leading to the loss of traditional lands, forced separation of families and loss of cultural identity (Mindframe, 2015). Prior to colonisation, traditional Aboriginal culture provided and supported Aboriginal people with optimal conditions for mental health through physical, social, emotional, cultural and spiritual aspects of wellbeing. Traditionally, mental health from an Aboriginal cultural perspective was understood collectively and linked to 'all aspects of life, community, spirituality, culture and country' (Parker & Milroy, 2014, p. 26).

Aboriginal and Torres Strait Islander people experience higher rates of SEWB problems due to some mental disorders compared with other Australians (Gee et al., 2014). The terminology 'social and emotional wellbeing (SEWB)' is preferred by Indigenous people when describing their mental health as it has a holistic and cultural connotation in contrast to the Western clinical view of mental health (ATSISPEP, 2015). **Mental health** is used mainly by non-Indigenous people when describing mental

mental health A state of wellbeing in which each individual realises their own potential, is able to cope with the normal stresses of life, to work productively and to make a contribution to their community (WHO, 2018).

health disorders (mental illnesses) or problems such as mood/psychotic/substance misuse disorders, crisis reactions, anxiety, depression, post-traumatic stress, self-harm and psychosis. Life experiences that impact Indigenous SEWB are grief and loss, trauma, self-harm, and suicidal thoughts and behaviours (HealthInfonet, 2020). Globally, suicide rates within Indigenous populations are consistently higher than for non-Indigenous populations (Cantor & Neulinger, 2000; Chandler & Lalonde, 1998; Chandler et al., 2003; Procter, 2005).

The burden of disease for mental illnesses is somewhat equally present in both Indigenous and non-Indigenous suicides, with alcohol and substance misuse obvious in Indigenous suicide cases. Many Indigenous people experience mental healthcare by means of hospitalisation in acute mental health wards, rather than by accessing services (health, medical, mental and specialist) in a preventative way and equally, like non-Indigenous people, through their general practitioner. What is evident among many Indigenous people is the type and level of chronic diseases being managed that contribute to early death and psychological distress and trauma (Kanowski, Jorm & Hart, 2009). While relationship issues, often recognised as a major stressful event, are commonly shared between Indigenous and non-Indigenous people (Kõlves, Potts & De Leo, 2015), there is evidence to support that there is a higher level of simultaneous exposure to multiple life stressors for Indigenous people (ABS, 2013). Such exposures include the death of a family member or friend, serious illness, inability to get a job and mental illness (Dudgeon, Calma and Holland, 2017).

As with all data relating to the health and wellbeing of Indigenous people, suicide rates in particular must be interpreted with caution, as they are based on population estimates and hospitalisation and mortality rates, which under-estimate the true figures. The rates of suicide are substantially higher in Indigenous populations as they suffer a higher burden of emotional distress and mental illness than is experienced by the wider community.

Georgatos (2013a, p. 1; 2013b) claims that Australia's First Nations people are suiciding at the world's highest rates. As a society, Aboriginal peoples endure horrific statistics for incarceration, homelessness and suicide. Indigenous suicides account for 4.2 per cent of all deaths (Silburn et al., 2014). The difference between Australia's national suicide rate and Indigenous people's suicide rate is one of the world's worst, particularly for Aboriginal youth (Georgatos, 2015).

The Australian Bureau of Statistics (ABS, 2017) reports that suicide among children and young people aged between five and seventeen years (both Indigenous and non-Indigenous) continues to be the prominent cause of all child deaths. Young Indigenous Australians have one of the highest rate of suicide in the world (ABS, 2017), a common reality in many communities. Indigenous males aged from fifteen to nineteen years are more than four times and Indigenous females nearly six times more likely to die by suicide compared with their non-Indigenous counterparts. Distressingly, Indigenous children under fourteen years of age are nearly eight times more likely to die by suicide compared with their non-Indigenous counterparts.

In 2018, suicide was the leading cause of death for Aboriginal and Torres Strait Islander people, with a total of 169 (24.1 per 100,000) deaths by suicide recorded, a slight increase from 2017's reporting of 165 (24.2 per 100,000) (Figure 14.1). Of the total of 169 deaths, 129 were males and 40 were females, with a median age of 31.8 years for males and 26.0 years for females (ABS, 2018).

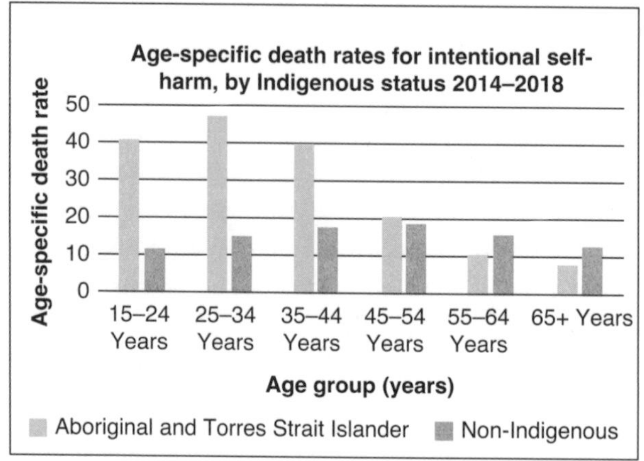

Figure 14.1 In 2018, the Indigenous suicide rate was over double that of other Australians
Sources: CBPATSISP (2020); Dudgeon, Holland & Walker (2019).

Figure 14.2 shows the age-specific death rate for intentional self-harm from 2015–19.

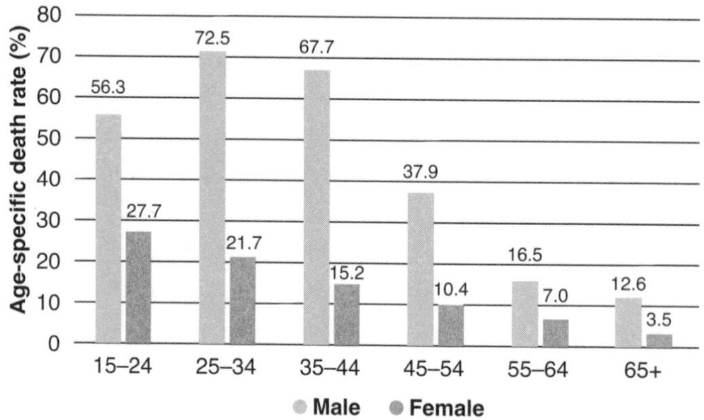

Figure 14.2 Age-specific death rate for intentional self-harm, by sex, 2015–19
Source: Reproduced from ABS (2019).

As Figure 14.3 shows, over a ten-year period, the number of Aboriginal and Torres Strait Islander suicides across the country since 2008, has increased by around 65 per cent.

Georgatos (2013b) undertook a global comparative analysis of suicide data and confirmed 'the prevalence of spates of suicides among Aboriginal Australian youth were the world's worst figures and these spates had become more prevalent and tragically setting higher medians year in and year out.' In the Aboriginal community of Mowanjum, in Western Australia, suicide was 100 times the national average. Aboriginal youth suicide in Australia is higher than any country globally, with the exception of Greenland. The epidemic and vulnerability of Aboriginal and Torres Strait Islander younger people to suicide is reflected in the demographics: the median age

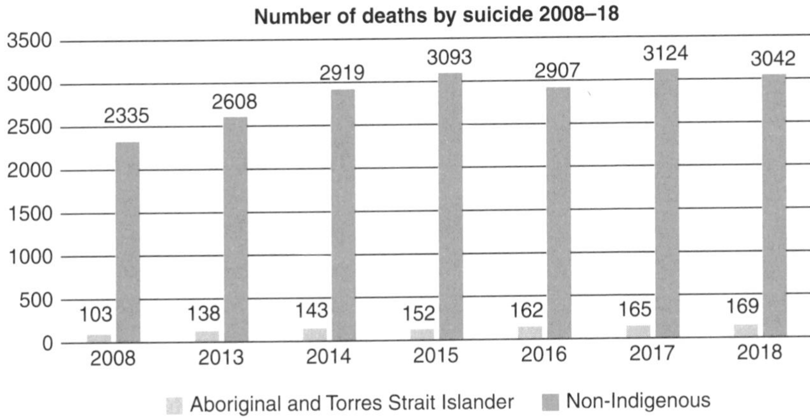

Figure 14.3 Over a ten-year period, the number of Aboriginal and Torres Strait Islander suicides across the country since 2008, has increased by around 65 per cent

Sources: Dudgeon & Luxford (2017); Dudgeon, Holland & Walker (2019).

of death by suicide for Aboriginal people is 21 years, compared with non-Aboriginal people at 37 years (Brown, 2014) (see Figure 14.4).

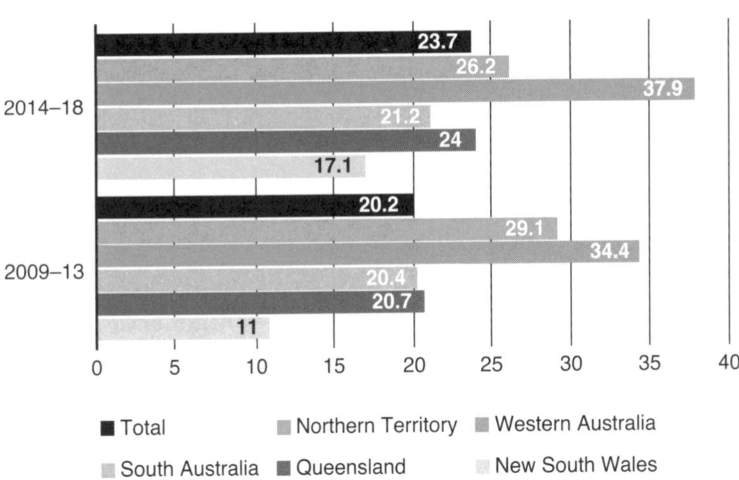

Figure 14.4 Standardised death rates for suicide for Aboriginal and Torres Strait Islander people by state or territory for the years 2009–13 and 2014–18

Source: Based on ABS (2018).

According to 2016 data, intentional self-harm is recognised as the fifth leading cause of death among Aboriginal and Torres Strait Islander people and death rates were twice as high compared with non-Indigenous populations (ABS, 2017). Intentional self-harm for 15–24 and 25–35 year-olds was the leading cause of death for Aboriginal and Torres Strait Islander people in 2012–16. It was further identified that intentional self-harm was much higher in the 25–34 and 35–44 years age groups, particularly for females.

While the suicide rate for people aged over 45 years is lower than for younger cohorts, it is difficult to draw conclusions from the data as fewer Aboriginal and

Torres Strait Islander people live to an age of over 65 years. When a suicide occurs within an Aboriginal and Torres Strait Islander community, there are wide-reaching impacts affecting immediate and extended family members, including those beyond the community. Each Aboriginal and Torres Strait Islander community is closely related and under-represented in the population, with a range of underlying social and health problems compounded by the ongoing cycle of trauma, grief and loss that becomes intergenerational. Therefore, **cluster suicides** can occur simply because Aboriginal and Torres Strait Islander communities are more closely connected; as a result, they become more obvious when trauma, grief and loss are continually being experienced (Kelly, Barnett & Dudgeon, 2009). The nature of cluster suicides means that 'they can unfold over time and alongside existing relationship networks, further compounding and extending the grief, loss and distress experienced by survivors of suicide (i.e. the families and communities)' (Kelly, Barnett & Dudgeon, 2009, p. 7; Ugle et al., 2009). In their analysis of Aboriginal suicides, Hunter and colleagues (2001) identified that clusters of suicides were occurring in particular communities at certain points of time and more frequently than across the general population. This clearly demonstrates that an urgent response is needed for suicide prevention strategies to address risk at the community level, rather than just at the individual level (Pink & Allbon, 2008; Hunter, 2007).

cluster suicides A number or chain of completed suicides in a discrete period of time and within a specific area (town or region), which are connected or said to have a 'contagious' element. Suicide is not itself 'contagious'.

Factors contributing to Indigenous suicides

While overall negative life experiences contribute to poor SEWB, substance abuse (misuse), sexual abuse and trauma contribute to suicide. The additional factors of intergenerational trauma, cumulative acute poverty and a lack of basic human rights continue to impact Aboriginal families and many communities today, and must be considered within this framework. Aboriginal and Torres Strait Islander people continue to experience the negative effects of colonisation and government-imposed policies that were detrimental to the existence of this population and culture. Aboriginal and Torres Strait Islander people were expected to conform to a society with Western ideologies, with the loss of their own culture, traditions and practices, resulting in extended social and health problems and positioning them as a disadvantaged group.

Specific factors associated with the legacy of colonisation that disproportionally impact the SEWB of Indigenous people include 'unresolved grief and loss, trauma and abuse, domestic violence, removal from family, substance misuse, family breakdown, cultural dislocation, racism and discrimination, and social disadvantage' (SHRG, 2004, p. 9). These contribute to the development of **psychological distress** and associated heightened suicide risk (Kelly et al., 2009).

psychological distress A term used to describe a range of symptoms and experiences of a person's internal life that are commonly held to be troubling, confusing or out of the ordinary.

The many traumas and physical illnesses suffered by Indigenous people have caused and continue to cause significant emotional stress, loss and grief for individuals, families and communities (Kitchener, Jorm & Kanowski, 2008). Psychiatrist Paul Brown (2014), working in the field of suicide with Aboriginal and non-Aboriginal communities in Western Australia, Victoria, Queensland and the Northern Territory, hypothesises that over the last ten years Aboriginal suicides have increasingly been related to violence and secularisation; he believes individuals are either driven or abandoned to suicide. In Aboriginal cultures, Brown argues, secularisation is equal to Westernisation. In his local analysis of suicides, he refers to First and Second Nation Australians as the historical-past and contemporary-present, and to historical risk factors for suicides, as they relate to loss of land and culture, trans-generational trauma, grief and loss, racism and social exclusion.

Invasion and subsequent colonisation caused a range of major impacts on the physical wellbeing and SEWB of Indigenous people in Australia. Some of the fundamentals of devastation were the bringing in of new diseases; massacres; removing people from their ancestral land, resulting in psychological distress and spiritual despair; and large groups of Aboriginal people being placed onto reserves, settlements and missions. This destroyed the Aboriginal way of life, leading to marginalisation and poverty. Dispossession and war upon Aboriginal people continued to take its toll on the health and wellbeing of Indigenous populations, denying them access to traditional foods, Country and practices, all of which affected their ability to carry out vital societal, legal and spiritual obligations (see Chapter 1 for further discussion). For Aboriginal and Torres Strait Islander people, colonial policies and practices from the past have unrelenting effects on health and wellbeing – evident in today's inequity in healthcare, economic, social, political, employment and educational outcomes. In spite of current policies aimed at addressing health inequalities for Indigenous people, not much has changed, as the dominant culture continues to create a welfare of dependency, a reliance on the provision of public sector resources and the means of delivery as opposed to Aboriginal control (Ward, 2015; Ward & Gorman, 2010). For these reasons, this public health issue should be approached with an understanding that social and emotional health and psychiatric disorders encompass oppression, racialism, environmental circumstances, economic factors, stress, trauma, grief, cultural genocide, psychological processes and ill-health (Mindframe, 2015).

QUESTIONS FOR REFLECTION

- How does Indigenous history over the last 200 years inform our understanding of suicide?
- What contributes to Aboriginal and Torres Strait Islander people having a high rate of suicide today?
- What group of Aboriginal people is predominantly affected by suicide? Why?

Social and emotional wellbeing vs Western concepts of mental health

Social and emotional wellbeing is about the freedom to communicate needs and feelings, the ability to love and be loved and the ability to cope with stress; it is about being able to relate, create and assert oneself and having options for change that help the development of a problem-solving approach (AHMAC, 2017). The terms 'social wellbeing' and 'emotional wellbeing' are defined differently by various cultural groups and individuals, over time and across the development continuum. The World Health Organization's Ottawa Charter for Health Promotion (WHO, 1986) proclaims that in order to achieve a level of satisfactory health, growth and development, an individual's basic needs must be met. These include peace, shelter, income, food, education, a stable ecosystem, sustainable resources, social justice and equity, all of which must be underpinned by a secure foundation. To achieve this state of health, individuals, families and communities must be allowed to develop free from harm or threat. Health for an individual or group is complete physical, mental and social wellbeing, and the ability to realise aspirations, satisfy needs, and change or cope with the environment (WHO, 1986). Health is understood as a resource for everyday life, not the objective of living.

Aboriginal and Torres Strait Islander peoples hold negative views of the terminology of mental illness and mental disorder. This has sometimes stemmed from negative experiences with mainstream health and welfare agencies, and also arises from the shame and stigma associated with the labelling of mental illness. The Indigenous concept of SEWB should be viewed differently from non-Indigenous concepts of mental health, which originate from illness and assume a clinical viewpoint. The Western concept emphasises the individual and their level of functioning, whereas from an Indigenous health viewpoint the emphasis is on belonging and connecting to everything around you, including the land, culture, spirit, ancestors, family and community (Commonwealth of Australia, 2017) (Figure 14.5).

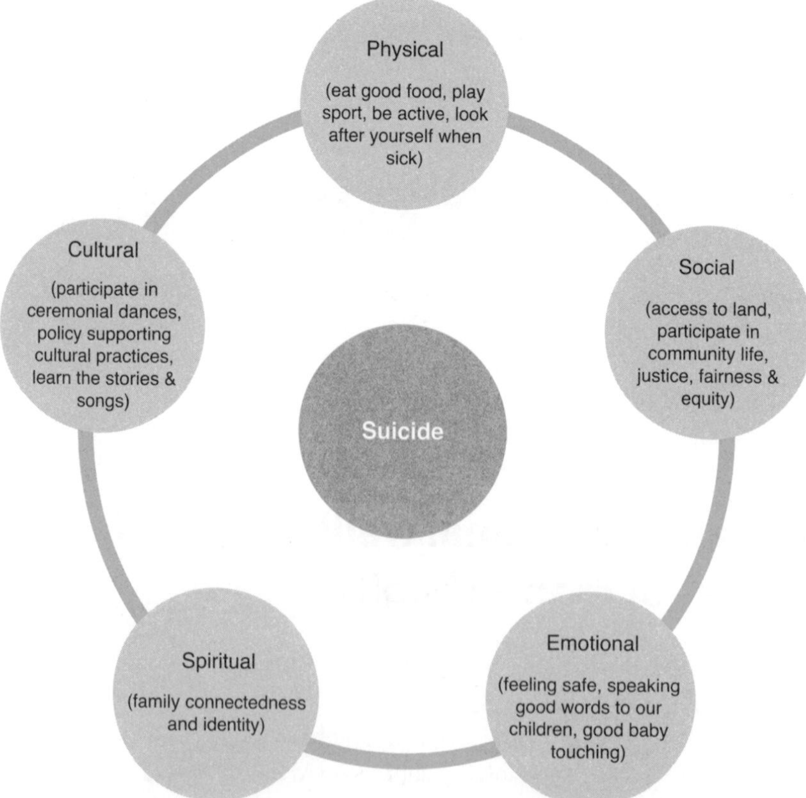

Figure 14.5 'If we don't have good social and emotional wellbeing (SEWB) (physical, social, emotional, spiritual and cultural depicts SEWB elements) we're at risk of mental ill-health and/or suicide.'

Source: Adapted from DHA (2020), p. 1.

From an Aboriginal perspective, holistic health and SEWB (mental health) all complement each other and can be described as encompassing mental, physical, cultural and spiritual health. Land, family and spirituality are central to wellbeing. 'Aboriginal and Torres Strait Islander peoples have great strengths, creativity and endurance and a deep understanding of the relationships between human beings and their environment' (SHRG, 2004, p. 6). Family and kinship are central, as are the bonds of reciprocal affection, responsibility and caring (Kelly, Barnett & Dudgeon, 2009, p. 17).

Aboriginal people and communities are in a constant state of grief and loss, mourning for the loss of loved ones who have died. It is very commonplace for many Aboriginal families to experience a high number of trauma events and funerals simultaneously in many communities, and people will travel long distances out of respect to support families (Ugle et al., 2009).

As explained above, Aboriginal and Torres Strait Islander understandings of SEWB and mental illness are different from those of mental health service providers in Australia. The National Consultancy Report on Aboriginal and Torres Strait Islander Mental Health, *Ways Forward* (Swan & Raphael, 1995), recognises that mental health and wellbeing are integrally linked to a 'whole-of-life' concept, not just a 'whole-body' one. Cultural wellbeing is steeped in harmonised interrelations – spiritual, environmental, ideological, political, social, economic, mental and physical. It is crucial to understand that while the harmony of these interrelations is disrupted, Aboriginal ill-health will persist (NSWMHC, 2013). Aboriginal health is holistic in the sense that a person's health is not considered to be separate from the community's health, and is part of a life–death–life cycle.

To understand the relationship of secularisation and suicide, we need an appreciation of traditional Aboriginal life, in which the ancestral land and the Dreaming were central. Aboriginal people were more than hunters and gatherers; they had sophisticated systems of agriculture and aquaculture, and practices such as fire-sticking (Pascoe, 2014). Community life was rich and varied, with marriage, children and life in tribal groups encompassing large families. People spoke in their traditional languages (tongue) and had rich cultural heritage and intimate knowledge of their land. Aboriginal people did everything in a natural way rather than a Western way. Knowledge of the land and its resources was unique and intimate, and was utilised for food sources, building of transport (such as boats for sea and river faring communities), tools for hunting and the making of medicinal preparations for health. The land's resources and the knowledge that was passed down from generation to generation were used for birthing practices, fixing broken bones, healing wounds and dealing with a whole range of physical ailments.

Aboriginal people encountered the Western way of life at a time when Western society itself was shifting from communalism to individualism. Over the last 200 years, White Australia has 'been trying controlling Aboriginal people through manipulated and self-absorbed policies that exists in a Western cultural framework' (Brown, 2014). Conflict has not only been between blacks and whites; it has also been intergenerational and intra-familial within Aboriginal culture. Intra-individual conflict was equally devastating (Brown, 2014). French sociologist René Girard (in Brown, 2014) argues that Indigenous populations fell prey to Western ways – resulting in the same social ills and adoption of narcissistic habits of self-destruction, such as suicide, alcoholism and crime. For that reason, regeneration or recolonisation of the land, art and culture within diverse communities across Australia, with an emphasis on young people and families, would bring to a halt the progress of increasing suicides, crime and substance misuse. Brown (2014) argues that 'community justice programs are far too downstream, public housing results in suffering consequent upon displacement and kinship networks, relationships and social and cultural needs are overlooked'. Suicide prevention programs from this perspective suggest that suicide is a medical condition mostly due to depression and can 'only be solved by putting pressure on youth and their communities to either prevent or treat clinical mood disorder[s]'. These programs do not work because they 'do not address the core issues of violence and secularisation' (Brown, 2014).

Contemporary understanding of Indigenous social and emotional wellbeing

Aboriginal and Torres Strait Islander health is holistic and encompasses SEWB elements of mental health, physical, social, cultural and spiritual health, which are central to wellbeing through cultural connection to land, family and spirituality (Kelly, Barnett & Dudgeon, 2009, p. 3). Family and kinship are dominant in Aboriginal understandings and ways of doing, in the broader concepts of family and in the connections with shared roles of affection, responsibility and compassion. The challenges in addressing Aboriginal and Torres Strait Islander mental health must be considered in this wider context of health and wellbeing.

Many of the social risk factors for suicide and the connections to SEWB for Indigenous people are tenuous (Elliot-Farrelly, 2004). The causes of suicide need to be analysed further in discussions with Indigenous people and their communities, based on a framework that encompasses a broad and holistic view of the history and of the social and lifestyle issues confronting Indigenous people. Intent is not always obvious, yet in the context of Aboriginal people suicides can often be impulsive and associated with intoxication with either drugs or alcohol (Elliot-Farrelly, 2004; Hunter et al., 2001; Tatz, 1999; Ward, 2019. There is a need to develop and design suicide-prevention strategies specifically to suit Aboriginal people and their communities (Elliot-Farrelly, 2004) and to reflect the cultural differences in how Indigenous people view mental health, suicide and suicidal behaviours.

SEWB and mental health problems can affect anyone, and they are becoming more common among Aboriginal people (Hunter, 2007). A culturally safe solution is therefore needed, one that employs multidimensional strategies that build on existing community strengths and provide counselling and social support for families in crisis situations. These culturally safe services must also provide continuity of care across the lifespan (AHMAC, 2017).

The loss of a life from suicide has a considerable impact on the family and the wider community, resulting in disruption to SEWB for Aboriginal people (De Leo, Sveticic & Milner, 2011). The high rates of Indigenous suicide are not only associated with the interplay of risk and protective factors, but also with broader social, economic and historic factors. Therefore, improving the SEWB of people would reduce the occurrence of suicides for Aboriginal and Torres Strait Islanders (QMHC, 2015).

Contemporary violence

In contemporary times, risk factors for suicide relate to psychiatric disorders, stressful life events and substance abuse, all of which are entrenched in high levels of social disadvantage of unemployment, homelessness, incarceration and family issues (Brown, 2014). In colonial times, violence was related directly to dispossession and oppression, in the form of armed assault upon Aboriginal populations across the country. More recently, Brown (2014) identifies the following as classes of violence as contributing to risk:

- domestic violence
- bullying in schools and the workplace
- interpersonal, gang, crowd and communal violence
- violent persecution of minority groups
- institutional and structural violence.

In Aboriginal societies today, the kind of bullying behaviour being experienced on a face-to-face level can relate to the colour of someone's skin, appearance and dress, being new in the community, cultural connection and cultural identity. Bullying can be experienced through negative experiences online and on social media platforms, with perpetrators referred to as trolls or keyboard warriors, who intimidate, threaten, exclude gossip about and make fun of people (Brown, 2014).

QUESTIONS FOR REFLECTION

- What historical factors contribute to poor SEWB?
- What is the difference between SEWB and mental health?
- What are some of the social factors that contribute to suicide in Indigenous communities?

Cultural safety in suicide prevention

Providing services to support SEWB requires a comprehensive, interdisciplinary approach that considers a holistic view of health, as discussed earlier in this chapter. Access to mental health services must encompass more than simply availability or geographic location, but also include the appropriateness, affordability and acceptability of the service. Providers of mental health services must have a comprehensive understanding of Aboriginal and Torres Strait Islander issues as they relate to mental health, to ensure the delivery of culturally safe SEWB healthcare (IAHA, 2012).

Historically, Aboriginal and Torres Strait Islander people have continually been exposed to various policies different from those for the mainstream population; this has resulted in different social risk factors being experienced by both groups. There is a view of mental health service delivery being overly focused on problems and deficits, individually focused and narrowly oriented toward a medical perspective. A high proportion of Aboriginal people have complex levels of physical illnesses and psychological distress, predisposing them to significant mental health problems, as well as a high death rate (Kanowski, Jorm & Hart, 2009). Limited access to education and knowledge of how to deal with crises while managing their SEWB health problems makes things worse. Mental health strategies need to be developed by Indigenous people to better provide communities and people with services and programs enabling them to recognise, respond to and prevent mental health problems and suicidal behaviours (Swan & Raphael, 1995). The National Strategic Framework for Aboriginal and Torres Strait Islander People's Mental Health and Social and Emotional Wellbeing 2017–2023 recognises the need to increase levels of literacy and awareness regarding mental health within the wider community (Commonwealth of Australia, 2017).

The complexity of needs in Aboriginal communities present a significant challenge to health services, and the Mental Health Commission of New South Wales notes that:

> The complex inter-relationship of cultural, social, economic, historical, individual and environmental factors influencing the mental health and social and emotional wellbeing of Aboriginal people is well documented, as is the collective distress and trauma that exist as underlying stressors to Aboriginal people's lives. Adding to this complexity is the social, cultural and geographical diversity of Aboriginal people and the inappropriateness of a 'one size fits all' approach.
>
> (MHCNSW, 2013, p. 8)

The lack of culturally safe SEWB health services has also been documented, with the National Inquiry into the Human Rights of People with Mental Illness finding that 'mental health professionals had little understanding of Aboriginal culture and society, resulting frequently in misdiagnosis and culturally unsafe treatment', and that 'existing mainstream mental health services were inadequate and culturally inappropriate for Aboriginal people' (cited in MHCNSW, 2013, p. 8).

In its nine guiding principles, the National Strategic Framework for Aboriginal and Torres Strait Islander People's Mental Health and Social and Emotional Wellbeing 2017–2023 includes the principles that 'Self-determination is central to the provision of Aboriginal and Torres Strait Islander health services' and 'Culturally valid understandings must shape the provision of services and must guide assessment, care and management of Aboriginal and Torres Strait Islander people's health, particularly mental health issues' (Commonwealth of Australia, 2017, p. 3). Risk factors for Aboriginal and Torres Strait Islanders' SEWB include traumatic experiences, domestic violence, cultural dislocation and ongoing grief (SHRG, 2004).

Land is central to community connections including the spiritual and emotional wellbeing of Indigenous individuals, families and communities (Kelly, Barnett

& Dudgeon, 2009). Protective factors can relate to a number of influences such as 'connection to land, culture, spirituality, ancestry and family and community' (Kelly, Barnett & Dudgeon, 2009, p. 2). In the face of adversity, these influences can assist Aboriginal and Torres Strait Islander people with resilience and recovery to lessen the impact of stressful situations on SEWB.

The National Strategic Framework for Aboriginal and Torres Strait Islander Peoples' Mental Health and Social and Emotional Wellbeing 2017–2023 reaffirms and extends on health as a multidimensional concept that recognises the strengths, resilience and diversity of Aboriginal and Torres Strait Islander peoples and their communities (Commonwealth of Australia, 2017).

Aboriginal and Torres Strait Islander cultures must be understood in view of their origins, and the differences in their history, lifestyles, families, communities, values and beliefs in relation to health and wellbeing, mental health and suicide. Each group or community is different in how these aspects are considered and valued by Aboriginal and Torres Strait Islander people and how they are interpreted by the wider health system. When this is acknowledge and addressed within communities and across Australia, health service provision will improve (Dudgeon et al., 2010).

QUESTIONS FOR REFLECTION

- What are the five principles of cultural safety in nursing?
- How do the principles of cultural safety inform your nursing practice and care of Aboriginal and Torres Strait Islander people?

It is evident in the literature, and supported by the voices of many Aboriginal and Torres Strait Islander people that there is a difference between cultural and Western frameworks of health and medicine, and current approaches do not allow for both worldviews to be aligned or be treated as complementary to the overall health of an individual and community. For instance, a holistic view of a hospital or facility will be difficult to take in a community in which the majority of the health services are established around a Western framework and understanding of health and medicine. In this context, a range of factors may prevent Aboriginal or Torres Strait Islander people from accessing health-related services. These include poor levels of literacy, which can hinder an understanding of how the health system works and the processes for each area – for example, if the process for accessing an emergency department is not entirely understood or inappropriately communicated. Aboriginal or Torres Strait Islander people may also continue to have negative associations with hospitals and health facilities based on their lived experiences, which continue to create barriers.

When providing mental healthcare, it is essential that health professionals are culturally aware of how an individual or community understands mental health and what it means to them when their loved ones become unwell. Being aware of how culture and traditional practices impact mental health is equally important, as behaviours can influence mental health situations. Furthermore, acknowledging the role of family and community members in supporting individuals in crisis and how these can be strengthened through strong relationships with health professionals are further strategies that can be used to ensure safe cultural care is provided (Cox & Taua, 2012 and also discussed in-depth in Chapter 3).

The National Strategic Framework for Aboriginal and Torres Strait Islander Peoples' Mental Health and Social and Emotional Well Being 2004–2009 (SHRG, 2004) recognises the diversity of Aboriginal and Torres Strait Islanders, their cultures, their histories and in many instances their different needs. The Framework further recognises as a priority the need to support Aboriginal and Torres Strait Islander people to effectively deal with, and triumph over, the effects of past policies and practices. Enjoying a high level of SEWB can be described as a person feeling good about their lifestyle and the way they feel. Feeling connected to family and community and exercising control of your choices and environments can help achieve these high levels (SAAHP, 2005, p. 4). SEWB is everybody's business – all sectors of society, community, individual and family. But, SEWB and mental health problems for Aboriginal people are not entirely recognised or understood across the Australian healthcare system.

SEWB and mental health problems can affect any person in society, and are becoming more common (Hunter 2007; Kelly, Barnett & Dudgeon, 2009; NMHC, 2014). Cultural and spiritual aspects contribute to Aboriginal and Torres Strait Islander people's understanding of health and mental health, and can influence how people present and develop symptoms when they become unwell. Health professionals and clinicians must understand these aspects to be able to provide effective, individualised care and treatment in a safe and culturally appropriate way. A holistic approach to health, where coordination of a client's needs and total care takes priority, must take into consideration the economic and social conditions that affect physical and emotional wellbeing. Healthcare must take into account physical, environmental, cultural and spiritual factors if it is to help people to achieve SEWB (Beyondblue, 2016).

The National Strategic Framework for Aboriginal and Torres Strait Islander Peoples' Mental Health and Social and Emotional Wellbeing 2017–2023 (Commonwealth of Australia, 2017) continues to advocate and support the early work originating from the *Ways Forward* report by Swan and Raphael (1995). This report was instrumental in highlighting Aboriginal and Torres Strait Islander mental health and SEWB. The new framework is developed to guide new developments in Aboriginal and Torres Strait Islander mental health and wellbeing reforms. The Australian Government is now working towards strengthening the health system's approach to mental health service delivery to and treatments for Aboriginal and Torres Strait Islander people through a stepped care model. This approach is vital to enhancing service integration and navigation of the larger health system (Commonwealth of Australia, 2017, p. 11). For the purposes of this chapter, the action areas set out in the Framework will support your direction and approach to mental health and SEWB for Aboriginal and Torres Strait Islander people.

Action area 2: Promote wellness

Outcome 2.1: Aboriginal and Torres Strait Islander communities and cultures are strong and support social and emotional wellbeing and mental health.

Rationale: Communities can be sources of support and resilience that promote SEWB when community organisation and functioning is culturally-informed and provides for cultural practice and transmission. For optimal social and emotional wellbeing in individuals and families, empowering communities to heal and to revitalise culture and cultural practices may be required.

Outcome 2.2: Aboriginal and Torres Strait Islander families are strong and supported.

Rationale: Families are pivotal to the wellbeing of individuals and communities, including through the transmission of culture. The way in which families operate can also help family members cope with disadvantage and stressful life experiences. Aboriginal and Torres Strait Islander people can view family structures and relationships differently and child rearing can be practised more collectively.

(Commonwealth of Australia, 2017, pp. 20–21)

QUESTIONS FOR REFLECTION

Refer to the National Strategic Framework for Aboriginal and Torres Strait Islander Peoples' Mental Health and Social and Emotional Wellbeing 2017–2023 (Commonwealth of Australia, 2017) as you answer the following questions. Consider service delivery and treatments when preparing your response.

- Describe what an Aboriginal Community Controlled Health Service is within a community setting.
- For Outcomes 2.1 and 2.2, identify five key strategies that would support the implementation of this in an Aboriginal Community Controlled Health Service (ACCHS).
- For Outcomes 2.1 and 2.2, outline in 300 words how you would involve Aboriginal and Torres Strait Islander people and list some of the potential outcomes.
- How do these outcomes support communities in their strategies for suicide prevention?

CASE STUDY

Marla

Marla is a ten-year-old Aboriginal girl living with her family in a three-bedroom state housing townhouse in a large city. She has two brothers aged six years and six months respectively. In the last twelve months, she has suffered the loss of her

(cont.)

maternal grandmother (aged 54 years) through chronic illness, her father (aged 30 years) from an acute myocardial infarction and a male cousin (aged sixteen years) from suicide. Three years ago, her sister died from sudden infant death syndrome aged thirteen months. Marla has lost all interest in attending school and has been spending most of her time at home helping her mother with the baby. Previously, she had been described as a pleasant student and achieved average grades, with good physical health and normal developmental milestones.

Marla's mother is concerned about her school refusal, and admits her school attendance has also been patchy over recent years. She is concerned about the school reporting the family to child welfare services and has reluctantly accepted the referral to child and adolescent mental health services for assessment.

Marla's family is supported by an extensive family kinship system with several aunties and paternal grandparents, and there are often additional relatives staying in the home. Marla presents as shy and stays close to her mother, often fussing over the baby. She says very little in the interview but admits she enjoys staying home to look after her brother. She denies most symptoms presented to her, but has trouble sleeping and usually ends up in her mother's bed at night. She displays little emotion but brightens up when interacting with her baby brother. She appears disinterested in the toys in the room, makes very little eye contact and refuses to stay without her mother present in the room.

Source: Extract reproduced with permission from Milroy (2014, p. 375).

QUESTIONS FOR REFLECTION

- What are the key considerations in addressing trauma and loss?
- Identify some strategies for working with Marla and her family.
- How would you support cultural connections?

CASE STUDY

Brandon

Brandon is a fourteen-year-old Aboriginal adolescent from a small remote community. He had been acting strangely for some time, but more recently had become aggressive towards his family. Brandon had been using marijuana quite heavily over recent months, had disturbed sleep and often walked around the house at night. He was seen talking to himself, sometimes shouting abuse and isolating himself in his room. He had threatened to kill everyone if they didn't leave him alone.

He was taken to the health centre and subsequently evacuated under the Mental Health Act to an authorised mental health adolescent in-patient unit for assessment for psychosis. On admission to the ward, he was quiet and guarded, mostly staring at the floor. He ignored most questions, but at times would look around the room suspiciously and stated on several occasions he wanted to go home. At times Brandon would pace around the room clenching his fists and banging his head on the wall.

He was given some sedation and over the next few days appeared to settle. He admitted to hearing several voices, one was his deceased grandfather calling his name and the others he didn't recognise but they said bad things about him and his family. He was worried he was going to be punished at night when he was asleep, but couldn't say what he had done wrong. These symptoms had been getting worse over a six-month period and he had used the marijuana to try to 'chill out' but it appeared to make things worse. He had thought about hanging himself but had not acted on these thoughts.

Source: Extract reproduced with permission from Milroy (2014, p. 377).

QUESTIONS FOR REFLECTION

- What are the main health priorities for this patient?
- What are the cultural considerations for this patient?
- What are the cultural protocols for Aboriginal people and communities about which you need to be aware?
- When conducting an assessment on Brandon, what types of questions would you ask him and his family?
- As a beginning health professional, how would you assist an Aboriginal person contemplating suicide?
- What services or resources would you refer the patient to in this situation?

Conclusion

Despite the high incidence of suicides in Indigenous communities, there continues to be a need for more research into the understandings and definitions of suicidal behaviour specific to Aboriginal and Torres Strait Islander people and their communities (SPA, 2009). It is evident that the loss of a life from suicide considerably impacts the family and the wider community, which in turn disrupts SEWB mental health (De Leo, Sveticic & Milner, 2011). Additionally, an adequate understanding of Aboriginal suicides in Aboriginal communities requires an appreciation of the historical and cultural context of those communities.

It is very important to understand and recognise from an Aboriginal and Torres Strait Islander perspective how health and mental health are defined, and how they depend on many different factors. It is also important to acknowledge that health is holistic and that it sits within a SEWB framework (AIHW, 2009).

Further social risk factors within Aboriginal populations would be better understood in terms of lifestyle rather than classifying them among mainstream risk factors, with a need for suicide-prevention strategies that address risk at the community level, rather than that of the individual (Hunter, 2007, cited in Ward, 2019). This means approaching people at a community level with community resources and facilities that would allow them to identify points of crisis, including those in crisis, which is central to implementing effective preventative measures.

This became evident in the Yarrabah Aboriginal community, where life-promotion officers were engaged and worked with community to identify people at risk. As a result, education and training was provided to workers to assist young people in crisis while closing the alcohol outlet to further reduce risk behaviours and increase pride and cultural connectivity (Procter, 2005). Suicide among Aboriginal and Torres Strait Islander people and communities must be considered in the context of history, intergenerational trauma, racism, colonisation, dispossession and policies of exclusion and economic disadvantage.

Learning activities

1. What is the link between SEWB and social determinants of health for Indigenous Australians?
2. From the perspective of an IHW, a nurse or mental health nurse, where does cultural safety begin?
3. When is mental health intervention justified?
4. What is the difference between Aboriginal and Torres Strait Islanders' concepts of health and a mainstream understanding of health?

FURTHER READING

ATSISPEP (2015). *Aboriginal and Torres Strait Islander Suicide Prevention Evaluation Project: Analysis using unpublished National Coronial Information System data. Fact Sheet 1. Note: Rates have been adjusted to account for cases with unknown Indigenous status.* Retrieved from www.atsispep.sis.uwa.edu.au

Commonwealth of Australia (2017). *National Strategic Framework for Aboriginal and Torres Strait Islander Peoples' Mental Health and Social and Emotional Wellbeing 2017–2023.* Canberra: DPMC. Retrieved from www.niaa.gov.au/sites/default/files/publications/mhsewb-framework_0.pdf

Department of Health (2016). *Cultural Respect Framework 2016–2026.* Canberra: Australian Government. Retrieved from www1.health.gov.au/internet/main/publishing.nsf/Content/indigenous-crf

Visit the companion website at www.cambridge.org/highereducation/isbn/9781108794695/resources to see further online resources.

REFERENCES

ABS (2013). *Family Stressors: Australian Aboriginal and Torres Strait Islander Health Survey, First Results, Australia, 2012–13.* Canberra: ABS. Retrieved from www.abs.gov.au/ausstats/abs@.nsf/Latestproducts/C0E1AC36B1E28917CA257C2F001456E3?opendocument

ABS (2017). *Causes of Death, Australia, 2016.* Canberra: ABS. Retrieved from: www.abs.gov.au/AUSSTATS/abs@.nsf/allprimarymainfeatures/52FFCC3AC316644DCA2583130014217F?opendocument

ABS (2018). *Causes of Death, Australia, 2018: Intentional Self-harm in Aboriginal and Torres Strait Islander People.* Canberra: ABS. Retrieved from: Retrieved from www.abs.gov.au/ausstats/abs@.nsf/Lookup/by%20Subject/3303.0~2018~Main%20Features~Intentional%20self-harm%20in%20Aboriginal%20and%20Torres%20Strait%20Islander%20people~4

ABS (2019). *Causes of Death, Australia, 2019: Intentional Self-harm in Aboriginal and Torres Strait Islander People.* Canberra: ABS. Retrieved from: www.abs.gov.au/statistics/health/causes-death/causes-death-australia/latest-release#intentional-self-harm-suicide-in-aboriginal-and-torres-strait-islander-people

AHMAC (2017). *Aboriginal and Torres Strait Islander Health Performance Framework: 2017 Report.* Canberra: AHMAC. Retrieved from www.niaa.gov.au/sites/default/files/publications/2017-health-performance-framework-report_1.pdf

AIHW. (2009). *Measuring the social and emotional well-being of Aboriginal and Torres Strait Islander peoples.* Cat. no. IHW 24. Canberra: AIHW.

ATSISPEP (2015). *Aboriginal and Torres Strait Islander Suicide Prevention Evaluation Project: Analysis using unpublished National Coronial Information System data. Fact Sheet 1. Note: Rates have been adjusted to account for cases with unknown Indigenous status.* Canberra: ABS. Retrieved from www.atsispep.sis.uwa.edu.au

Beyondblue (2016). *Inquiry into Aboriginal Youth Suicides.* Melbourne: Beyondblue. Retrieved from www.beyondblue.org.au/docs/default-source/policy-submissions/bw0404_wa-aboriginal-youth-suicide-inquiry97295baaf37161bc846eff0000e9d3fc.pdf?sfvrsn=9b583aea_0

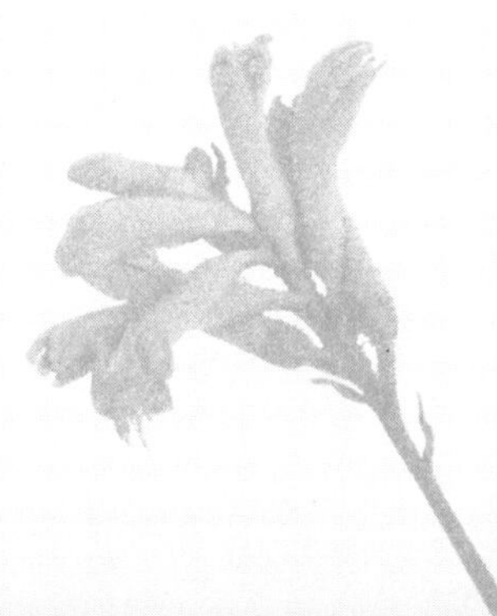

Brown, P. (2014). Aboriginal suicide. *The Stringer*, 2 November. Retrieved from https://thestringer.com.au/aboriginal-suicide-9001#.YAd4xOkzZXs

Cantor, C. & Neulinger, K. (2000). The epidemiology of suicide and attempted suicide among young Australians. *Australian and New Zealand Journal of Psychiatry*, 34, 370–87.

Cantor, C., Neulinger, K., Roth, J. & Spinks, D. (1998). *The Epidemiology of Suicide and Attempted Suicide Among Young Australians: A Literature Review Prepared for the National Health and Medical Research Council*, Canberra: NHMRC.

CBPATSISP (2020). Statistics. Retrieved from www.cbpatsisp.com.au/resources/statistics

Chandler, M.J. & Lalonde, C.E. (1998). Cultural continuity as a hedge against suicide in Canada's First Nations. *Transcultural Psychiatry*, 35, 191–219.

Chandler, M.J., Lalonde, C.E., Sokol, B.W. & Hallett, D. (2003). Personal persistence, identity development, and suicide: A study of Native and Non-Native North American adolescents. *Monographs of the Society for Research into Child Development*, 68(2): vi–viii.

Commonwealth of Australia (2017). *National Strategic Framework for Aboriginal and Torres Strait Islander Peoples' Mental Health and Social and Emotional Wellbeing 2017–2023*. Canberra: DPMC. Retrieved from www.niaa.gov.au/sites/default/files/publications/mhsewb-framework_0.pdf

Cox, L. & Taua, C. (2012). Cultural safety: Cultural considerations. In H. Forbes & E. Watt, (eds), *Jarvis's Physical Examination and Health Assessment*. Sydney: Elsevier, pp. 40–60.

De Leo, D., Sveticic, J. & Milner, A. (2011). Suicide in Indigenous people in Queensland: Trends and methods, 1994–2007. *Australia and New Zealand Journal of Psychiatry*, 45(7), 532–8.

DHA (2020). *Fact Sheet 16: Suicide Prevention in Indigenous Communities: Life is for Living*. Canberra: DHA.

Dudgeon, P., Calma, T. & Holland, C. (2017). The context and causes of the suicide of Indigenous people in Australia. *Journal of Indigenous Wellbeing Te Mauri – Pimatisiwin*, 1(2), 5–15. Retrieved from https://journalindigenouswellbeing.com/media/2018/07/82.65.The-context-and-causes-of-the-suicide-of-Indigenous-people-in-Australia.pdf

Dudgeon P., Holland C. & Walker R. (2019). *Fact Sheet 2 Indigenous Suicide Deaths 1981 to 2018*. Perth: CBPATSISP. Retrieved from www.cbpatsisp.com.au/wp-content/uploads/2020/03/Fact-Sheet-2.pdf

Dudgeon, P. & Luxford, Y. (2017). *Real Time Suicide Data: A Discussion Paper*. Canberra: ATSISPEP.

Dudgeon, P., Wright, M., Paradies, Y., Garvey, D. & Walker, I. (2010). The social, cultural and historical context of Aboriginal and Torres Strait Islander Australians. In N. Purdie, P. Dudgeon & R. Walker (eds), *Working Together: Aboriginal and Torres Strait Islander Mental Health and Wellbeing Principles and Practice*. Canberra: Commonwealth of Australia, pp. 25–42.

Elliot-Farrelly, T. (2004). Australian Aboriginal suicide: The need for an Aboriginal suicidology? *Australian e-Journal for the Advancement of Mental Health*, 3(3), 138–45.

Gee, G., Dudgeon, P., Schultz, C., Hart, A. & Kelly, K. (2014). Aboriginal and Torres Strait Islander social and emotional wellbeing. In P.Dudgeon, H. Milroy & R. Walker (eds), *Working Together: Aboriginal and Torres Strait Islander Mental Health*

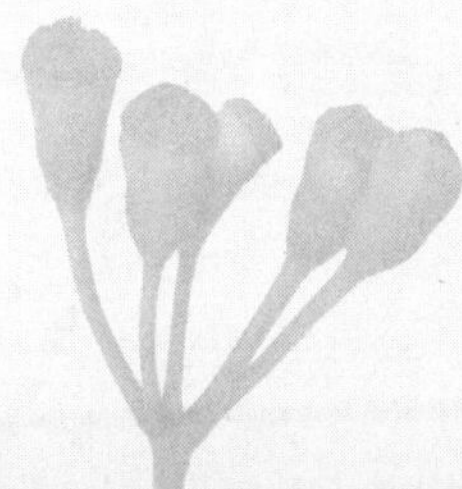

and Wellbeing Principles and Practice (2nd edn). Canberra: Commonwealth of Australia, pp. 55–69.

Georgatos, G. (2013a). 77 Aboriginal suicides in South Australia alone. *The Stringer*, 4 October. Retrieved from https://thestringer.com.au/77-aboriginal-suicides-in-south-australia-alone-4994#.YAd-lOkzZXs

Georgatos, G. (2013b). The Australian Aboriginal suicide epidemic. *Independent Australia*, 16 October. Retrieved from https://independentaustralia.net/australia/australia-display/the-australian-aboriginal-suicide-epidemic,5818

Georgatos, G. (2015). Understanding Australia's suicide crisis. *The Stringer*, 20 February. Retrieved from https://thestringer.com.au/understanding-australias-suicide-crises-9606#.YAd-cekzZXs

HealthInfoNet (2020). Social and emotional wellbeing. Retrieved from https://healthinfonet.ecu.edu.au/learn/health-topics/social-and-emotional-wellbeing

Hunter, E. (2007). Disadvantage and discontent: A review of issues relevant to the mental health of rural and remote Indigenous Australians. *Australian Journal of Rural Health*, 15, 88–93.

Hunter, E. & Milroy, H. (2006). Aboriginal and Torres Strait Islander suicide in context. *Archives in Suicide Research*, 10(2), 141–57.

Hunter, E., Reser, J., Baird, M. & Reser, P. (2001). *An Analysis of Suicide in Indigenous Communities of North Queensland: The Historical, Cultural and Symbolic Landscape*. Canberra: DHAC.

IAHA (2012). Media release, 10 October. Retrieved from https://iaha.com.au/iahas-media-release

Kanowski, L.J., Jorm, A.F. & Hart, L.M. (2009). A mental health first aid training program for Australian Aboriginal and Torres Strait Islander peoples: Description and initial evaluation. *International Journal of Mental Health Systems*, 3(1). Retrieved from https://doi.org/10.1186/1752-4458-3-10

Kelly, K., Barnett, L. & Dudgeon, P. (2009). *A Submission to the Australian Senate Community Affairs References Committee: Inquiry into Suicide in Australia*. Melbourne: AIPA.

Kelly, K., Dudgeon, P., Gee, G. & Glaskin, B. (2009). *Living on the Edge: Social and Emotional Wellbeing and Risk and Protective Factors for Serious Psychological Distress Among Aboriginal and Torres Strait Islander People*. Darwin: CRCAH.

Kitchener, B., Jorm, A. & Kanowski, L. (2008). *Aboriginal and Torres Strait Islander Mental Health First Aid Manual*. Melbourne: ORYGEN Research Centre, University of Melbourne.

Kõlves, K., Potts, B. & De Leo, D. (2015). Ten years of suicide mortality in Australia: Socio-economic and psychiatric factors in Queensland. *Journal of Forensic and Legal Medicine*, 36, 136–43.

MHCNSW (2013). *Yarning Honestly About Aboriginal Mental Health in NSW*. Sydney: MHCNSW.

Milroy (2014). Understanding the lives of Aboriginal children and families. In P.Dudgeon, H. Milroy & R. Walker (eds), *Working Together: Aboriginal and Torres Strait Islander Mental Health and Wellbeing Principles and Practice* (2nd edn). Canberra: Commonwealth of Australia, pp. 373–82.

Mindframe (2015). Aboriginal and Torres Strait Islander Australians. Retrieved from www.mindframe-media.info/for-media/reporting-mental-illness/priority-population-group

NMHC (2014). *The National Review of Mental Health Programmes and Services*. Sydney: NMHC.

Parker, R. (2010). Australia's Aboriginal population and mental health. *The Journal of Nervous and Mental Disease*, 198(1), 3–7.

Parker, R. (2012). Aboriginal and Torres Strait Islander mental health: Paradise lost? *Medical Journal of Australia*. 196(2), 89–90.

Parker, R. & Milroy, H. (2014). Aboriginal and Torres Strait Islander Mental Health: An Overview. In P.Dudgeon, H. Milroy & R. Walker (eds), *Working Together: Aboriginal and Torres Strait Islander Mental Health and Wellbeing Principles and Practice* (2nd edn). Canberra: Commonwealth of Australia, pp. 25–39.

Pascoe, B. (2014). *Dark Emu, Black Seeds: Agriculture or Accident?* Broome: Magabala Books.

Pink, B. & Allbon, P. (2008). *The Health and Welfare of Australia's Aboriginal and Torres Strait Islander Peoples*. Canberra:ABS & AIHW.

Procter, N.G. (2005). Parasuicide, self-harm and suicide in Aboriginal people in rural Australia: A review of the literature with implications for mental health nursing practice. *International Journal of Nursing Practice*, 11(5), 237–41.

QMHC (2015). *Queensland Suicide Prevention Action Plan 2015–17*. Brisbane: QMHC. Retrieved from www.qmhc.qld.gov.au/sites/default/files/wp-content/uploads/2015/09/Queensland-Suicide-Prevention-Action-Plan-2015–17_WEB.pdf

SHRG (2004). *National Strategic Framework for Aboriginal and Torres Strait Islander People's Mental Health and Social and Emotional Well-Being 2004–2009*. NRAIHX & NMHWG Health Council and National Mental Health Working Group.

Silburn, S., Robinson, G., Leckning, B., Henry,D., Cox, A. & Kickett, D. (2014). Preventing suicide among Aboriginal Australians. In P.Dudgeon, H. Milroy & R. Walker (eds), *Working Together: Aboriginal and Torres Strait Islander Mental Health and Wellbeing Principles and Practice* (2nd edn). Canberra: Commonwealth of Australia, pp. 147–64.

South Australian Aboriginal Health Partnership (2005). *Aboriginal Health – Everybody's Business: Social and Emotional Wellbeing. A South Australian Strategy for Aboriginal and Torres Strait Islander People 2005–2010*. Adelaide: SA Health. Retrieved from www.sahealth.sa.gov.au/wps/wcm/connect/3dbc7480434bc3e498bbdeba9c78a5ba/social_emot_wellbeing.pdf?MOD=AJPERES&CACHEID=ROOTWORKSPACE-3dbc7480434bc3e498bbdeba9c78a5ba-niRaWp9

SPA (2009). *Suicide and Self-Harm Among Gay, Lesbian, Bisexual and Transgender Communities: SPA Position Statement*. Sydney: SPA.

Swan, P. & Raphael, B. (1995). *Ways Forward: National Aboriginal and Torres Strait Islander Mental Health Policy National Consultancy Report*. Canberra: Australian Government Publishing Service.

Tatz, C. (1999). *Aboriginal Suicide is Different: Aboriginal Youth Suicide in New South Wales, the Australian Capital Territory and New Zealand: Towards a Model of Explanation and Alleviation*. Canberra: Criminology Research Council.

Tatz, C. (2011). Aborigines, sport and suicide in C.J. Hallinan & B. Judd (eds), *Indigenous People, Race Relations and Australian Sport*. Special edition of *Sport in Society*. London: Routledge.

Ugle, K. Glaskin, B., Dudgeon, P. & Hillman, S. (2009). *Discussion Paper on a Statewide Aboriginal Suicide Postvention Project*. Perth: Active Response Bereavement Outreach.

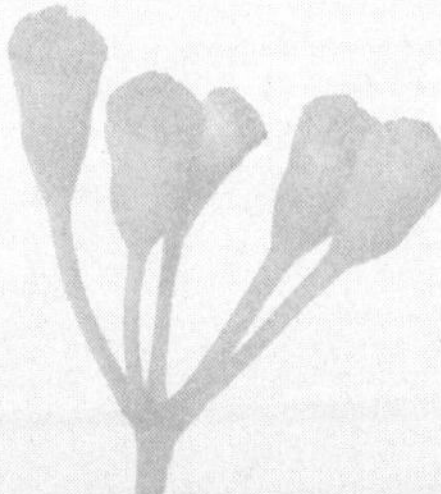

Ward, R. (2015). *Health and wellbeing.* In K. Price (ed.), *Knowledge of Life: Aboriginal and Torres Strait Islander Australia.* Melbourne: Cambridge University Press.

Ward, R. (2019). Suicide prevention: Exploring Aboriginal understandings of suicides from a social and emotional wellbeing framework. Unpublished PhD thesis, University of Southern Queensland.

Ward, R. & Gorman, D. (2010). Racism, discrimination and health services to Aboriginal people in South West Queensland. *Aboriginal and Islander Health Worker Journal,* 34(6), 3–5.

WHO (1986). *Ottawa Charter for Health Promotion.* Geneva: WHO.

WHO (2018). Mental health: strengthening our response. Retrieved from www.who.int/news-room/fact-sheets/detail/mental-health-strengthening-our-response#:~:text=Mental%20health%20is%20a%20state,to%20his%20or%20her%20community

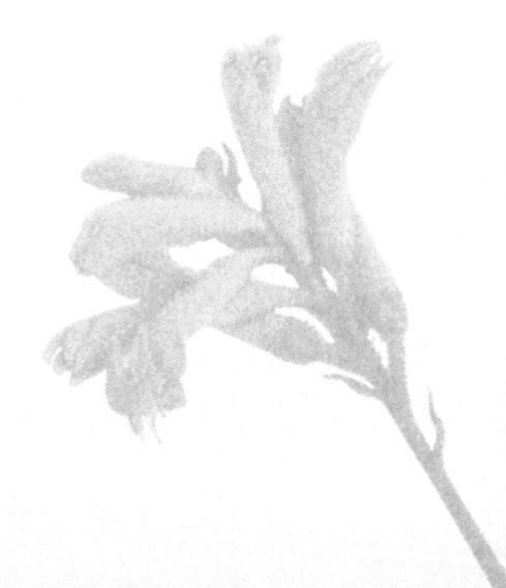

15

Indigenous child health

Donna Hartz and Jessica Bennett

LEARNING OBJECTIVES

This chapter will help you to understand:

- The national policies that guide Aboriginal and Torres Strait Islander children and family's health policy development, and program and service design
- The cultural safety and social considerations required in assessing and caring for Aboriginal and Torres Strait Islander children
- The initiatives and strategies that promote a healthy start to life for Aboriginal and Torres Strait Islander children
- The health screening and care initiatives aimed at promoting Aboriginal and Torres Strait Islander children's health

KEY WORDS

common Indigenous child health infections
infant and child mortality
traditional child-rearing practices
universal health screening
vulnerable families

Introduction

The quality of our health is largely determined by foetal development in pregnancy and the experiences and environments to which we are exposed in infancy and childhood. These factors shape and contribute to lifelong health effects that occur into adult life. While there is little and conflicted documentation about the health of Aboriginal and Torres Strait Islander children prior to the invasion, what is known is that Aboriginal and Torres Strait Islander children were few and precious, and their holistic health needs were met within their strong and extended family structures. Child mortality and morbidity were an accepted part of life in pre-invasion times; this is reflected in traditional birthing practices and women's business. Traditionally, our children learnt culture, food gathering, ceremony, kinship relationships, law, gender-specific work and other important values and structures throughout childhood. Post-invasion, the introduction of disease, the impacts of loss of traditional food sources due to dispossession of lands, and the fracturing and removal of traditional family and community structure all fuelled the increased Indigenous mortality and morbidity rates evidenced today (Boulton, 2016).

Currently, irrespective of age, Aboriginal and Torres Strait Islander children have higher rates of illness, hospitalisation and death, and are more likely to be exposed to stressful life events, than non-Indigenous children. Fundamental to improving the health of Aboriginal and Torres Strait Islander children are culturally safe initiatives incorporated into effective maternal and child health services such as health promotion, targeted screening, immunisation and access to specialist care and treatments in partnership with the family and community, resulting in some small gains. However, this is not enough and there is still a large disparity in the health and equity gap that needs urgent attention. The Australian Government acknowledges that the existing child and family health service system does not currently meet the needs of all Aboriginal and Torres Strait Islander children and their families (DPMC, 2019).

It is imperative that governments, health policy-makers and health professionals take stock of the current health outcomes and health practices, to seek a better way of understanding in gaining knowledge and implementing the best evidence-based practice and service delivery to Aboriginal and Torres Strait Islander families. Intrinsic in any health initiative is the incorporation of cultural safety, responsive health carers and community engagement, leadership and/or partnership. This chapter explores the basic tenets of Aboriginal and Torres Strait Islander infant and child health, and introduces the key considerations when providing care in varied settings.

National policies for the health of Aboriginal and Torres Strait Islander children and families

The Australian Government published the National Framework for Health Services for Aboriginal and Torres Strait Islander Children and Families in 2016. This framework provides culturally safe and evidence-based guidance for child and family health policy development, program design and service design for Australian Indigenous communities (Department of Health, 2016). It is recommended that this framework be used in conjunction with the National Framework for Universal Child and Family Health Services. The former framework recommends that any service delivery model should be integrated into primary health care; be local or regional and networked; be multidisciplinary and collaborative; provide continuity of care; provide holistic assessment; and be sufficiently flexible to meet the needs of the child and their family (Department of Health, 2016, p. 3).

Cultural and social considerations

A child's early attachment and bonding with a primary caregiver are fundamental to healthy human growth and development. The physical and emotional bond that typically forms between an infant and the caregiver in infancy is the means by which a child's primary needs are met and the moulding for future behaviours and relationships. This connection is a holistic foundation for subsequent social, emotional, and cognitive development, which is also culturally specific to the child and family. Any situation that impedes this can affect a child reaching optimal development.

traditional child-rearing practices Children have an extended kinship with a collective community responsibility, a high regard for the guidance of Elders, a freedom to explore the world and an engagement with culture and spirituality, all creating connection and a strong sense of identity (AIFS, 2020).

Traditional child-rearing practices in the Aboriginal and Torres Strait Islander community commenced with the babies and infants (up to eighteen months) staying intimately close to family by being carried in furs or bark initially, then on the shoulders of family members. The primary caregivers may have been all or any one of the immediate siblings, aunties or grandparents. In contrast, older children (beginning from eighteen months) were encouraged to develop self-reliance and independence, and were encouraged to freely explore their surroundings with the child learning from mishaps and gaining resilience (Smythe, 1878, cited in MacDonald, 2014).

In the modern eurocentric context, these behaviours could be interpreted as insecure attachment or inadequate caring/parenting from a non-Aboriginal and Torres Strait Islander perspective (Yeo, 2003). Alongside the ongoing impacts of colonisation, this perspective has contributed to the widespread disruption of secure attachment and positive parenting skills for Aboriginal and Torres Strait Islander people (Heath et al., 2011). In relation to this, Yeo (2003), p. 293) asserts that

> any assessment of bonding and attachment of Aboriginal and Torres Strait Islander children must take into account the historical, cultural and spiritual contexts. The impact of the sociopolitical history in Australia over the past 200 years continues and is still being experienced by the Aboriginal and Torres Strait Islander people.

Kinship is paramount to wellbeing for Aboriginal and Torres Strait Islander people. Although child-rearing practices differ between families and communities, generally the extended family contributes to raising children. The child's father and paternal uncles are considered fathers; the child's mother and maternal aunties are considered mothers; cousins may be considered as siblings; and close unrelated adults may also be considered as aunties or uncles. Parental responsibilities may be shared between several close relatives – kinship is fundamental (Lohoar, Butera & Kennedy, 2014).

In some situations, customary adoption occurs, where another family member will undertake the primary parenting role (Heath et al., 2011; Yeo, 2003). While it is more common in rural and remote areas of Australia, the household in which the child lives may host a large number of family members that live within the household as well as those who visit frequently (AIHW, 2020a). As a collective, Aboriginal and Torres Strait Islander families and communities are responsible for contributing to the safety and child-rearing practices of all children within the community.

Social determinants of health for Aboriginal and Torres Strait Islander people have been discussed throughout this book. In addition to considering and clarifying the individual child's cultural and kinship situation, other factors that may impact the integrity of such situations must be explored and considered, as a child's development is also shaped by their environment in the postnatal period and beyond (Moore et al., 2015). The following are some major life situations that may impact the child's health, their social and emotional wellbeing and their ability to access services:

- poverty, household unemployment and financial stress – affect ability to pay for food, clothing, school, health services, transportation, childcare, medicines and adequate housing
- remoteness – local services not available, lack of transportation, lack of childcare, lack of privacy in small community
- low levels of education – influence ability to understand the importance of healthcare or how to navigate funding or service provision
- lack of social support, strained/absent relationship with partner or family, leading to social isolation and difficulty taking child to appointments
- substance abuse, mental health issues and domestic violence – may all pose more urgent priorities, preventing the carer/s and children from attending care
- mistrust of health professionals, especially where there is previous removal of children due to welfare issues or a reputation for lack of racial/cultural understanding or presence of discrimination
- lack of language or culturally specific services or staff
- concurrent health issues/morbidities of the parent/carers – for anaemia, heart disease, kidney disease and poor nutrition.

Sources: Adapted from Best Start Resource Centre (2020) and Kikkawa (2015).

Chronic stress and trauma produced by life situations can impact the healthy growth of the baby, both during pregnancy and infancy and throughout childhood. Stress and anxiety during pregnancy have been linked to pre-term birth and low birthweight babies (Lima et al., 2018). Pre-term birth and low birthweight are associated with increased developmental delays and longer hospital admissions. Maternal nutritional deficits, as well as drug and alcohol use, can cause congenital anomalies. For example, alcohol use in pregnancy can cause Foetal Alcohol Spectrum Disorder (FASD), a condition characterised by physical anomalies but also lifelong developmental and behavioural issues. Perinatal depression, mental health issues, and drug and alcohol use all impact the ability of mothers and carers to promote a secure and positive attachment to their babies and infants. The support of such **vulnerable families** is essential to child and family social and emotional wellbeing. This is discussed later in the chapter.

vulnerable families Families with complex life and health needs requiring trauma-informed care that is culturally responsive.

Birth registration and Aboriginal and Torres Strait Islander identification

The importance of Aboriginal and Torres Strait Islander identification during health service care helps to promote appropriate data collection and health status reporting.

Health carers can play a pivotal role in asking about identification and opportunistically providing information and/or support in birth registration, as this plays a significant role in accessing services and facilities that impact on social and economic standing and important social and cultural determinants of health. The importance of this is evidenced by health policies that mandate health carers to ask whether a person identifies as Indigenous. NSW Health (2012) has developed a policy directive that outlines the requirements for accurate recording and collecting of identification for Aboriginal and Torres Strait Islander people.

Of even greater importance is the promotion of registration of babies at birth, including their Indigenous status. Griffiths et al. (2019) observe that unregistered births of Aboriginal and Torres Strait Islander Australians are higher than in the wider community, and applications for birth certificates are noticeably lower. In some communities, up to one-fifth of Aboriginal and Torres Strait Islander children under the age of 16 are not registered (Gibberd, Simpson & Eades, 2016).

Birth registration is essential, as this entitles a person to a birth certificate. This is one of the most important documents that establishes identity and is required to ensure appropriate and funded access to health services. Support for women – especially for those women who are most disadvantaged – is essential in registering their babies birth prior to discharge from maternity care (Gibberd et al., 2016). There are initiatives supporting parents and individuals, including disadvantaged or vulnerable people living in regional and remote Aboriginal and Torres Strait Islander communities, to obtain a birth certificate or register a unregistered birth – for example, the Western Australian Department of Justice hold a 'Open Day' Program for general birth registration (WA Department of Justice, 2019).

QUESTIONS FOR REFLECTION

- Can you identify the cultural determinants that may be impacted by a lack of birth registration?
- Can you identify other social or cultural determinants that may be impacted by a lack of birth registration?

Infant and child mortality

infant and child mortality The child mortality rate is defined as 'the number of deaths among children aged 0–4 years old as a proportion of the total number of children in that age group, presented as a rate per 100,000 population' (DPMC, 2020, p. 16).

Since British invasion, the mortality and morbidity rates of Aboriginal and Torres Strait Islander children have been hugely disparate from non-Indigenous children and largely unaddressed until relatively recently. In an attempt to redress this, in 2008 the Australian Government introduced the Closing the Gap initiative, which set out six target areas for improvement. This included reducing the **infant and child mortality** rate for children aged from birth to four years by 50 per cent by 2018. However, by 2018 the mortality rates of Aboriginal and Torres Strait Islander children compared with non-Indigenous children had not significantly decreased, with a small reduction of only 10 per cent (DPMC, 2019).

The 2018 data of Aboriginal and Torres Strait Islander infant and child mortality shows the death rate to be greater than twice the rate for these children's non-Indigenous counterparts: 146 Indigenous and 70 non-Indigenous per 100,000 children (AIHW, 2018, p. 316). The reported key factors associated with infant and child mortality include low birthweight and pre-term births, poor maternal health and high-risk maternal behaviours (smoking, alcohol, substance misuse). In addition, poor nutrition during pregnancy, poverty and socioeconomic hardships, and ensuing barriers to accessing health services are ongoing contributors (DPMC, 2019). The majority of deaths of children aged from birth to four years can be linked back to acquired morbidity in the perinatal period, with 86 per cent of all deaths in children under the age of one year (AIHW, 2020a). Other major causes include Sudden Infant Death Syndrome (SIDS) and other lethal sleeping accidents, congenital malformations, infection, injury, poisoning (McNamara et al., 2018) and drowning (Wallis et al., 2015).

On a broader age scale, the mortality rates for Indigenous children aged from one to fourteen years between 2015 and 2017 was two times higher than for non-Indigenous children. Indigenous children aged from one to fourteen years were more likely to die from injuries, cancer and nervous system disease, while those aged from fifteen to seventeen years old were more likely to die from transport fatalities and, tragically, suicide (AIHW, 2020a).

These statistics are not just numbers on a page: they represent the poor health outcomes of the lived experiences of many Aboriginal and Torres Strait Island families in our communities. As health professionals, we so often focus on the numbers and the problems; however, there is a lived story behind that number that health professionals need to reflect on and examine. These stories provide context to the statistics and the real faces and lives they represent, and they play an integral role in helping nurses and midwives to become culturally safe practitioners.

Providing a healthy start to life

Providing culturally safe care for Aboriginal and Torres Strait Islander babies, mothers and families at the beginning of life is paramount. The first five years of life lay down the foundations for healthy living, learning, behaviours and wellbeing. Access to culturally safe maternal and child health services can reduce the risk of poor health outcomes for Aboriginal and Torres Strait Islander mothers and their babies, children and families. Along with higher perinatal and infant mortality rates, Aboriginal and Torres Strait Islander babies also have higher morbidity rates than non-Indigenous babies, including low birthweight, prematurity and admission to special care nurseries and neonatal intensive cares units at birth (AIHW, 2019). To redress this, support needs to come from all levels of government, the healthcare sector and the community. Health policies and frameworks need to continue to identify and address the needs of vulnerable Aboriginal and Torres Strait Islander children and families in order to promote a healthier start to life (CEE, 2018). Strategies should include providing referrals to appropriate services, availability of culturally safe services in the community, improving health literacy and providing health professionals with appropriate training in cultural safety.

Initiatives aimed to promote a better start to life

One of the most impactful strategies promoting a healthy start to life has been the development of community co-designed birthing on Country service (this is discussed in greater depth in Chapter 8. These services have demonstrated promise in reducing the pre-term birth rate of Indigenous babies while providing culturally safe, individualised continuity of midwifery care, family support workers and wrap-around services (Kildea et al., 2019).

Two national strategies that have attempted to promote healthier outcomes for mothers and their infants are the New Directions program (AIHW, 2014) and the Australian Nurse Family Partnership Program (ANFPP) (Nguyen et al., 2018). These are culturally safe services, which provide access to or support during antenatal care; standard information about baby care; practical advice and assistance with breastfeeding, nutrition and parenting; monitoring of developmental milestones, immunisation status and infections; and health checks for Aboriginal and Torres Strait Islander preschool children (AIHW, 2014). The ANFPP provides home visits until the child's second birthday.

Another initiative is the Strong Fathers Strong Families program. This is an Australian Government initiative that aims to

> promote the role of Aboriginal and Torres Strait Islander fathers, partners, grandfathers and uncles, and encourage them to actively participate in their children's and family's lives, particularly in the antenatal period and early childhood development years.
>
> (Urbis, 2013, p. i)

The aims of this program vary between sites where it has been implemented, but broadly they include increased access for males to culturally appropriate health services and other childbearing, parenting and health-promotion programs; promotion of their ability to contribute positively to the health and wellbeing of the mother's pregnancy and healthy environment for their infant's health and development; and becoming role models for their family and community.

universal health screening A national framework of scheduled health service or practitioner visits from birth to school. This includes the monitoring of health, development and compliance with the national immunisation schedule.

Universal health screening and developmental monitoring

The National Framework for Universal Child and Family Health Services (NCHWS, 2011) provides guidance on the establishment of universal child and family health services. The framework recommends a schedule of periodic visits for children at their health service or with their healthcare providers from birth until school age. The schedule enables the monitoring of health, development and compliance with the national immunisation schedule. This schedule aligns with critical periods in child development and provides opportunities for age-appropriate parental/carer guidance and support.

Most states and territories provide a child health record for each baby at the time of birth and prior to discharge from care; this information about the baby's birth and health is recorded and is significant to their health. The records also outline to parents or carers the recommended schedule of health screening visits from birth and into childhood. The medical records have individual sections to record the child's health and illnesses, developmental progress and completed vaccinations. The NSW Health Personal Health Record, also known as the Blue Book, and Queensland Health's Red Book are comprehensive examples of such health records. These books provide information and resources to support parents and carers.

The initial contact by health workers with the new family is recommended at one to two weeks after birth. However, home visiting services are not always available or appropriate, particularly in rural and remote Aboriginal and Torres Strait Islander communities. For a variety of reasons, accessing comprehensive universal child and family health services may be hindered or inequitable. To address this, programs have been introduced to support Aboriginal and Torres Strait Islander families to receive culturally safe and recommended care. Additional support, screening, assessments and interventions should be undertaken in communities where children are more likely to have otitis media (regular otoscopy), nutritional deficiencies (weight and height measurement, anaemia screening, deworming programs) and skin infections (skin checks). These health conditions are discussed in greater depth in the following sections.

Most Aboriginal and Torres Strait Islander Community Health Services (ATICHSs) offer infant and child screening services and provide integrated health programs to address health priorities, support families, facilitate consultations and make referrals to relevant services (Department of Health, 2016). In some – mostly urban – areas, sustained home visiting is offered through the local health district or community services, and extended screening and visit schedules are specifically available for vulnerable population groups (ACHT-CACHS, 2012; Kimla et al., 2019). This care is delivered by Aboriginal Maternal and Child Health Services (AMCHS) or mainstream local health district maternal and child services. It is essential to ensure a 'one size fits all' approach is not used for Aboriginal and Torres Strait Islander children and families, as each community is diverse and has a range of health priorities and initiatives that suit the community's needs.

QUESTIONS FOR REFLECTION

- What programs are available in your area to support a healthy start to life for mothers and babies?
- What resource are available to parents and carers of Aboriginal and Torres Strait Islander children to support recommended screening and health promotion?
- Are hand-held records available for each child?
- What services are available in your local area to provide screening?
- Do you know how to refer to these services?

Supporting vulnerable families

Families need to feel culturally safe when accessing services. Culturally safe and/or community-controlled health services (CCHS) play an important role in delivering health care and providing much-needed support to vulnerable families. This is because of the historical intergenerational removal of children from parents and communities (Laverty, McDermott & Calma, 2017; McKenna, 2020). Building trust and positive active engagement in Aboriginal and Torres Strait Islander communities can contribute to the breakdown of health barriers for families and children. Along with an increased incidence of maternal mental, drug and alcohol health problems, a heightened fear of removal of babies and children into state custody is prevalent for Aboriginal and Torres Strait Islander families. This is well founded, with data indicating that in Australia in 2019, Aboriginal and Torres Strait Islander children were ten times more likely to be in out-of-home care (e.g. looked-after status) than non-Indigenous children (AIHW, 2020b).

It is important to reflect on the dispossession, disruption and cultural disconnection faced by Aboriginal and Torres Strait Islander people since colonisation. The forced removal of children and the subsequent trauma that was caused by the inhuman treatment have resulted in dysfunctional family relationships and disadvantaged childhood upbringing. Aboriginal and Torres Strait Islander children who were brought up in boarding homes and on missions were not provided with the basic fundamental human care and did not experience affectionate and nurturing care from parents and family. When an individual is not given the right to a childhood, symptoms such as an absence of attachment and a lack of effective modelling of parenting skills can occur (Newton, 2018). Aboriginal and Torres Strait Islander children in out-of-home care have higher rates of mental health and developmental needs, with key attributing factors trauma and inadequate attachment (AIHW, 2020b; Shmerling et al., 2019). Trauma-informed care that is culturally responsive and culturally healing is a path that can enable vulnerable families to improve the general health and wellbeing of their infants and family (Atkinson, 2013; Kickett, Chandran & Mitchell, 2019. In caring for Aboriginal and Torres Strait Islander children, the following practice points are useful for promoting family integrity and dignity:

- Ask who is in the child's extended kinship structure and who is the primary carer for the child. The parent or carer accompanying the child may not be the primary carer: family-centred care is key for culturally responsive practice.
- Discuss and involve the parent/carer/family in the process of exploring or investigating care options.
- Find out about any issues affecting the family and their environment. Background issues may explain the medical presentation.
- Provide honest and balanced information about care options to the parents/family, especially when vulnerabilities are identified.
- Be familiar with your local Aboriginal and Torres Strait communities for current projects or initiatives that can support vulnerable children and their families.
- Self-reflect on your personal biases, prejudices and worldviews, to ensure culturally safe care is given. It is important to draw on your learnt knowledges and previous experiences.

- Include the designated Aboriginal and/or Torres Strait Islander health worker or liaison worker or, if they are absent, a community Elder who may be able to advocate for the family.

Promoting the health of Aboriginal and Torres Strait Islander children

Certain health issues are more common in Indigenous Australian children than in their non-Indigenous counterparts. These include **common Indigenous child health infections** such as otitis media and skin infections, as well as more invasive conditions, including bloodstream infections, pneumonia and bronchiectasis. These infections can have ongoing lifelong consequences and contribute to the burden of disease for a vulnerable population.

common Indigenous child health infections These include otitis media, skin infections, gut and parasitic infections, bloodstream infections, pneumonia and bronchiectasis. These can have ongoing lifelong consequences.

Aboriginal and Torres Strait Islander children are over-represented among severely ill children admitted to Australian hospitals and intensive care units (ICUs). Health service providers need to provide access to culturally appropriate information on health promotion, illness and injury prevention. Health promotion should be co-designed and community-based by Aboriginal and Torres Strait Islander people, which is evidenced through the ongoing widening of the health gap (Conte et al., 2019). Higher level health services and hospitals, along with primary healthcare facilities, usually have a network structure with defined care pathways that include Aboriginal and Torres Strait Islander-specific services or healthcare workers. This section looks at common health issues relevant to Aboriginal and Torres Strait Islander children.

Immunisation

The Australian Government's Immunise Australia Program has promoted improvement in vaccination rates for one-, two- and five-year-olds. This program has played a critical role in reducing infections caused by vaccine-preventable infections and is one of the most effective ways of protecting Australia's children from diseases. The recent Immunise Australia data indicate a substantial improvement to over 97 per cent of all Aboriginal and Torres Strait Islander children being fully immunised by the age of five years in 2017 (CEE, 2018). This rate is comparable to the rates for the general population of school-age children. One strategy that has aided the improvement rate of vaccination coverage is the 'Save the Date to Vaccinate' campaign and smartphone app. Currently, the Australian federal government initiative, 'No jab, No pay', withholds welfare payments from families whose children who are not fully immunised.

PRACTICE POINT

- Ask about the immunisation status of Aboriginal and Torres Strait Islander children in your care. If it is non-compliant, be opportunistic and discuss with the parents and carers the benefits of immunisation and offer relevant vaccinations, if clinically appropriate (i.e. there are no contraindications).

Nutrition

The Australian Infant Feeding Guidelines provide health professionals with evidence-based information on feeding of newborns and infants (NHMRC, 2012). Breastfeeding confers optimal nutritional and immunology requirements for babies and infants. Higher breastfeeding rates have been reported among Aboriginal and Torres Strait Islander women in rural and remote communities, with 80 per cent of babies being breastfed at one or more times in infancy compared with those living in urban setting (ABS, 2012). The benefits of breastfeeding address many of the disparate health conditions afflicting Aboriginal and Torres Strait Islander children. Breastfed infants have lower incidences of gastroenteritis, necrotising enterocolitis, gastro-esophageal reflux, respiratory infections, asthma, otitis media, allergies and diabetes (NHMRC, 2012). Exclusive breastfeeding may be protective of cognitive function in particular language skills, psychomotor development and behavioural problems, and improve motor development (Grace et al., 2017). Health workers need to be culturally safe in promoting the benefits of breastfeeding in communities. Women who use infant formula to feed their babies should be made aware of the implications of the cost associated with bottle-feeding and the health implications for their babies when water supply quality is questionable, as well as the need to maintain hygiene standards in bottle and equipment cleansing and storage of milk products (NHMRC, 2012).

Malnourishment and anaemia are common occurrences in Aboriginal and Torres Strait Islander infants, and rates are much higher than in the general population during a child's first year of life. Poor nutrition during infancy affects early growth and development, which impact health and learning for life. Promotion of nutrition and breastfeeding practices should be embedded into Aboriginal and Torres Strait Islander health promotion. Low birthweight, chronic infection, parasite infestation, and delayed and inadequate access to a balanced dietary intake all contribute to nutritional deficits (Bar-Zeev et al., 2013). Conversely, obesity is also an issue for Aboriginal and Torres Strait Islander children (AHMAC, 2017, p. 143).

QUESTIONS FOR REFLECTION

- Is your health facility breastfeeding friendly? This means it has a breastfeeding policy and provides quiet areas for mothers to nurture their babies and young children, or to express and store breastmilk if required.
- What health promotion is visible and available around the benefits of breastfeeding to mothers and infants?

Oral health

Aboriginal and Torres Strait Islander children have higher rates of dental cavities, with higher incidences in rural and remote areas. Oral health refers to more than just the health of teeth; it also includes the health of the muscles, bone and gum tissue. The higher rates of low oral health are attributed to poor dental hygiene, inadequate diets and a lack of fluoridated water due to the consequences of colonisation. Improved nutrition can promote better oral hygiene status; however, in rural and remote communities an appropriate diet is not always accessible. Twenty-five per cent of Aboriginal and Torres Strait Islander children experience tooth decay before primary school (AHMAC, 2017, p. 59). The promotion of brushing teeth twice a day with fluoridated toothpaste – especially in areas where there is no access to fluoridated water – was suggested by NSW programs in schools with community consultation and education (Dimitropoulos et al., 2018). In 2019, tooth decay of Aboriginal and Torres Strait Islander children was reported as being 61 per cent in primary teeth and 36 per cent in secondary teeth, compared with rates of 41 per cent and 23 per cent respectively in non-Indigenous children (AIHW, 2020a). During early childhood, oral health habits should include routine and regular dental check-ups.

Infections

Infectious processes in Aboriginal and Torres Strait Islander infants and children are a leading cause of mortality, and occur at twice the rate of non-Indigenous children. Commonly reported infections include pneumococcal, meningococcal and Group A streptococcus, which occur despite modern vaccination regimes. These infective organisms cause acute and chronic diseases that impact health, growth and development. Aboriginal and Torres Strait Islander children with severe, life-threatening infections have been reported as three time more likely to be admitted to ICUs than non-Indigenous children. Of those admitted to an ICU, a third are associated with pre-existing conditions from birth, chronic illnesses, cancer and burns, and the majority of these are infants (40 per cent) and young children (33 per cent) (Ostrowski et al., 2017). The following sections provide a brief summary of common health conditions afflicting Aboriginal and Torres Strait Islander children.

Ear health

Rates of recurrent and chronic ear infections – in particular otitis media (middle ear infection) and resultant hearing impairment – are high in Aboriginal and Torres Strait Islander children (approximately 65 per cent) (AHMAC, 2017, p. 69). Otitis media is 2.4 times more likely to occur in Indigenous children than in non-Indigenous children, with infection rates as high as 90 per cent in remote communities among children up to the age of five years (Edwards & Moffat, 2014). Associated factors for ear infections include household overcrowding, environmental cigarette smoke, premature birth, bottle feeding, poverty and poor nutrition. Infections can begin very soon after birth and continue into adolescence, with hearing loss contributing to developmental delays included speech and learning and, in the longer term, unemployment (Closing the Gap Clearinghouse, 2014). Sadly, studies in the Northern Territory found an association with hearing impairment and Aboriginal youth offending (56 per cent for boys; 37 per cent for girls) (He et al., 2019) and adult imprisonment (Vanderpoll & Howard, 2012).

Pneumococcal and haemophilus influenza type B (Hib) vaccinations and short-term use of antibiotics can help to reduce the number of otitis media episodes. Screening at birth for risk factors and ongoing routine child health checks that incorporate ear and hearing assessment promotes timely treatment and management in the healthcare setting. All babies in Australia should be screened for congenital hearing problems in the first month of life. Health promotion to raise awareness of the impact of household smoking on ear infections is integral to promoting improved outcomes (Closing the Gap Clearinghouse, 2014). More information and resources can be found at Care for Kids. An example of a program aimed at screening, preventing and treating ear infections and hearing loss is Queensland Health's Statewide Aboriginal and Torres Strait Islander Ear Health Deadly Ears Program.

CASE STUDY

Deadly Ears program

The Deadly Hearing team provides an example of a comprehensive ear health program, which consists of:

- working in eleven partner locations across rural and remote Queensland where we deliver frontline clinical services and build local capacity
- coordinating policy and practice changes across the health, early childhood and education sectors
- delivering workforce training and professional development for healthcare professionals and educators
- undertaking research to improve the prevention, treatment and management of middle ear disease and its impacts on early childhood development.

The Deadly Ears Program consists of four teams:

- the Primary Health Team – which provides training and professional development, and sector-level support to healthcare professionals and service providers
- the Allied Health Team – which provides audiology, speech pathology and occupational therapy services and support to children and families, as well as to allied health, early years and education professionals and services to identify and manage hearing loss and other impacts associated with middle ear disease
- the Ear Nose and Throat (ENT) Outreach Team – which provides specialist outreach ENT clinics and surgeries for Aboriginal and Torres Strait Islander children with otitis media and associated conductive hearing loss
- the Administration Team – which provides support to the other teams so they can do their work.

Source: Reproduced from CHQHHS (2020).

Respiratory health

Rates of acute respiratory infection and short and long-term morbidity rates remain substantially higher for Indigenous than for non-Indigenous children, and respiratory episodes are ten times more likely (Basnayake, Morgan & Chang, 2017; Torzillo & Chang, 2014). Asthma affects 12 per cent of Aboriginal and Torres Strait Islander children aged from birth to fourteen years compared with 8 per cent of non-Indigenous children, and is more likely to affect children in urban and rural areas (ABS, 2019). Asthma can coexist with more than one chronic disease and requires access to appropriate health services for management. It can also impact a child's ability to attend school (O'Grady et al., 2018). Overcrowding, non-compliance with immunisation schedules, exposure to passive smoking and infant formula feeding are known for their contribution to increased risk and spread of respiratory illnesses, and the exacerbation of asthma. Education follow-up and community inclusion can improve long-term asthma outcomes. Aboriginal and Torres Strait Islander children are also prone to acquiring pneumonia and influenza. The immunisation programs are essential, and NSW Health currently funds free influenza vaccination clinics for all children aged from six months to five years of age (CEE, 2018).

Skin health

Impetigo and scabies are endemic in remote Aboriginal and Torres Strait Islander communities. These skin infections can have long-term and serious morbidity by promoting opportunistic systemic bacterial infections that cause diseases like glomerulonephritis and acute rheumatic heart disease (ARHD) (Quilty, Kaye & Currie, 2017). ARHD is caused by acute rheumatic fever, an illness that if untreated affects the heart, joints, brain and skin, and can lead to permanent damage to the heart valves (Australian Indigenous HealthInfoNet, 2020c). Skin infections can also impact the child's quality of life and affect school attendance (Thomas et al., 2017).

Scabies is a parasitic infestation of the skin where the tiny mites burrow into the upper layers of the skin, causing intensely itchy lesions. This can lead to crusted scabies (a form of scabies where there is a main source of infection in the community containing millions of mites), which is highly infectious (McMullan et al., 2016). Children presenting with recurrent scabies infections should have an environmental assessment undertaken to exclude sentinel household contacts that have crusted scabies. One successful program, the East Arnhem Scabies Control Program, was able to improve episodes of recurrent scabies. Its management protocol used active case findings to identify people with crusted scabies. The cases were then treated, either in hospital or in the community, and had regular one- to four-weekly skin checks and regular use of kerolytic cream and moisturisers, as well as scabies (acaricide) cream two to four times weekly (Lokuge et al., 2014).

Impetigo is a highly contagious skin condition characterised by fluid-filled red sores that pop easily and leave a yellow crust; it occurs on the face, neck and hands of young children and infants. The sores may be accompanied by an itchy rash and swollen lymph nodes. Children who wear diapers also tend to get impetigo around the diaper area. Impetigo is caused by both *Streptococcus pyogenes* and *Staphylococcus aureus*, and is commonly associated with scabies infestation (Bowen et al., 2014). Impetigo is caused by skin-to-skin contact, sharing of towels, bedding and toys with an individual who has the disease, insect and animal bites, and cuts and abrasions. Overcrowding increases the risk of exposure to the condition and makes clearing up the disease more difficult in settings where reinfection is more likely to occur.

Impetigo usually gets better within around two to three weeks by regular cleansing of the sores with soap and water. The main treatments prescribed are antibiotic creams or antibiotic tablets, which can reduce the length of the illness to around seven to ten days and can lower the risk of the infection being spread to others. Health promotion is a key to reducing infection and complications. A community-based media health-promotion strategy aimed at children and youth is the Indigenous hip hop Project Merredin 'Gotta Keep it Strong'.

Gastrointestinal infection and parasitic infestation

Aboriginal and Torres Strait Islander children in regional and remote areas are more likely to have gastrointestinal issues that affect their nutritional and general health status. Gastrointestinal infection is closely linked to the social determinants of health and, where there are deficits, requires proactive approaches by all levels of government to prevent disease (Ali, Foster & Hall, 2018). Acute infections affecting the ability of the stomach and intestinal tract are more commonly preventable; however, in these circumstances they are not easily escapable for Aboriginal and Torres Strait Islander children. Hospitalisation is 50 times higher for gastrointestinal infections in the most disadvantages areas compared with the least disadvantaged (CEE, 2018). Parasitic gut infestation is common, and often there can be multiple species present – both worms and protozoans.

Giardiasis is a very prevalent intestinal protozoan parasite, particularly in young children, and is seen mostly in remote areas. Giardiasis is spread through drinking contaminated water and person-to-person contact, food and soil. It can also be contracted through contaminated bodies of water and swimming pools. In some states or territories, giardiasis is a notifiable infection. Prevention can be promoted through education on proper sanitation, clean drinking water (boiling drinking water where contaminated) and good personal hygiene practices. Giaridiosis is treated with metronidazole (Flagyl) (Asher et al., 2014). Other common parasitic infections are hookworm, threadworm and roundworm. Hookworm causes internal blood loss, leading to iron deficiency anaemia as well as loss of appetite, reduced gut absorption and intestinal digestion. While decreasing in prevalence, hookworm infection is likely to affect children living in rural and remote areas. Roundworms and threadworms live in the gut and can be contracted via soil and dirt. Common over-the-counter antihelminth medications can treat these (Davies et al., 2013).

QUESTIONS FOR REFLECTION

- What are the prevalent health conditions, if any, in your local health area?
- Do you know what the current screening and treatment procedures are for these health conditions?

Accidents and hospitalisation

Indigenous children have higher rate of unintentional hospitalisation than non-Indigenous children, with the higher discrepancies due to falls from playground equipment, burns, poisoning and teenage assaults (AIHW, 2016, 2020a; Moller et al.,

2016). During 2016–17, Aboriginal and Torres Strait Islander children from birth to fourteen years of age were considerably more likely than non-Indigenous children to be hospitalised from injury. During 2015–17, the leading causes of hospitalisation leading to death were land transport accidents, accidental drownings and threats to breathing (AIHW, 2020a). The most common cause of injury in young children was falls, with the main cause being falls from play equipment. For teenagers – both boys and girls – there were higher rates of admission for assault and intentional self-harm. Girls were seventeen times and boys four times more likely than non-Indigenous teenagers to have been injured through assault (AIHW, 2016). Drowning was also 44 per cent higher than for non-Indigenous children, with a survival rate of 90 per cent (Wallis et al., 2015).

A systematic review of Australia's youth found suicide rates among Aboriginal and Torres Strait Islander children were rising substantially (Dickson et al., 2019). The review found limitations in the literature answering why suicide is increasing among the communities; however, it outlined how to monitor and prevent the phenomenon. Culturally targeted injury-prevention measures aimed at injury mechanism and age groups are required to reverse this situation. Examples of programs aimed at reducing unintentional injury and hospitalisation can be found at online at HealthInfoNet (see online resource section of the companion website). An overview of some key programs is provided below.

Blacktown Aboriginal Safety Promotion Program

This program includes the following projects:

- the Home Safe Home project, which conducted safety audits in homes to identify and reduce the impact of physical hazards
- the Ngarra Safety in the Local Environment project, which conducted safety audits in pubs and clubs to reduce the impact of unsafe drinking and driving
- the Keeping Aboriginal Youth Safe project, which supported young Aboriginal people to obtain and keep their drivers licence.

(Australian Indigenous HealthInfonet, 2020b)

Aboriginal Child Car Restraint Information Workshop WALGA RoadWise program

This program addressed the non-use of seatbelts and child car restraints among some Aboriginal people in the Pilbara region of Western Australia. Aboriginal ambassadors were trained to share information on child car restraints with their family members and their communities, and workshops were conducted to help raise awareness and prevention of road trauma in the communities

(Australian Indigenous HealthInfonet, 2020a)

Headspace centres

Headspace runs 100 centres across Australia that act as 'a one-stop shop' for young people (twelve- to 25-year-olds) who need help with mental health, physical health (including sexual health), alcohol and other drugs, or work and study support (headspace, 2020). The headspace website contains useful information for children, youth, communities and health providers to help prevent and support children and youth at risk of suicide.

Providing Aboriginal and Torres Strait Islander integrated and networked services

The following case study is an example of an urban model of primary health care promoting optimal child health.

CASE STUDY

La Perouse Community Health Service Pediatrics Clinic, Sydney

A collaborative community-based outreach service at La Perouse Community Health Service, Sydney provides care aimed at reducing health risk factors, and screening and intervention for developmental and medical problems commencing during pregnancy and early in life. This is a partnership and collaboration between the Prince of Wales Hospital, Sydney Children's Hospital, the Royal Hospital for Women and the La Perouse community.

Tanisha is a seventeen-year-old Aboriginal and Torres Strait Islander pregnant woman who has been raised by her mother's sister, Aunty Gloria, since her mother's death ten years ago in southeastern Sydney. Tanisha finds out from her friends and other aunties in the community that there is a local maternity service available for Aboriginal and Torres Strait Islander women. She books in with the Malabar Community Midwifery Link Service. At her first visit, she meets with a midwife and an Aboriginal and Torres Strait Islander health education officer, who coordinate her care needs. The midwives coordinate and ensure an obstetrician, paediatrician, social worker and any other required relevant healthcare professional provide care as indicated. A child and family health nurse and Aboriginal liaison and education officer also meet with Tanisha to plan her transition to motherhood. During the course of her pregnancy, the social worker ensures she has financial support and practical support from a female doctor, who monitors her health due to her age, and a psychiatrist with whom she is able to discuss losing her mother as a child and any other issues that arise. She finds the local La Perouse community clinic convenient and private. She is also able to meet other young mums and takes part in art group where she paints her story on a plaster cast of her pregnant belly.

After discharge from hospital after the birth of her baby girl, Ella, Tanisha has early home visiting focusing on both baby Ella and Tanisha's progress. Ella was found to have congenital hearing loss that was diagnosed in hospital during the routine audiometry test. Tanisha continues to attend the mothers' group at the clinic where her Child and Family Health Nurse is available to provide ongoing support to her and her baby girl. She knows that at the La Perouse Community Health Centre she can also receive information about baby care, practical advice and assistance with breastfeeding, nutrition and parenting, monitoring of the baby's developmental milestones, immunisation status and infections, and health checks before starting school. The integrated service also provides paediatric clinics, hearing clinics and referral to hospital and emergency department follow-up if Tanisha or Ella needs it. Tanisha and Ella are able to have ongoing support for Ella's hearing needs until the age of sixteen years.

For more information on this service see Gardner et al. (2016).

QUESTIONS FOR REFLECTION

- What care components of La Perouse Community Paediatric Clinic will promote Ella's health and wellbeing?
- What services exist in your area to support a young mother and her growing children?

Conclusion

Prior to invasion, Aboriginal and Torres Strait Islander children were few and precious, and their holistic health needs were met within their strong and extended family structures. Child mortality and morbidity were an accepted part of life, and child-rearing practices promoted resilience. Post-invasion, the introduction of disease, loss of traditional food sources due to dispossession of lands and the fracturing of traditional family and community structure fuelled an increase in mortality and morbidity rates (Boulton, 2016).

While some gains have been made in improving Aboriginal and Torres Strait Islander children's health, a disparate gap still exists (Department of Health, 2016). Many strategies are in place to promote improvements: targeted maternal and child health services, health promotion, targeted screening, immunisation and access to specialist care and treatments in partnership with the family and their communities.

As a clinician, it may seem insurmountable that you can have an impact on this situation. However, it is important to recognise the resilience and strengths of Aboriginal and Torres Strait Islander people to know what is right for their people and support them in this evolving society. Awareness will lead to safety of cultural practice while practising and engaging with the community. Understand the intergenerational trauma that impacts health and social situations, and promote initiatives that support Aboriginal and Torres Strait Islander people to maintain family and kinship integrity and traditions. Practical strategies have been laid out in this chapter to promote child and infant health. As an individual, you can help families to access initiatives and services to promote health and wellbeing by ensuring that they are enabled – ask, include, explain, support, refer and care by being a culturally safe practitioner.

Learning activities

1. What are the prevalent health conditions, if any, in your local health area? Do some research and make a list. Do you know the current screening and treatment for these health conditions?
2. In the immediate area where you work, what Aboriginal and Torres Strait Islander services or liaison people are available to support your Aboriginal or Torres Strait Islander families and your clinical practice? Do you know the contact details of your local Aboriginal and Torres Strait Islander liaison officer/worker? Do you know how to refer a child to these services?
3. Ask about the immunisation status of the Aboriginal and Torres Strait Islander children in your care. If non-compliant, be opportunistic and discuss with the parents and carers the benefits of immunisation. Offer relevant vaccination if clinically appropriate – that is, if there are no contraindications.

FURTHER READING

AIHW (2020). *Australia's Children*. Canberra: AIHW. Retrieved from www.aihw.gov.au/reports/children-youth/australias-children

Davis, M. (2019). *Family is Culture. Final Report of the Independent Review into Aboriginal Out-of-home Care in NSW.* Sydney: NSW Government. Retrieved from www.familyisculture.nsw.gov.au/__data/assets/pdf_file/0011/726329/Family-Is-Culture-Review-Report.pdf.

Family Matters (2019). *The Family Matters Report 2019: Measuring Trends to Turn the Tide on the Over-representation of Aboriginal and Torres Strait Islander Children in Out-of-home Care in Australia.* Retrieved from www.familymatters.org.au/wp-content/uploads/2020/02/1097_F.M-2019_LR.ƒupdated.pdf.

Visit the companion website at www.cambridge.org/highereducation/isbn/9781108794695/resources to see further online resources.

REFERENCES

ABS (2012). Breastfeeding. In *Australian Health Survey: Health Service Usage and Health Related Actions, 2011–12*. Canberra: ABS. Retrieved from www.abs.gov.au/ausstats/abs@.nsf/Lookup/6664B939E49FD9C1CA257B39000F2E4B.

ABS (2019). *National Aboriginal and Torres Strait Islander Health Survey, 2018–2019: Asthma and Chronic Obstructive Pulmonary Disease*. Canberra: ABS. Retrieved from https://www.abs.gov.au/statistics/people/aboriginal-and-torres-strait-islander-peoples/national-aboriginal-and-torres-strait-islander-health-survey/latest-release#asthma-and-chronic-obstructive-pulmonary-disease

ACHT – CACHS (2012). *Aboriginal Child Health Schedule Rationale Document: Child and Adolescent Statewide Policy*. Perth: Western Australian Government.

AHMAC (2017). *Aboriginal and Torres Strait Islander Health Performance Framework 2017 Report*. Canberra: AHMAC.

AIFS (2020). *Strengths of Australian Aboriginal Cultural Practices in Family Life and Child Rearing*. Retrieved from https://aifs.gov.au/cfca/publications/strengths-australian-aboriginal-cultural-practices-family-life-and-child-r/export

AIHW (2014). *New Directions: Mothers and Babies Services: Assessment of the program Using nKPI Data December 2012 to December 2013*. Canberra: AIHW.

AIHW (2016). *Hospitalised Injury in Aboriginal and Torres Strait Islander Children and Young People 2011–13*. Canberra: AIHW.

AIHW (2018). *Australia's Health 2018*. Canberra: AIHW.

AIHW (2019). *Australia's Mothers and Babies 2017 – in Brief*. Canberra: AIHW.

AIHW (2020a). *Australia's Children*. Canberra: AIHW.

AIHW (2020b). *Child Protection Australia 2018–19*. Canberra: AIHW.

Ali, S.H., Foster, T. & Hall, N.L. (2018). The relationship between infectious disease and housing maintenance in Indigenous Australian households. *International Journal of Environmental Research and Public Health*, 15(12), 2827.

Asher, A.J., Holt, D.C., Andrews, R.M. & Power, M.L. (2014). Distribution of Giardia duodenalis assemblages A and B among children living in a remote Indigenous community of the Northern Territory, Australia. *PLOS One*, https://journals.plos.org/plosone/article/metrics?id=10.1371/journal.pone.0112058.

Atkinson, J. (2013). *Trauma-informed Services and Trauma-specific Care for Indigenous Australian Children*. Resource sheet no. 21. Canberra: AIHW & AIFS.

Australian Indigenous HealthInfoNet (2020a). *Aboriginal Child Car Restraint Information Workshop WALGA RoadWise Program*. Perth: Australian Indigenous HealthInfoNet.

Australian Indigenous HealthInfoNet (2020b). *Blacktown Aboriginal Safety Promotion Program*. Perth: Australian Indigenous HealthInfoNet.

Australian Indigenous HealthInfoNet (2020c). *Overview of Australian Indigenous and Torres Strait Islander Health Status, 2019*. Perth: Australian Indigenous HealthInfoNet.

Bar-Zeev, S.J., Kruske, S.G., Barclay, L.M., Bar-Zeev, N. & Kildea, S.V. (2013). Adherence to management guidelines for growth faltering and anaemia in remote dwelling Australian Aboriginal infants and barriers to health service delivery. *BMC Health Services Research*, 13, 250.

Basnayake, T.L., Morgan, L.C. & Chang, A.B. (2017). The global burden of respiratory infections in Indigenous children and adults: A review. *Respirology*, 22: 1518–28.

Best Start Resource Centre (2020). *Reducing the Impact: Working with Pregnant Women Who Live in Difficult Life Situations*. Retrieved from www.beststart.org/resources/anti_poverty/pdf/REDUCE.pdf

Boulton, J. (2016). Disrupting demography: Population collapse and rebound. In J. Boulton with G. Macdonald (eds), *Aboriginal Children, History and Health*. New York: Routledge, pp. 119–35.

Bowen, A.C., Tong, S.Y., Chatfield, M.D. & Carapetis, J.R. (2014). The microbiology of impetigo in Indigenous children: Associations between Streptococcus pyogenes, Staphylococcus aureus, scabies, and nasal carriage. *BMC Infectious Diseases*, 14(1), 727.

CEE (2018). *Aboriginal Kids – A Healthy Start to Life: Report of the Chief Health Officer 2018*. Sydney: NSW Ministry of Health. Retrieved from www.health.nsw.gov.au/hsnsw/Publications/chief-health-officers-report-2018.pdf

CHQHHS (2020). *Deadly Ears*. Retrieved from www.childrens.health.qld.gov.au/chq/our-services/community-health-services/deadly-ears

Closing the Gap Clearinghouse (2014). *Ear Disease in Aboriginal and Torres Strait Islander Children*. Resource sheet no. 35. Canberra: AIHW & AIFS.

Conte, K.P., Gwynn, J., Turner, N., Koller, C. & Gillham, K.E. (2019). Making space for Aboriginal and Torres Strait Islander community health workers in health promotion. *Health Promotion International*, doi:10.1093/heapro/daz035

Davies, J., Majumdar, S.S., Forbes, R.T.M., Smith, P., Currie, B.J. & Baird, R.W. (2013). Hookworm in the Northern Territory: Down but not out. *Medical Journal of Australia*, 198(5), 278–81.

Department of Health (2016). *National Framework for the Health Services for Aboriginal and Torres Strait Islander Children and Families*. Canberra: Australian Government.

Dickson, J.M., Cruise, K., McCall, C.A. & Taylor, P.J. (2019). A systematic review of the antecedents and prevalence of suicide, self-harm and suicide ideation in Australian Aboriginal and Torres Strait Islander Youth. *International Journal of Environmental Research and Public Health*, 16(17), 3154.

Dimitropoulos, Y., Holden, A., Gwynne, K., Irving, M., Binge, N. & Blinkhorn, A. (2018). An assessment of strategies to control dental caries in Aboriginal children living in

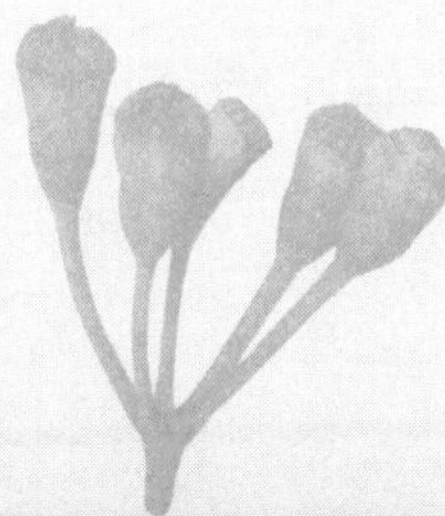

rural and remote communities in New South Wales, Australia. *BMC Oral Health*, 18(177). doi:10.1186/s12903-018–0643-y

DPMC (2019). *Closing the Gap Prime Minister's Report 2019*. Canberra: Commonwealth of Australia. Retrieved from www.niaa.gov.au/sites/default/files/reports/closing-the-gap-2019/sites/default/files/ctg-report-20193872.pdf?a=1.

DPMC (2020). *Closing the Gap: Prime Minister's Report 2020*. Canberra: Commonwealth of Australia.

Edwards, J. & Moffat,C,D. (2014). Otitis media in remote communities. *Australian Nursing and Midwifery Journal*, 21(9): 28.

Gardner, S., Woolfenden, S., Callaghan, L. ... Zwi, K. (2016). Picture of the health status of Aboriginal children living in an urban setting of Sydney. *Australian Health Review*, 40(3), 337–344.

Gibberd, A.J., Simpson, J.M. & Eades, S.J. (2016). No official identity: A data linkage study of birth registration of Aboriginal children in Western Australia. *Australian and New Zealand Journal of Public Health*, 40(4), 388–94.

Grace, T., Oddy, W., Bulsara, M. & Hands, B. (2017). Breastfeeding and motor development: A longitudinal cohort study. *Human Movement Science*, 51: 9–16.

Griffiths, K., Coleman, C., Al-Yaman, F. ... Madden, R. (2019). The identification of Aboriginal and Torres Strait Islander people in official statistics and other data: Critical issues of international significance. *Statistical Journal of the IOAS*, 35, 91–106.

He, V.Y., Su, J.-Y., Guthridge, S., Malvaso, C., Howard, D., Williams, T. & Leach, A. (2019). Hearing and justice: The link between hearing impairment in early childhood and youth offending in Aboriginal children living in remote communities of the Northern Territory, Australia. *Health & Justice*, 7(1): 16.

headspace (2020). Our centres. Retrieved from https://headspace.org.au/our-services/our-centres.

Heath, F., Bor, W., Thompson, J. & Cox, L. (2011). Diversity, disruption, continuity: Parenting and social and emotional wellbeing amongst Aboriginal peoples and Torres Strait Islanders. *Australian and New Zealand Journal of Family Therapy*, 32(4), 300–13.

Kickett, G., Chandran, S. & Mitchell, J. (2019). Woon-yah Ngullah Goorlanggass – caring for our children: A culturally strong, therapeutic kinship care for Aboriginal children, young people and their families. *Developing Practice: The Child, Youth and Family Work Journal*, 52: 25–39.

Kikkawa, D. (2015). *Multiple Disadvantage and Major Life Events in Report from Wave 5*. Canberra: Department of Social Services.

Kildea, S., Gao, Y., Hickey, S. ... Roe, Y. (2019). Reducing preterm birth amongst Aboriginal and Torres Strait Islander babies: A prospective cohort study, Brisbane, Australia. *EClinicalMedicine*, 12, 43–51.

Kimla, K., Nathanson, D., Woolfenden, S. & Zwi, K. (2019). Identification of vulnerability within a child and family health service. *Australian Health Review*, 43: 171–7.

Laverty, M., McDermott, D.R. & Calma, T. (2017). Embedding cultural safety in Australia's main health care standards. *Medical Journal of Australia*, 207(1), 15–16.

Lima, S., El Dib, R.P., Rodrigues, M., Ferraz, G., Molina, A.C., Neto, C., de Lima, M. & Rudge, M. (2018). Is the risk of low birth weight or preterm labor greater when maternal stress is experienced during pregnancy? A systematic review and meta-analysis of cohort studies. *PlOS One*, 13(7), e0200594.

Lohoar, S., Butera, N. & Kennedy, E. (2014). *Strengths of Australian Aboriginal Cultural Practices in Family Life and Child Rearing.* Canberra: AIFS.

Lokuge, B., Kopczynski, A., Woltmann, A. … Prince, S. (2014). Crusted scabies in remote Australia, a new way forward: Lessons and outcomes from the East Arnhem Scabies Control Program. *Medical Journal of Australia*, 200(11), 644–8.

MacDonald G. (2014). Traditions of Aboriginal parenting. In J. Boulton (ed.), *Aboriginal Children: History and Health.* New York: Routlege, pp. 40–76.

McKenna, B. (2020). Cultural safety: There is no turning back. *Journal of Psychiatric and Mental Health Nursing*, 187, 164–73.

McMullan, B.J., Bowen, A., Blyth, C.C. … Turnidge, J. (2016). Epidemiology and mortality of Staphylococcus aureus bacteremia in Australian and New Zealand children. *JAMA Pediatrics*, 170(10), 979–86.

McNamara, B., Gubhaju, L., Jorm, L. … Eades, S. (2018). Exploring factors impacting early childhood health among Aboriginal and Torres Strait Islander families and communities: Protocol for a population-based cohort study using data linkage (the 'Defying the Odds' study). *BMJ Open*, 8: e021236.

Moller, H., Falster, K., Ivers, R., Falster, M.O., Clapham, K. & Jorm, L. (2016). Closing the Aboriginal child injury gap: Targets for injury prevention. *Australian and New Zealand Journal of Public Health*, 41(1), 8–14.

Moore, T.G., McDonald, M., Carlon, L. & O'Rourke, K. (2015). Early childhood development and the social determinants of health inequities. *Health Promotion International*, 30(2), 102–15.

NCHWS (2011). *National Framework for Universal Child and Family Health Services.* Canberra: Department of Health. Retrieved from www.health.gov.au/internet/main/publishing.nsf/content/AFF3C1C460BA5300CA257BF0001A8D86/$File/NFUCFHS.PDF

Newton, B.J. (2018). Understanding child neglect in Aboriginal families and communities in the context of trauma. *Child & Family Social Work*, 24(2), 218–26.

Nguyen, H., Zarnowiecki, D., Segal, L., Gent, D., Silver, B. & Boffa, J. (2018). Feasibility of implementing infant home visiting in a Central Australian Aboriginal community. *Prevention Science*, 19(7), 966–76.

NHMRC (2012). *Infant Feeding Guidelines.* Retrieved from www.eatforhealth.gov.au/sites/default/files/files/the_guidelines/n56b_infant_feeding_summary_130808.pdf

NSW Health (2012). *Aboriginal and Torres Strait Islander Origin: Recording of Information of Patients and Clients.* Retrieved from www1.health.nsw.gov.au/pds/ActivePDSDocuments/PD2012_042.pdf

O'Grady, K., Hall, K., Bell., A., Chang, A. & Potter, C. (2018). Review of respiratory diseases among Aboriginal and Torres Strait Islander children. *Australian Indigenous Health Bulletin*, 18(2): 1–32.

Ostrowski, J.A., MacLaren, G., Alexander, J. … Schlapbach, L.J. (2017). The burden of invasive infections in critically ill Indigenous children in Australia. *Medical Journal of Australia*, 206(2), 78–84.

Quilty, S., Kaye, T.S. & Currie, B.J. (2017). Crusted scabies in Northern and Central Australia – now is the time for eradication. *Medical Journal of Australia*, 206(2), 96.

Shmerling, E., Creati, M., Belfrage, M. & Hedges, S. (2019). The health needs of Aboriginal and Torres Strait Islander children in out-of-home care. *Journal of Paediatric Child Health*, 56(3), 384–8.https://doi.org/10.1111/jpc.14624

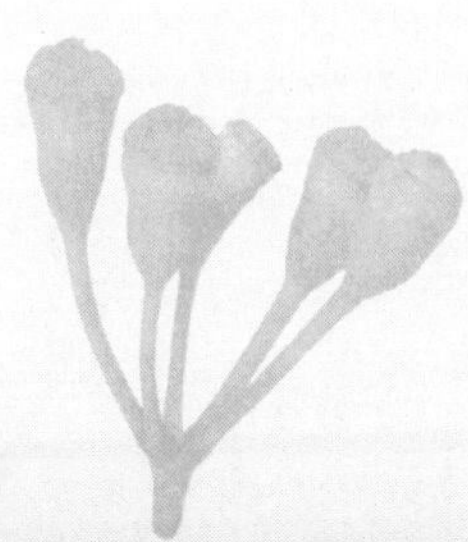

Thomas, S., Crooks, K., Taylor, K., Massey, P.D., Williams, R. & Pearce, G. (2017). Reducing recurrence of bacterial skin infections in Aboriginal children in rural communities: new ways of thinking, new ways of working. *Australian Journal of Primary Health*, doi:10.1071/PY16135

Torzillo, P.J. & Chang, A.B. (2014). Acute respiratory infections among Indigenous children. *Medical Journal of Australia*, 200(10), 559–60.

Urbis (2013). *A Descriptive Analysis of the Strong Fathers Strong Families Programme: Final Report.* Canberra: Department of Health.

Vanderpoll, T. & Howard, D. (2012). Massive prevalence of hearing loss among Aboriginal inmates in the Northern Territory. *Indigenous Law Bulletin*, 7(28), 3–7.

WA Department of Justice (2019). *Annual Report 2019/2020.* Retrieved from www.wa.gov.au/sites/default/files/2020–09/Department-of-Justice-Annual-Report-2019–2020_0.pdf

Wallis, B.A., Watt, K., Franklin, R.C. & Kimble, R.M. (2015). Drowning in Aboriginal and Torres Strait Islander children and adolescents in Queensland (Australia). *BMC Public Health*, 15, 795.

Yeo, S.S. (2003). Bonding and attachment of Australian Aboriginal children. *Child Abuse Review*, 12(5), 292–304.

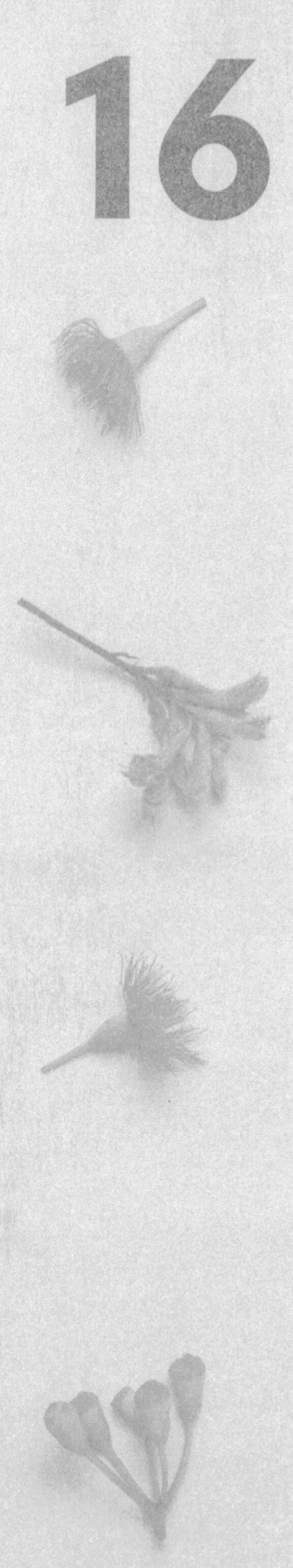

16 Caring for our Elders

Bronwyn Fredericks and Linda Deravin

With acknowledgement to Doseena Fergie

LEARNING OBJECTIVES

This chapter will help you to understand:

- Perspectives on Aboriginal and Torres Strait Islander ageing and aged care and the important contributions made by our Elders
- Relevant policies and strategies in caring for our Elders
- Providing culturally safe care to older Aboriginal and Torres Strait Islander people
- The role of nurses in advocating for appropriate care for older Aboriginal and Torres Strait Islander people

KEY WORDS

cultural determinants of health
dementia
Elder
human rights
palliative care
patient-centred care

Introduction

This chapter explores the health and wellbeing of older Aboriginal and Torres Strait Islander peoples and the factors that need to be considered in relation to their care, including chronic conditions, a shorter lifespan and culturally safe and appropriate aged care. Older Aboriginal and Torres Strait Islander people and their families make conscious decisions around care, and the role of nurses is to support individuals and their families in making informed decisions. Reasons are presented that explain why some Aboriginal and Torres Strait Islander people may be viewed by various health professionals as being non-compliant or disengaging in the health system and in relation to their ongoing care, including palliative care, when in fact they are making conscious choices that can be culturally defined and seen as a cultural determinant of health.

Elders and older Aboriginal and Torres Strait Islander people

It is important to remember that there can be vast differences between Aboriginal and Torres Strait Islander **Elders**. In this chapter, the term 'Elders' collectively represents Aboriginal and Torres Strait Islander people who are highly respected keepers of knowledge, which may or may not include cultural knowledge about customs, beliefs, ceremony, creation stories, historical stories, language and other knowledges. Historically, it was Aboriginal and Torres Strait Islander Elders who passed on knowledge to the younger generations. Elders were the carriers and transmitters of knowledge to future generations, and are respected across both Aboriginal and Torres Strait Islander peoples and communities. In some communities, Elders are held in very high esteem and may be seen as living treasures for the knowledge they hold and the teachings they have to offer.

Elder Being an Aboriginal or Torres Strait Islander Elder is not defined by gender or age. Elders are recognised because they have earned respect through being custodians of knowledge or lore, or through wisdom, experiences and actions. Not all communities are the same in the way they define Elders.

Elders within Aboriginal and Torres Strait Islander communities across Australia have lived under the harshest of the Acts of Administration, discussed in Chapters 1 and 2. Many of our community Elders over the age of approximately 60 years were born and lived on missions and reserves, having been forcibly removed there. Families were often split up and placed on different reserves or missions. Stolen wages are a very common theme through the lived experiences of our Elders, as is the removal of their children. This phenomena is known as the 'Stolen Generations' (AHRC, 2009).

Age structure of Indigenous and non-Indigenous Australians

It has been established in earlier chapters that Aboriginal and Torres Strait Islander Australians are the most socially and economically disadvantaged group in Australia and have the poorest health status compared with non-Indigenous Australians (AIHW, 2019b). Data show that there have been some improvements in life expectancy and lower rates of chronic disease; however, Indigenous women and men still have lower life expectancy and higher rates of chronic disease than non-Indigenous women and men (ABS, 2018). It is important to understand the impact of early onset of chronic disease and an anticipated earlier need for care, including in-home care and the possibility of residential care, along with a shorter life-expectancy.

As shown by the data in Figure 16.1, there are two distinct and obvious differences in the age structure between Indigenous and non-Indigenous Australians. First, there are proportionately fewer Aboriginal and Torres Strait Islander Elders and older people in comparison to non-Indigenous older people and the number dramatically declines by the age of 45 onwards. Second, the Indigenous population has a relatively young age structure. In 2016, the median age was 23 years, compared with 37.8 years for the non-Indigenous population (ABS, 2018). Over one-third (34 per cent) were aged under 15 years, compared with 18 per cent of non-Indigenous people. In the older population, Indigenous Australians represent 4 per cent of people over the age of 65 years compared with 16 per cent in the non-Indigenous Australian population (AIHW, 2019b). Australia now has more non-Indigenous centenarians than ever before; sadly, this is not the case for Indigenous Australian Elders and older people.

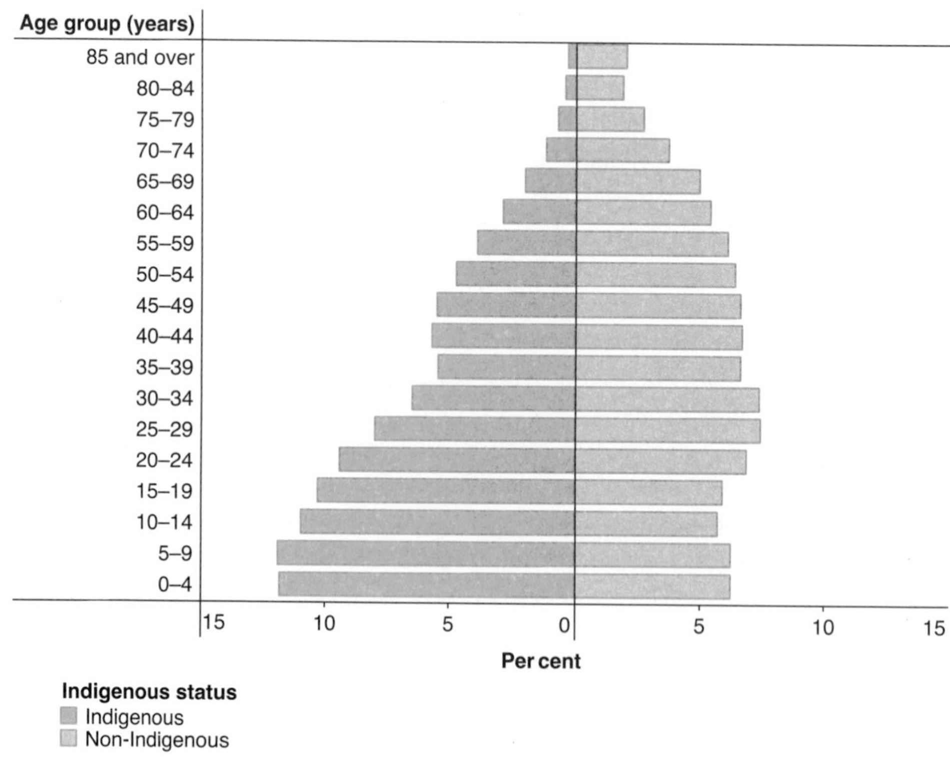

Figure 16.1 Age structure of the Australian population by Indigenous status, 30 June 2016

Source: Reproduced from AIHW (2019b), based on ABS (2018).

In this regard, Elders within the Aboriginal and Torres Strait Islander community may be particularly well looked after and respected (Best & Drummond, 2018). This is not the case in all communities, where it might be difficult to provide the level of care required for people with complex and competing chronic conditions within the home or community environment, particularly in some regional, rural and remote communities.

Some Aboriginal and Torres Strait Islander people may be referred to as 'Aunty' or 'Uncle' as a sign of respect for their knowledge and the legacy they have lived (Best & Drummond, 2018). Yet caution needs to be taken about calling everyone by these terms. Not all older Aboriginal and Torres Strait Islander people are regarded as Elders, and not all Aboriginal and Torres Strait Islander people like being called 'Aunty' or 'Uncle', either because they don't see themselves in this way or they don't like to be called by these terms by everyone. It is best to ask a person what they like to be called or how they wish to be referred to.

On 13 February 2008, the former Prime Minister Kevin Rudd with the Leader of the Opposition, Brendan Nelson, carried an empty *coolamon*, the symbol of the tragic removal of Aboriginal children, and handed it to the Speaker of the House of Representatives in the Australian Parliament on behalf of the 'Stolen Generations'. The *coolamon* is generally understood to be a carrying vessel. More than 200 years of intergenerational stress and trauma had been experienced across Aboriginal Australia prior to that symbolic act. Reynolds (2000) emphasised that history and circumstances affect health, and that over the past 220 years Indigenous Australians had suffered accumulating and persisting trauma. These effects are further exacerbated by exposure to continuing high levels of stress and trauma, including multiple bereavements and other losses (Ferguson, Baker et al., 2016).

Many Elders and older members of the Aboriginal and Torres Strait Islander community today have been negatively affected by the policies of the past, individually or within their families and community (Dudgeon & Walker, 2011; Dudgeon et al., 2010; Zubrick, 2014). They may still have issues connected with the ongoing impact of these insidious policies and with unresolved trauma, which compounds their health issues. Additionally, older members of the community may have multi-generational caring roles that can involve being the primary carer for their grandchildren and great-grandchildren. So who cares for the Elders and older members of the Aboriginal community?

CASE STUDY

Elder Ivy Molly Booth

Aboriginal Elder Ivy Molly Booth, who gifted us the name of this book, is an example of a living treasure. She is also the matrilineal grandmother of the Odette Best. Ivy Booth nee Darby is the Elder of the Wakgun people of the Gurreng Gurreng Nation. Her Country extends north along the Burnett River, west as far as Mundubbera and north to Eidsvold along the Dawes Range to Cania Gorge, then east to Mirriamvale and Baffle Creek. The land then extends south, down to Mt Perry and to the Burnett

(cont.)

River. Ivy Booth was born at Camboon Station and removed to Taroom Aboriginal Settlement in the early 1920s, before again being removed to Woorabinda Mission when it commenced in 1927. She is the only surviving original dormitory girl of Woorabinda. At Woorabinda, Ivy Booth met and married her husband, Clancy Booth, a Boonthamurra man.

In 2014, a group of young people retraced the footsteps of their ancestors, who were forced to walk more than 200 kilometres from Taroom to Woorabinda over 90 years ago. Ivy Booth was there to meet the walkers (Whop, 2014). She is great-great-grandmother to a large and extended family in Rockhampton, Queensland and further afield. Ivy Booth is at least 102 years old. She still lives in her own home and is supported to do so by her family and community.

QUESTIONS FOR REFLECTION

- How may Elders do you think there might be of such an age in Australian society?
- What do you think would need to be considered in caring for Ivy Booth?
- What would be the role of the nurse in such care?
- What do you think the situation would be if Ivy Booth were not in her own home with the support of her family?
- Why might Ivy Booth be considered a living treasure?

The issues discussed above and the needs of Elders and older community members were further emphasised in Australia during the development of the Aboriginal and Torres Strait Islander Health Plan 2013–2023, which states that:

> Older Aboriginal and Torres Strait Islander people should have the option to choose their environment where they feel most comfortable to age particularly if affected by ill-health and disability.
>
> (Commonwealth of Australia, 2013, p. 38)

human rights Recognising the inherent value of each and every person, regardless of background, where someone lives, what someone looks like, what they think and what they believe (AHRC, 2013).

patient-centred care Health care that is respectful of, and responsive to, the preferences, needs and values of patients and consumers.

This plan encourages a **human rights** approach to Indigenous ageing, promoting **patient-centred care** and decision-making, and respect for the inherent dignity of older people. The Australian Government has pledged its commitment to the *United Nations Declaration on the Rights of Indigenous Peoples* (United Nations, 2007), which promotes awareness, recognition and implementation of the human rights of Indigenous peoples and must report to the United Nations on how it does this.

This is relevant in health service planning, given the current statistics on chronic disease extracted from the 2018 National Aboriginal and Torres Strait Islander Health Measures Survey (NATSIHMS) (ABS, 2019). This is the largest biomedical survey of Aboriginal and Torres Strait Island peoples. The latest report provides the following information:

- Four in ten people had at least one chronic condition.
- The incidence of asthma was significantly higher in non-remote areas (17 per cent) and twice that for those living in remote areas (9 per cent).

- One-quarter of people surveyed reported having a mental or behavioural condition.
- There was an increase in anxiety (17 per cent) and depression (13 per cent) from the 2012–13 report with almost one in ten people reporting that this condition was affecting their daily living.
- Heart disease was the leading cause of death; this rose from 4 per cent in 2012–13 to 5 per cent in 2018–19.
- Participants living in remote areas were two-and-a-half times more likely to have signs of chronic kidney disease than their counterparts in the urban setting (3.4 per cent compared with 1.4 per cent).

The three common diseases of cardiovascular disease, diabetes and chronic kidney disease are not only risk factors themselves, but the comorbidity between them is more common for Aboriginal and Torres Strait Islander people compared with non-Indigenous people. Issues of care are compounded for all people living in isolated and remote communities, and include the cost of food (Ferguson , O'Dea et al., 2016; Power et al., 2020) and a range of other problems (Hellsten, 2014; Langton & Perkins, 2008; SCRGSP, 2016).

QUESTIONS FOR REFLECTION

- What are the issues for Elders and older people living in isolated or remote communities (for example, in Bourke, NSW or Mornington Island or Saibai Island, Queensland or Halls Creek, Western Australia or another community)?
- If you were a Registered Nurse in such a community, what issues of care would you need to consider?
- What would the impact of living in a remote locality be on the Elder or older person?
- What would the impact be on the community?

Health policy and strategy in caring for our Elders

The Council of Australian Governments (COAG) acknowledged that statistics like those derived from the NATSIHMS need to improve, even though this would take a number of years to achieve. The Council emphasised that for appropriate and effective interventions to be applied in order to decrease preventable deaths, healthcare services needed to be available, accessible and culturally safe. They additionally recognised that Aboriginal and Torres Strait Islander community controlled health services (CCHS) are able to ensure a better outcome than mainstream services because they would reduce unintentional racism, access barriers and improve health outcomes. Chapter 6, which focuses on CCHSs, addresses these issues. The World Health Organization (WHO) has recognised the need for a human rights dimension in aged-care plans – one that requires the employment of Indigenous Australian health workers in the aged-care workforce to ensure culturally safe and respectful service. To support this strategy, there is also an immediate need to provide education and support to the existing aged care workforce in providing culturally safe care (Deravin-Malone, 2017). Even so, other considerations need to be taken into account when caring for the needs of Indigenous Australians. Australian Bureau of Statistics (ABS, 2016) data collection recognised that Indigenous Australians are more likely than non-Indigenous Australians to have provided care. Most of these carers are women, who are unpaid but support family and friends with a disability, mental illness, chronic condition, terminal illness or who are frail. Of these women, the majority of primary carers are mothers aged between 45–54 years, followed by other female relatives. More of these women require assistance for their own self-care needs due to chronic disease than their non-Indigenous counterparts who may be caring for their older relatives (ABS, 2016).

Few Indigenous Australians identify as carers, although many have significant responsibilities of care that impact their ability to maintain a job and receive an adequate level of income to support themselves and others. They may also be unaware of the kinds of support available to them, so services may not be able to respond to them if there is little communication between organisations and services, and people engaged in a range of caring roles. In such situations, carers may experience a lack of information and receive little opportunity for health education and health literacy. For people living in rural or remote areas, there is the added issue of social isolation and location barriers when trying to access health and welfare services.

A recent study undertaken in the greater Rockhampton region of Central Queensland (Fredericks et al., 2016) explored people's experiences and perceptions of living with chronic conditions. It involved interviewing and workshopping with Indigenous people with chronic conditions and their carers, along with healthcare providers. The research identified a number of issues as well as strategies for improving the care of Aboriginal and/or Torres Strait Islander people with chronic conditions. The strategies included having culturally safe communication to build knowledge about the understanding of chronic conditions and preventative care. It is well recognised that when health services are culturally welcoming and increase their cultural safety across all areas of their service delivery, they will establish stronger rapport with their Indigenous clients, including their older Indigenous clients. These clients will then feel more welcome and access the service when needed and without concern and fear. This helps to build strong relationships over time between Elders and older Indigenous people, their carers, and family members and health services.

Aboriginal and Torres Strait Islander people with chronic conditions also articulated that they worry about and fear for their future in relation to health and the impact of the **cultural determinants of health** and social determinants, such as housing, income, education and employment (Fredericks et al., 2016). This may be even more of an issue for Aboriginal and Torres Strait Islander people due to many experiencing chronic diseases at an earlier age, and hence many will still be in the workforce or looking for employment. All these factors influence the decisions Aboriginal and Torres Strait Islander Elders and older people make about where and how they will live, and about their future care options. Thus, for health services, health providers and nurses to make a real difference to the health and care of Elder and older Aboriginal and Torres

cultural determinants of health Features by which basic differentiation of culture is possible. Examples include race, ethnicity, country of origin and language.

Strait Islander people, there needs to be a recognition and understanding of these interconnecting issues. There is a need to work across the contexts of individual lives and groups within the broader Indigenous community.

QUESTIONS FOR REFLECTION

- What might be some of the issues for Elders and older people living near you?
- What might be some of the interconnecting issues?
- As a nurse, how would you raise these and begin to explore and address the care options?
- Think about how you would work with other nurses, and other health professionals and services. What could improve the ways in which you might do this?

Culturally safe care

In Australia, Aboriginal and Torres Strait Islander people can access aged-care services from the age of 50, rather than 70 years and over as for other Australians. This is in response to the early onset of chronic conditions that affect people at a younger age. There may be Aboriginal and Torres Strait Islander people across a broad spectrum of ages and with a diversity of care needs accessing aged-care services or living within aged-care facilities in the general community. In 2018, there were 1700 Aboriginal and Torres Strait Islander people in permanent residential aged-care facilities (AIHW, 2019b). Approximately 49 per cent of Aboriginal and Torres Strait Islander people over the age of 75 years were living in aged care facilities. Within the 65–75 years age group, Indigenous Australians were twice as likely to be in residential care compared with non-Indigenous Australians. Indigenous Australians were also more likely to use supported community-based services, with Indigenous Australians being three times more likely to use home support and seven times more likely to use home care AIHW, 2019b). This clearly demonstrates that care for our older population is heavily reliant on community-based services.

In some communities, community members have advocated for, organised and established specific aged-care services for Aboriginal and Torres Strait Islander Elders and older people. There may be non-government organisations (NGOs) established for this specific purpose or they may be sponsored by existing Aboriginal and Torres Strait Islander or broader community organisations. Throughout Australia, programs and services such as the Multi-Purpose Service (MPS) program and the National Aboriginal and Torres Strait Islander Flexible Aged Care Program (NATSIFACP), as well as other programs referred to as Home and Community Care (HACC), provide care to our Elders. Aged-care packages are delivered into people's homes. Also available are centre-based respite care, residential hostels (which have some personal care) and nursing homes that specifically service Aboriginal and Torres Strait Islander people. There are standards and processes to follow with administering all of these (see AAQA, 2015, 2016). These are operated as culturally safe services, incorporating culturally safe practices, and they are in high demand. As such, and with the slight improvements in life expectancy within the Indigenous population, there is an increasing older population and an increasing pressure to care for Elders and older people.

The Royal Commission into Aged Care Services' 2019 interim report highlighted that the provision of culturally safe services is limited. Those that do exist are generally developed by Aboriginal Communities in response to the lack of provision in mainstream services (Tracey & Briggs, 2019). There are not enough services and facilities, and those that do exist can be located a long way from where people have lived for most of their lives and from where their family and other community members still live. This in itself can provide additional stress and affect social and emotional wellbeing when individuals are disconnected from their family members and cultural supports.

A government initiative that supports care of our Elders in the aged care sector, detailed in *Action to Support Older Aboriginal and Torres Strait Islander People: A Guide for Consumers* (ACSCDS, 2019) – clearly outlines the care our Elders want when engaging with aged care services. Most importantly, our Elders wish to have the following key principles of care:

- easily accessible information regarding their choices so that they can make informed decisions
- the active involvement in all aspects of their care planning
- access to culturally safe aged care services, regardless of location
- a preference to live on Country wherever possible with the support of aged care services
- an aged care system that is aware of the impact of harmful colonisation policies and its associated trauma caused by the forced separation of children from their families
- aged care services not being linked with organisations that supported the removal of children from families and thus retraumatising those who are the survivors of colonisation practices.

(ACSCDS, 2019)

CASE STUDY

Family/communal responsibility towards Elders

In this case study, Sarina shares some of her understandings about her mother and her father, and how they as a family would benefit from all knowing more about Alzheimer's and dementia. This was shared through research undertaken by Doseena Fergie, which explored care of older Indigenous Australians. In the discussion with Doseena, Sarina highlighted how she had attended a health education session with others, which included both Indigenous and non-Indigenous people. This took place when her mother was first diagnosed and enabled her to gain insight and information in how she could best assist her mother and then later her father. She has continued to participate in regular health education sessions.

Sarina shares her perceptions of the health education session with health professionals and with people who attended in the role of carers. She also explores the differences between how Indigenous and non-Indigenous people look at health communication and care. She articulates that health and wellbeing from an Indigenous perspective is relationship-based, that much time is put into developing relationships and connection and that everyone in the family who has a role with the person needing care and who supports the support-people and carers would be involved in receiving information. This would enable everyone within the immediate family and broader extended family to know what is happening and what needs to happen with regard to her mother and father. When family members don't attend the health education sessions, they can be unsure or confused about the health condition and what needs to happen regarding care. When everyone attends and is clear and together in knowing, it can result in appropriate care, including culturally safe care.

Sarina said:

> I have a concern about Mum. I noticed her memory loss, her incontinence was getting worse; she did not have a 'care' factor, which was the biggest thing. Dad knew about Alzheimer's but not dementia and the various stages until lately.
>
> It was good to see Indigenous people in health education. They were still communicating whether they knew each other or not – we are family. Whereas the white people [in the first health education session] were individuals, even though they get all the services. For us to have something similar we are flowing. How we are yarning is different. [Sarina is referring to the flow of the conversation once the relationship of family or how people are connected is made, and how it assists in gaining access to information.]
>
> Families are so big. If I can get them together they would be so interested. How do you involve the whole family in what I know about dementia? Our Elders put up a front and teach us all different – they are proud people and display to others that they are good because they know …
>
> The communal responsibility as a family is not the same as it was when some of our Elders that we are looking after were young. We are a product of our global society. If the family were there in the seminar they would have understood.

QUESTIONS FOR REFLECTION

- What are some considerations for culturally safe care that are indicated in this case study?
- What is the advantage of including both Indigenous and non-Indigenous people in education sessions regarding culturally safe care?
- What could potentially be some of the issues that may arise when people come from different cultural backgrounds?

Dementia

dementia Now referred to as a neurocognitive disorder (NCD) (APA, 2013), is the result of chronic or progressive damage to the brain (Forman & Pond, 2015).

Dementia is a broad term that includes specific chronic conditions such as Alzheimer's disease, Lewy body disease, vascular dementia and frontotemporal disease (Deravin & Anderson, 2019). Alzheimer's Australia indicates that the prevalence of dementia within the Aboriginal and Torres Strait Islander population for people 45 years and over was 12.4 per cent compared with a rate of 2.6 per cent in the wider Australian population in 2007 (Alzheimer's Australia, 2007). More recent statistics on the prevalence of dementia within the Aboriginal and Torres Strait Islander population are not available; however, as our Elders are living longer and previous statistics show our Elders have dementia at five times higher than the wider population, as a chronic condition the impact for our Elders is significant. In addition, dementia is found in more younger Indigenous people compared with the broader Australian population (AIHW, 2011) and this rate is expected to increase as life expectancy in the Indigenous population also improves (Garvey et al., 2011). Research in rural and remote areas suggests that rates are higher than in the non-Aboriginal population but poorly detected among communities. The 2009–212 Koori Growing Old Well Study indicates that dementia has an earlier onset among the Indigenous population, given the high risk factors that include chronic comorbidities (Arkles et al., 2010). At 5.2 times higher than for other Australians, this is significant. The research showed that Alzheimer's is the most common form of dementia found within the Indigenous population and that dementia is also more prevalent in Indigenous males compared with women in the broader population (Alzheimer's Australia, 2007). In 2017, dementia was the second leading cause of death Australia wide (AIHW, 2019a).

There are mixed understandings of dementia and the behaviours resulting from dementia. For example, people can be concerned when a person with dementia behaves in certain ways or does not behave in the way people expect them to. Moreover, it can be particularly distressing and traumatic for individuals, families and communities when people have cultural, family or other obligations that they cannot fulfil due to dementia. Some Aboriginal people might refer to what is happening to a person as being 'out of balance' or having a 'sick spirit' (Alzheimer's Australia, 2006); other community members will struggle with understanding, while others will have be aware of the impacts of dementia. There is a range of understandings and beliefs about dementia in the Aboriginal and Torres Strait Islander population, just as there is in the broader population.

It is important to encourage people to seek an assessment and to also care for others who they think might have dementia. Assessments should be carried out in ways that consider all issues and take into account other health conditions that are being managed. What must be considered in any assessment process is the fear that may be present from past interactions with the medical system and experiences of child removal. These fears, along with a lack of understanding about dementia, can be a barrier for Elders in accessing assistance and can cause further trauma (Arkles et al., 2010; Sherwood, 2013). These fears are in addition to the other issues that may be experienced, which are similar to those of non-Indigenous Australians.

The following case study will extend your thinking about your role as a nurse, the mix of services with which you might work and the care options for individuals that you might need to consider.

CASE STUDY

Alfred and Sonia

In the case study below, Alfred shares with the interviewer how he is trying to understand and manage the care of his wife, Sonia, along with himself. His daughter, Melissa, discusses how she is trying to ensure the care of both her mother and her father. Because his daughter, Melissa, is present, Alfred refers to his wife as Mum.

ALFRED: Either way, how I'm affected by dementia myself and what I have to deal with Mum … What freedom have I got? … the thought of when I'm outside doing what I like and then the phone rings and I have to rush in. Mum can't get to it. We have to accept it and battle on as best we can.

MELISSA: Dementia is a new ball game for Dad. At least Darlene [a carer] went to a workshop and that info has helped him. Now he can see the changes in Mum. For example, repetition. I've got to have the patience to deal with it and be educated and see how Mum fits in. Be different if Darlene lived here. Twenty years ago, Alzheimer's was on his mind and not dementia. He never dreamed of learning about dementia but now Mum has it and Dad is confronted with it. It's a large thing to adjust myself to it.

ALFRED: Learning is easily done but actually *doing* is difficult, especially when I am by myself. If I've got a question about something, I've got no one there to ask until the carer comes.

MELISSA: Dad's mind is in two ways because he wants to be outside as well as inside. Dad has a routine set in his mind before he goes to sleep. But now, in the morning, he has learnt to change the routine. He reasons it out if he has to deal with Mum.

ALFRED: Routine has been drilled into you from being in the army. When I was growing up is was how you went about life – look for something to do, keep yourself busy, don't be lazy. Planning before you go to sleep about tomorrow but knowing that it could change in the morning. For others – why can't they get into a routine and get up and do things? Now the whole structure of living has gone out the door. TV is an example where people adopt that this is how you go about life. We need to help them to see and do things in an organised way. This is a problem with today's working class and youth – like doing 100 kilometres an hour in an 80 kilometre an hour zone so, as a driver, I go a roundabout way and not in peak traffic. You make adjustments. But you're still learning as an Elder. The only advantage with us is that we learnt respect – how you conduct yourself – from our parents and grandparents. Today, violence that's displayed on TV and social media has increased. To put fear into people to get what they want – there's a lack of respect for Elders. When it comes to young people today we think, 'Why are they doing all this stuff?'

(cont.)

Unemployment has a lot to do with this. When they're introduced to the dole – they use it and get up to mischief. They bring it on themselves.

MELISSA: We lack a well-established welfare organisation with field officers to go out and find out the community's needs, come back and discuss it, and then have the resources to do it. We can't do it if you don't know.

QUESTIONS FOR REFLECTION

- What is being described and experienced in this case study?
- What was your first response to what is being discussed? How would you manage your emotions in order to ensure cultural safety within these situations?
- How might you respond to this situation if you were the nurse who was being made aware of the issues raised? Explain your plan of action.

The role of the nurse in end-of-life care

As discussed in earlier chapters, increasing numbers of Aboriginal and Torres Strait Islander people now live in Australia's urban, peri-urban and regional areas. Some Indigenous people may still live on Country, but this number is decreasing due to a range of factors. During their later years, many Aboriginal and Torres Strait Islander people seek to return to their homelands – their Country – to spend their last years. Some people may be able to travel back to their Country for a visit, or to relocate, but for others it may be too difficult due to a range of reasons. Sometimes, despite the difficulty and lack of treatment and care options, some people will choose to go home. This is deemed to be a higher priority than remaining in the urban or regional centre to receive treatment (Indigenous Palliative Care Project, 2009). This may be hard to understand and confrontational to healthcare providers, including nurses who seek to offer care and treatment during the later period of life. Great care needs to be taken in not assuming that everyone thinks in the same way about **palliative care** and treatment, and in recognising that all Aboriginal and Torres Strait Islander people are different in how they will manage this period of time. Respect is vital in all interactions during this time.

palliative care High-level care for the terminally ill and their families, especially that provided by an organised health service.

If a person and their family decides that it is time to go home, back to Country, community health providers, CCHOs and other services all have an important role to play. It will be important to work in partnership with other health providers and to collaborate with the individuals concerned and their families and communities. The role of the nurse is partly that of a facilitator here, supporting brokerage of the care and treatment during this period of time. The nurse can enable a culturally safe way and assist in a dignified and respectful passing or they can hinder, disable and disempower during what can be a difficult time. This can be difficult for the nurse and medical staff too but it can also be intensely rewarding and support you to significantly grow in your nursing practice with Aboriginal and Torres Strait Islander people.

QUESTIONS FOR REFLECTION

- Consider how you view your own end of life. Have you thought what you want for yourself?
- Talk to your own loved ones and ask them what they want for themselves. Is it different from your own ideas or are they the same?
- Consider now how you would best advocate for and work with other nurses with different ideas about end of life and its care in supporting you and your family members. Explain your plan.

Conclusion

This chapter has examined what is meant by Elders in Aboriginal and Torres Strait Islander Australia. It has further examined dementia, human rights, patient-centred care and chronic disease. Importantly, it also discusses palliative care for those seeking to go back to Country at end of life – what this may mean for Aboriginal and Torres Strait Islander peoples and some of the challenges that this may present to you, as a nurse – specifically, the challenge to practise in a culturally safe way that respects the histories of, and provides the unique care needed by, our Elders.

Learning activities

1. Can you identify any aged-care services specifically for Aboriginal and Torres Strait Islander people in your region?
   - Why are they needed? What roles do they fulfil?
   - What might need to be considered in catering for Aboriginal and Torres Strait Islander men or women, considering what you know from earlier chapters?
   - Do these services meet the needs of people from varying cultural, gendered, sexual identities? Different religious beliefs? Different food and language or communication needs? If so, how? If not, why not?
2. What are some reasons why Indigenous men and women may choose to attend services that are available to all older people in preference to an Indigenous-specific service for older people?
3. How best might you assist a family if its members are preparing to support an Elder or older Aboriginal and Torres Strait Islander person to travel back to their community after some time away?

Resources and networks to assist you

- Australian Indigenous HealthInfoNet http://www.healthinfonet.ecu.edu.au
- National Aboriginal and Torres Strait Islander Flexible Aged Care Program
- Quality Framework for the National Aboriginal and Torres Strait Islander Flexible Aged Care Program
- My Aged Care: Aboriginal and/or Torres Strait Islander people

FURTHER READING

ACES & Harvey, K. (2003). *Aboriginal Elders' Voices: Stories of the 'Tide of History'. Victorian Indigenous Elders' Life Stories & Oral Histories.* Melbourne: Aboriginal Community Elders Service and Language Australia.

ACSCDS (2019). *Actions to Support Older Aboriginal and Torres Strait Islander People: A Guide for Consumers.* Canberra: Commonwealth of Australia.

Cotter, P.R., Condon, J.R., Barnes, T., Smith, L.R. & Cunningham, T. (2012). Do Indigenous Australians age prematurely? The implications of life expectancy and health conditions of older Indigenous people for health and aged care policy. *Australian Health Review*, 36(1), 68–74.

Visit the companion website to see at www.cambridge.org/highereducation/isbn/9781108794695/resources further online resources.

REFERENCES

AAQA (2015). *National Aboriginal and Torres Strait Islander Flexible Aged Care Program. Quality Review.* Canberra: AAQA.

AAQA (2016). *National Aboriginal and Torres Strait Islander Flexible Aged Care Program. Quality Standards Self-assessment tool.* Canberra: AAQA.

ABS (2016). *National Aboriginal and Torres Strait Islander Social Survey 2014–15.* Canberra: ABS.

ABS (2018). *Estimates of Aboriginal And Torres Strait Islander Australians, June 2016.* Canberra: ABS. Retrieved from www.abs.gov.au/ausstats/abs@.nsf/mf/3238.0.55.001

ABS (2019). *National Aboriginal and Torres Strait Islander Health Survey, 2018–19.* Retrieved from www.abs.gov.au/ausstats/abs@.nsf/mf/4715.0

ACSCDS (2019). *Actions to Support Older Aboriginal and Torres Strait Islander People: A Guide for Consumers.* Canberra: Department of Health. Retrieved from www.health.gov.au/sites/default/files/actions-to-support-older-aboriginal-and-torres-strait-islander-people-a-guide-for-consumers_0.pdf.

AHRC (2009). Track the history timeline: The stolen generations. Retrieved from www.humanrights.gov.au/track-history-timeline-stolen-generations

AHRC (2013). What are human rights? Retrieved from https://humanrights.gov.au/about/what-are-human-rights

AIHW (2011). *Indigenous Australians in Aged Care.* Canberra: AIHW. Retrieved from www.aihw.gov.au/aged-care/residential-and-community-2011

AIHW (2019a). *Dementia.* Canberra: AIHW. Retrieved from www.aihw.gov.au/reports-data/health-conditions-disability-deaths/dementia/overview

AIHW (2019b). *Profile of Indigenous Australians.* Canberra: AIHW. Retrieved from www.aihw.gov.au/reports/australias-welfare/profile-of-indigenous-australians

Alzheimer's Australia (2006). *Beginning the Conversation: Addressing Dementia in Aboriginal and Torres Strait Islander Communities. Workshop Report, 8–9 November.* Adelaide: Alzheimer's Australia. Retrieved from www.fightdementia.org.au/understanding-dementia/aboriginal–torres-strait-islander-groups.aspx

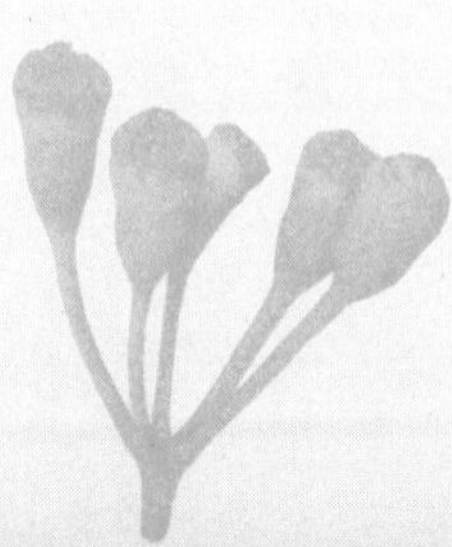

Alzheimer's Australia (2007). *Dementia: A Major Health Problem for Indigenous People. Briefing Prepared for Parliamentary Friends of Dementia.* Retrieved from www.healthinfonet.ecu.edu.au/key-resources/bibliography?lid=1171

APA (2013). *Diagnostic and Statistical Manual of Mental Disorders* (5th edn). Arlington, VA: APA.

Arkles, R.S., Jackson, P.L.R., Robertson, H., Draper, B., Chalkey, S. & Broe, G.A. (2010). *Ageing, Cognition and Dementia in Australian Aboriginals and Torres Strait Islander Peoples.* Sydney: Neuroscience Research Australia and Muru Marri Indigenous Health Unit, University of New South Wales.

Best, O. & Drummond, A. (2018). Working with Australian Aboriginal and Torres Strait Islander Elders. In K. Scott, M. Webb and S. Sorrentino (eds), *Long-term Caring: Residential, Home and Community Aged Care* (4th edn). Sydney: Mosby Elsevier.

Commonwealth of Australia (2013). *National Aboriginal and Torres Strait Islander Health Plan 2013–2023.* Canberra: Commonwealth of Australia. Retrieved from www1.health.gov.au/internet/main/publishing.nsf/content/B92E980680486C3BCA257BF0001BAF01/$File/health-plan.pdf

Deravin, L. & Anderson, J. (eds) (2019). *Chronic Care Nursing: A Framework for Practice* (2nd ed.). Melbourne: Cambridge University Press.

Deravin-Malone, L. (2017). Indigenous Australians living longer still the gap remains. *Australian Nursing & Midwifery Journal*, 24(7), 41.

Dudgeon, P. & Walker, R. (2011). The health, social and emotional wellbeing of Aboriginal women. In R. Thackrah, K. Scott & J. Winch (eds), *Indigenous Australian Health and Cultures: An Introduction for Health Professionals.* Sydney: Pearson Education.

Dudgeon, P., Wright, M., Paradies, Y., Garvey, D. & Walker, I. (2010). The social, cultural and historical context of Aboriginal and Torres Strait Islander Australians. In N Purdie, P. Dudgeon & R. Walker (eds), *Working Together: Aboriginal and Torres Strait Islander Mental Health and Wellbeing Principles and Practice.* Canberra: DHA.

Ferguson, M., Baker, A., Young, S. & Procter, N. (2016). Understanding suicide among Aboriginal communities. *Australian Nursing & Midwifery Journal*, 23(8), 36.

Ferguson, M., O'Dea, K., Chatfield, M., Moodie, M., Altman, J. & Brimlecombe, J. (2016). The comparative cost of food and beverages at remote Indigenous communities, Northern Territory, Australia. *Australian and New Zealand Journal of Public Health*, 40, S21–26.

Forman, D. & Pond, D. (2015). *Care of the Person with Dementia: Interprofessional Practice and Education.* Melbourne: Cambridge University Press.

Fredericks, B., Daniels, C., Kinnear, S., Mann, J. & Croftwarcon, P. (2016). *Exploring Aboriginal and Torres Strait Islander Knowledge, Experiences and Perceptions of Chronic Health Conditions in the Greater Rockhampton Region.* Rockhampton: CQUniversity. Retrieved from http://acquire.cqu.edu.au:8080/vital/access/manager/Repository/cqu:13182

Garvey, G., Simmonds, D., Clements, V. … Beattie, E. (2011). Understanding dementia amongst Indigenous Australians. *Aboriginal and Islander Health Worker Journal*, 35(2), 16–18.

Hellsten, D. (2014). Caring for our Elders. In O. Best and B. Fredericks (eds), *Yatdjuligin: Aboriginal and Torres Strait Islander Nursing & Midwifery Care.* Melbourne: Cambridge University Press.

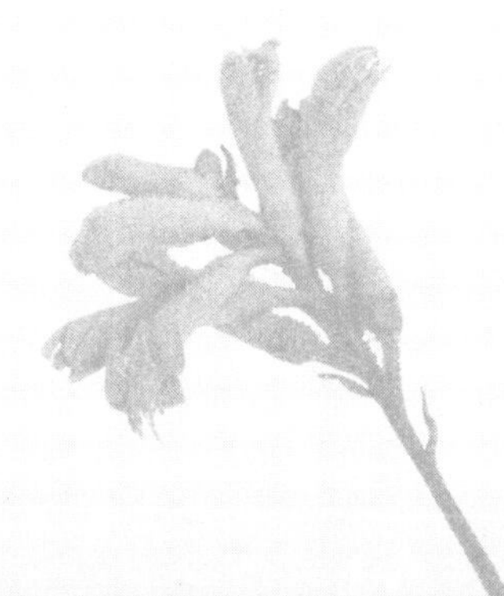

Indigenous Palliative Care Project (2009). *Providing Culturally Appropriate Palliative Care to Aboriginal and Torres Strait Islander Peoples. Resource Kit.* Canberra: Australian Government, National Palliative Care Program. Retrieved from www.caresearch .com.au/caresearch/tabid/86/Default.aspx.

Langton, M. & Perkins, R. (eds). (2008). *The First Australians: An Illustrated History.* Melbourne: Melbourne University Press.

Power, T., Wilson. D., Best, O., Brockie, T., Bearskin, L., Millender, E. & Lowe, J. (2020). COVID-19 and Indigenous Peoples: An imperative for action. *Journal of Clinical Nursing*, 29(15–16), 2737–41.

Reynolds, H. (2000). *Why Weren't We Told? A Personal Search for the Truth About Our History*. Ringwood: Penguin.

SCRGSP (2016). *Overcoming Indigenous Disadvantage: Key Indicators 2016.* Canberra: Productivity Commission.

Sherwood, J. (2013). Colonisation – It's bad for your health: The context of Aboriginal health. *Contemporary Nurse*, 46(1), 28–40.

Tracey, R. & Briggs, L. (2019). *Royal Commission into Aged Care Quality and Safety: Interim Report – Neglect.* Retrieved from https://agedcare.royalcommission.gov .au/publications/Documents/interim-report/interim-report-volume-1.pdf

United Nations (2007). *United Nations Declaration on the Rights of Indigenous Peoples.* Geneva: United Nations. Retrieved from www.un.org/development/desa/ indigenouspeoples/declaration-on-the-rights-of-indigenous-peoples.html

Whop, M. (2014). Indigenous youngsters walk 200 kilometres from Taroom to Woorabinda, retracing ancestors' steps. *ABC News*, 10 July. Retrieved from www.abc.net.au/news/2014–07–10/indigenous-youngsters-retrace-the-steps-of-their-ancestors/5586440

Zubrick, S.R., Shepherd, C.C., Dudgeon, P., Gee, G., Paradies, Y., Scrine, C. & Walker, R. (2014). Social determinants of social and emotional wellbeing. In P. Dudgeon, H. Milroy & R. Walker (eds), *Working Together: Aboriginal and Torres Strait Islander Mental Health and Wellbeing Principles and Practice* (2nd ed.). Canberra: AIHW, pp. 93–112.

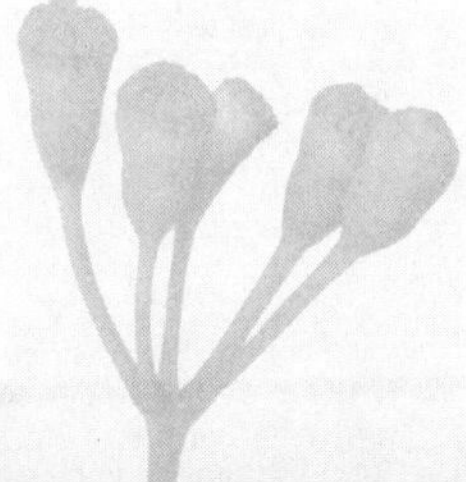

Index